The politics of vaccination

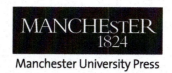

Manchester University Press

SOCIAL HISTORIES OF MEDICINE

Series editors: David Cantor and Keir Waddington

Social Histories of Medicine is concerned with all aspects of health, illness and medicine, from prehistory to the present, in every part of the world. The series covers the circumstances that promote health or illness, the ways in which people experience and explain such conditions and what, practically, they do about them. Practitioners of all approaches to health and healing come within its scope, as do their ideas, beliefs and practices, and the social, economic and cultural contexts in which they operate. Methodologically, the series welcomes relevant studies in social, economic, cultural and intellectual history, as well as approaches derived from other disciplines in the arts, sciences, social sciences and humanities. The series is a collaboration between Manchester University Press and the Society for the Social History of Medicine.

Previously published

The metamorphosis of autism: A history of child development in Britain *Bonnie Evans*

Payment and philanthropy in British healthcare, 1918–48 *George Campbell Gosling*

The politics of vaccination

A global history

Edited by Christine Holmberg, Stuart Blume and Paul Greenough

Manchester University Press

Published by Manchester University Press

Altrincham Street, Manchester M1 7JA

www.manchesteruniversitypress.co.uk

British Library Cataloguing-in-Publication Data
A catalogue record for this book is available from the British Library

Library of Congress Cataloging-in-Publication Data applied for

ISBN   978 1 5261 1088 6   hardback

ISBN   978 1 5261 1090 9   paperback

First published 2017

Typeset in 11 on 12 pt Arno Pro Regular
by Toppan Best-set Premedia Limited
Printed in Great Britain
by Lightning Source

Contents

Figures and tables

Figures

Tables

Contributors

Christine Holmberg is the director of a research group on 'health services research' with a particular focus on risk, health decision-making, illness experience and science and technology studies at the Institute of Public Health, Universitätsmedizin Berlin, Germany. She holds a doctorate from the Humboldt-University Berlin in Anthropology and a Master of Public Health in Epidemiology from the University of Illinois at Chicago. Her most recent publications include 'Gaining Control over Breast Cancer Risk: Transforming vulnerability, uncertainty, and the future through clinical trial participation – a qualitative study', published in *Sociology of Health and Illness* (2015).

Stuart Blume is Emeritus Professor of Science & Technology Studies at the University of Amsterdam and a member of the Department of Anthropology. He worked previously at the University of Sussex, the OECD in Paris, the London School of Economics, and in various British government departments, including the Cabinet Office (1975–77), and from 1977 to 1980 as Research Secretary of the Committee on Social Inequalities in Health (the 'Black Committee'). From 2009 to 2012 he was 'Professor 2' at SUM, University of Oslo, Norway; and in 2013–14 Prometeo fellow at the University of Cuenca, Ecuador. Publications include *Insight and Industry: The Dynamics of Technological Change in Medicine* (Cambridge MA: MIT Press, 1992) and (with Sidsel Roalkvam, Desmond McNeill et al.) *Protecting the World's Children. Immunisation Policies and Practices* (Oxford University Press, 2013).

Paul Greenough is Emeritus Professor of South Asian history at the University of Iowa and also has an appointment in the Department of Community and Behavioral Health. He has published numerous chapters and articles on the social history of disease, welfare and environment in Bengal and India. He is the founding director of his university's Global Health Studies Program and the author or co-editor of four books, including *Nature in the Global South: Environmental Projects in South and Southeast Asia* (Duke University Press, 2004) and *Against Stigma: Global Studies in Caste and Race Since Durban* (Orient Black-Swan, 2009).

Niels Brimnes is Associate Professor in history and South Asian studies at Aarhus University, Denmark. He is currently head of the Department of History. He has written a number of articles on the introduction of western medicine in early colonial India and on the history of tuberculosis control in the twentieth century, both in India and on a global scale. He has recently published *Languished Hopes. Tuberculosis, the State and International Assistance in Twentieth-century India* (Orient BlackSwan, 2016).

Dora Vargha is lecturer in medical humanities at the Department of History and Centre for Medical History at the University of Exeter. Her work explores global health history from an Eastern European perspective. She has published work on the Cold War politics of polio in Hungary, the history of internationalism and disability history. She is founding editor of Central and Eastern European History of Medicine Network.

Eun Kyung Choi is a Research Professor at the Institute of Medical History and Culture at Seoul National University Hospital. She graduated from Seoul National University College of Medicine and received a PhD in History of Medicine. She also teaches History of Medicine and Medical Humanities in Seoul National University and Kangwon National University. Her recent publications are (with Young A. Lee), 'The Body Image and Medical Knowledge of the Korean Public in the 1930s through the Medical Advice Column 'Jisang byeongwon (Hospital on Paper) ', *Journal of the Korean History of Science Society,* 37(1) (2015), pp. 235–64; and 'Mobilization of Medical Professionals and Establishment of Physical Standards for Conscription in 1950s–1960s South Korea', *The Journal of Humanities,* 36(4) (2015), pp. 231–58.

Young-Gyung Paik is an Associate Professor at Korea National Open University and has an appointment also in the Science, Technology and Policy Program at Korea Advanced Institute of Science and Technology. She has published widely on the development of medical technologies and its gendered implications in South Korea. She has contributed chapters to *New Millennium South Korea: Neoliberal Capitalism and Transnational Movements* (Routledge, 2010) and *Reconfiguring Reproduction: Feminist Health Perspectives on Assisted Reproductive Technologies* (Zubaan Books, 2015).

Ana María Carrillo is a historian of medicine at the Department of Public Health of the Faculty of Medicine of the National Autonomous University of Mexico. She has published more than sixty articles and chapters on the history of epidemics and public health in nineteenth- and twentieth-century Mexico. Her book about the birth of public health in Mexico is in press. She is a member of the National System of Researchers.

Jaime Larry Benchimol is a senior researcher at the Casa de Oswaldo Cruz, Oswaldo Cruz Foundation; professor with the Graduate Program in the History of Science and Health at the Casa de Oswaldo Cruz; and professor with the Graduate Program in Living Conditions and Health Situations in Amazonia at the Leônidas e Maria Deane Institute in Manaus. He was science editor of *História, Ciências, Saúde – Manguinhos* from January 1997 to March 2015 and continues to serve on the journal's editorial board. His research and teaching focus chiefly on the history of the life sciences and the history of tropical medicine and public health. He continues to be interested in an earlier research subject, urban history.

Julia Yongue is a professor in the Faculty of Economics of Hosei University in Tokyo, Japan. Her research combines the histories of business, pharmacy and the impact of health policy on the development of the pharmaceutical industry in Japan. Her most recent work is a co-edited volume, *Encyclopedia of Pharmaceutical History*, published in Japanese in 2016. She currently serves as a council member of the Japanese Society for History of Pharmacy and the Business History Society of Japan.

Andrea Stöckl is a medical sociologist/anthropologist at the Norwich Medical School at the University of East Anglia. She has published on the politics of vaccination policies, especially in Europe and in Great Britain, with a focus on women's health issues. Her other interests lie in the ethics of care, the emotional aspects of care and controversial surgery on women, such as hymen reconstruction and female genital mutilation. She is interested on the intersections of ethics and social lives.

Anna Smajdor is Associate Professor of Practical Philosophy at the University of Oslo. Her research interests cover a range of ethical questions related to developments in biomedical science and she has published widely in this field. She is the co-author (with Ruth Deech) of *From IVF to Immortality: Controversy in the Era of Reproductive Technology* (Oxford University Press, 2008).

Britta Lundgren is Professor of Ethnology at the Department of Culture and Media Studies at Umeå University, Sweden. She has been the Dean of the Faculty of Arts and the founder and director of the National Graduate School for Gender Studies and has also led the interdisciplinary research programme 'Challenging Gender'. She has published works on friendship, grief and mourning, family and gender, academic culture, and the disciplinary history of ethnology. Her interest now lies in the field of medical humanities and she is working on a four-year project focusing the A(H1N1) pandemic – Epidemics, Vaccination and the Power of Narratives – financed by the Marcus and Amalia Wallenberg Foundation in Sweden.

Martin Holmberg is an MD and associate professor specialising in infectious diseases. He has worked many years as a clinical doctor and then as senior medical officer at the National Board of Health and Welfare, the authority that was responsible for pandemic preparedness and for coordinating the response to the A(H1N1) 2009 pandemic. He is now retired but is serving as a medical expert in the project, Epidemics, Vaccination and the Power of Narratives, at Umeå University.

Elisha P. Renne is a professor in the Department of Afroamerican and African Studies (DAAS) and in the Department of Anthropology at the University of Michigan, Ann Arbor. She has published numerous articles and chapters on African ethnology and infectious disease; fertility and reproductive health; gender relations; and the anthropology of development. She has also authored or co-edited seven books, which include *Population and Progress in a Yoruba Town* (Edinburgh University Press, 2003) and *The Politics of Polio in Northern Nigeria* (Indiana University Press, 2010).

William Muraskin is Professor of Urban Studies, Queens College, City University of New York. He is the author of five books on the politics surrounding the formation of international health policy concerning vaccine development and delivery for the children of the South: *Polio Eradication and Its Discontents: A Historian's Journey Through an International Public Health (Un)Civil War* (Orient BlackSwan, 2012); *The Crusade to Immunize the World's Children: the Origin of the Bill and Melinda Gates Children's Vaccine Program and the Birth of the Global Alliance for Vaccines and Immunization* (Global BioBusiness Books, 2005); *Vaccines for Developing Economies: Who Will Pay?*, edited, rearranged, and supplemented by William Muraskin (The Albert B. Sabin Vaccine Institute, 2001); *The Politics of International Health: the Children's Vaccine Initiative and the Struggle to Develop Vaccines for the Third World* (State University of New York Press, 1998); and *The War Against Hepatitis B: a History of the International Task Force on Hepatitis B Immunization* (University of Pennsylvania Press, 1995). Most of his funding over the years has been from the Rockefeller Foundation.

Acknowledgements

The editors would like to thank the Fritz-Thyssen-Foundation who funded the international conference on the development and change of immunisation throughout history – socio-political development and the implementation of new medical practices that took place in Berlin, Germany in April 2011. We would also acknowledge additional funding received for the conference from the European Science Foundation through the network 'Standard drugs and drug standards. A comparative historical study of pharmaceuticals in the twentieth century'. The idea of the book and the collaboration of the authors started at this conference. We thank Dr Marion Hulverscheidt with whom we received funding for the conference in Berlin and who was a co-chair of the meeting and important discussant in shaping the book. To discuss and reflect on the chapters and to finalise the book, the authors received funding from the Society of Social History of Medicine to conduct a workshop on 'Vaccination between Research, Health Politics, and Nation: Lessons learned from historical examples on vaccination campaigns and vaccination development' held at the East Anglia University Medical School in Norwich, UK in October 2013. We also would like to thank the anonymous reviewers for their comments on an earlier version of the book. Finally, we thank those who helped us bring the book into shape for publication: in particular Juliana Thon, Iris Maertens, Julie Slater, and Ashley Witcher.

Introduction

Paul Greenough, Stuart Blume and Christine Holmberg

Government-organised vaccination campaigns are political projects that presume to shape the immunity of whole populations.[1] Like other pervasive expressions of state power – taxing, policing, conscripting – mass vaccination arouses anxiety in some people but sentiments of civic duty and shared solidarity in others. As a rule, controversy clings to immunisation programmes,[2] and different social formations – classes, urban elites, ethnic and confessional majorities and minorities, specialised workforces, refugees, provincial antagonists of capital cities – have at different times and places disputed, evaded or actively opposed state-led vaccination. Nonetheless, in most communities vaccines have come to be accepted as the most effective means for halting the spread of communicable diseases. People now tend to demand public health immunisation, and the development of new vaccines, for example against HIV, malaria and Ebola, are eagerly awaited. But compliance is always an issue. A key premise of this collection is that a state's ability to produce, or at least distribute, large quantities of vaccine, as well as its ability to manage the necessarily awkward intrusion into healthy bodies, have at different times and places strengthened or weakened social cohesion.

This book's eleven chapters and afterword document key campaigns against major infections since 1800 (but mostly after 1950) in Europe, South and East Asia, West Africa and the Americas. Throughout, the authors explore relationships among vaccination, vaccine-making and the discourses and debates on citizenship and nationhood that

accompanied mass campaigns. Two bold, not wholly unfamiliar gener-
alisations emerge:

- A government's capacity to manufacture its own vaccines has frequently played a role in building and sustaining national sovereignty.
- The success or failure of a vaccination campaign has notable effects
on the inner formation of participants' sense of community and
citizenship.

As will be seen, mass immunisation should not be considered a neutral
practice; it requires assessment in its relation to state power, national
identity and the individual's sense of obligation to self and others.

What's new in this book?

While historians have explored the evolution of public health in different parts of the world, and of vaccination as a key component, few have
located vaccination in relation to twentieth- and twenty-first-century
political milestones like colonial nationalism, decolonisation, the Cold
War, the rise of economic neo-liberalism and recent geo-political shifts.
This collection gives a comparative overview of immunisation at different times in widely different parts of the world and under different
types of political regime.

Five of the chapters are set in the last fifty years.[3] Four others pay
particular attention to the development and manufacture of vaccines,
because the capacity to produce the vaccines that publicly run programmes required was long taken as a sign of sovereign responsibility
and authority – an authority that is being relinquished in many countries, going back to the the 1980s.[4]

The remaining chapters hark back to earlier episodes of vaccination
controversy in the nineteenth and twentieth centuries. An afterword
relates disturbing shortcuts taken by an elite fraternity of global health
leaders that has launched the major disease eradication and immunisation programmes since the 1980s.[5]

Core themes in the chapters include immunisation as an element
of state formation; citizens' articulation of seeing (or not seeing) their
needs incorporated into public health practice; allegations that development aid is inappropriately steering third-world health policies;
and an ideological shift that regards vaccines more as profitable

commodities than as essential tools of public health. Each chapter has been written by a specialist trained in appropriate languages and literatures. Taken together they encompass vaccination, not only as a public health measure, but also as a source of disruptions that evoke abstract outcomes, such as a sense of shared solidarity (or of outrage over violations of bodily integrity), the glow of humanitarian achievement (or disgust with first-world hubris), or neo-liberal satisfaction that bargaining when sourcing vaccines results in thrift and efficiency (or in patriotic regret that a nation's manufacturing capacity is swiftly draining away). Above all they suggest that immunisation is a novel historical lens through which to view changes in 'society' and 'nation' over time.

Vaccine politics in historiographical perspective

The collection builds on a solid body of literature that links the nineteenth-century advent of public health immunisation to the consolidation and emergence of nation-states. For example, as Peter Baldwin has argued, smallpox vaccination in the early 1800s served to demonstrate the willingness of small, newly formed German states to protect their citizens.[6] On the other hand, assertive localism in Britain, motivated by a reluctance to experience vaccination at the hands of outsiders and officials, led to serious provincial opposition, as Deborah Brunton argues in her survey of public immunisation in England, Wales, Scotland and Ireland.[7] Christoph Gradmann and Volker Hess have shown that statistics, epidemiology and bacteriology were allied sciences closely linked in Europe to the proliferation of vaccines as vital tools for the new profession of public health.[8] Bacteriological research after 1890 was directed by public policy to develop new vaccines, sera and antitoxins, and both state laboratories and private pharmaceutical companies began to produce them for governments.[9] There have been too few studies, however, of the 'networks of innovation' required for vaccine research and development, a notable exception being Louis Galambos's history of the firm Merck, Sharpe and Dohme.[10]

In the USA robust private manufacture of vaccines after 1900 was accompanied by 'breathless coverage' of scientific benefits in the press; but there were occasional disasters, and by 1902 the Public Health

Service was empowered to inspect pharmaceutical products and regulate their sales.[11]

Bacteriological thinking and associated technologies and practices were put to use far beyond Europe and North America, largely to protect expanding imperial interests. Colonial medical and public health policies in the later nineteenth century have attracted considerable attention.[12] Most of these accounts terminate with a colony's independence. A few other authors address inter-colonial health collaborations and international health organisations, such as the Health Office of the League of Nations and the International Red Cross.[13] Myron Echenberg has written a detailed study of responses to the plague pandemic that went around the world in 1894–1901.[14] Bacteriological research into cholera, malaria and plague was launched in this period in colonial North Africa and tropical Asia by British, French and Dutch microbiologists. Several vaccine institutes were established in late Victorian India, well before many European countries, in response to plague, cholera and other diseases. As Ilana Löwy and Pratik Chakrabarti have shown, more than half a dozen Indian vaccine institutes conducted research and also produced vaccines and sera against cholera and plague but also against rabies, tetanus, diphtheria, smallpox, typhoid and snakebites.[15] Despite this long record of institutional research, Anil Kumar has found that colonial research policies before Independence in 1947 failed to lay the foundation for a sustainable path for vaccine development and production in an independent India.[16]

In the early decades of the twentieth century private foundations – notably the Rockefeller Foundation and the Pasteur Institute – contributed heavily to the establishment of bacteriological research in much of Asia, Latin America and in parts of Africa.[17] Anne-Marie Moulin has examined the Pasteur Institute's global 'adventure of vaccination' in the nineteenth and twentieth centuries in several books and articles.[18] Latin American scholars have examined the activities of the Pasteur Institute and the Rockefeller Foundation in the Americas,[19] although national accounts are few and Mexico and Brazil have received most historical attention.[20] Ana Maria Carrillo, among other Mexican scholars, has discussed the establishment of the Instituto Bacteriólogico Nacional in Mexico City in 1905, which maintained close ties with the Parisian Pasteur Institute.[21] This institute, like its peers in India, combined basic research with the production of vaccines and sera, although its work was severely disrupted by the Mexican revolution of 1910–17. Mariola Espinosa's recovery of the domestic American origins of the US war on Spain in Cuba in 1898 moves the familiar story of the American army's sanitary imperialism and yellow fever eradication in a new direction.[22]

For the period 1914–50 there is a paucity of accounts of public health outside Europe and North America.[23] After the disruptions due to world wars and global depression, the late 1940s and 1950s saw three large-scale processes – the post-war reconstruction and Cold War ideological conflict, decolonisation and the advent of the World Health Organization (WHO) – that rearranged the supply–demand relationship for vaccines between the West and the rest of the world.

These inter-connections are sketched in James Colgrove's history of immunisation politics in twentieth-century USA, in Randall Packard's outline of 'post-colonial medicine', and in Tania Keefe and Mark Zacher's overview of a the new post-war global governance in which constituents are 'united by contagion'.[24] The role of the WHO in immunisation politics throughout this period is very complex, but it should be noted that a bacteriological and biological unit carried forward to the WHO from the League of Nations, and the WHO has maintained the responsibility for standardising and evaluating the world's diversity of vaccinal products.[25]

The eradication of smallpox by vaccination was envisaged by Edward Jenner as early as 1802, but success was only achieved after the WHO launched a determined global vaccination programme in 1966. The technical and organisational resources for this triumph are surveyed in a monumental official history that includes a dozen distinct regional and country narratives;[26] however, this volume touches only lightly on the policy shifts and political accommodations that made eradication possible. A stream of monographs and memoirs have examined these matters in India in depth; the focus on India is justified by the fact that 30–40 per cent of all the smallpox in the world was found in that country in 1967 at the inception of the intensified Smallpox Eradication Programme (SEP).[27] In the final stage of the South Asia SEP (1973–75) the WHO flew a sizeable number of foreign (mainly American) physician-epidemiologists into the region to close the ledger once and for all.[28] Paul Greenough has described instances of coercion during this last phase in India and Bangladesh, although William Foege, the lead epidemiologist for the South Asia programme, has denied that coercion was required for eradication.[29] The smallpox campaign's success was subsequently hailed as proof not only that eradication was possible, but also that globally coordinated action offered hope for finishing off a number of other diseases. It also inspired the launch of the WHO's worldwide Expanded Programme of Immunisation (EPI) in 1974, and it was effectively cited to justify the launch of the global polio eradication programme in 1988.[30]

Public health histories since smallpox eradication

Contemporary funders, organisers and managers of immunisation campaigns in both the developed and developing countries are well aware of widespread public scepticism if not opposition. While physical attacks on vaccinators, though not unknown are rare, opposition to vaccination has become common. Increasing numbers of well-educated parents in prosperous countries, each with its unique history of state–citizen encounters, now question the benefits of vaccination for their children.[31]

The editors consider the unwinding and comparing of these histories to be instructive, and they hope the collection will be a bridge between history, the qualitative social sciences and the public health community. While most of the chapters that follow have a critical tone, this should not be taken to imply any rejection of the benefits that vaccines have brought, or a denial of the millions of lives that have been saved.

As editors, our view is that the policies and practices that determine how vaccines are used can only be strengthened by critical analysis and by acknowledgement of past failings. As Anne-Marie Moulin has observed, 'the concept of public resistance to immunisation campaigns [can be] replaced by acceptability, which suggests that selecting the procedures to employ when immunising a given population is a hypothesis that should be evaluated based on history'.[32]

Of the many developments affecting public health since the 1970s, two are particularly significant for understanding the current role of vaccination. One is the gradual erosion of the concept of 'international health' (implying the cooperation of sovereign nations in tackling health problems) and its replacement by the concept of 'global health'. Scholars differ in their interpretations of this trend. On the one hand, the political and legal scholar David Fidler underlines changes in the mechanical facts of pathogenic transmission, especially the rapidity with which dire infections (e.g. SARS, Avian flu, Ebola) spread from place to place through air travel; his conclusion is that effective responses require the subordination of national sovereignties and jurisdictions to global authorities.[33] On the other hand, anthropologists and medical historians, digging deeper, draw connections among 'emerging diseases', 'global health' and new forms of great-power security interests;[34] it is argued that the WHO has 'reposition[ed] itself as a credible and highly visible contributor to the rapidly changing field of global health'.[35] What is clear is that the global health concept helps legitimate the authority of supranational institutions and programmes. William Muraskin, almost alone among historians, has analysed the emerging structures and incentives that compel many developing countries to line up behind global priorities – in particular global eradication and other immunisation programmes – while reluctantly scaling back their own, locally defined health needs.[36]

A second development is the emergence of claims by individuals, collectivities and humanitarian organisations to the 'right to health', which implies that governments should become accountable for public health measures to 'the highest attainable standard'.[37] A further dimension of health rights is the obligation to interrogate and confront public health authorities whenever they institute arbitrary programmes of surveillance and compulsion.[38] If in the classic liberal framework, bioethics favours autonomy and individual choice, proponents of the new subdiscipline of 'public health ethics' argue for the priorities and perspectives of collectives and communities.[39] Public health ethics argues, for example, that high levels of vaccination coverage ('herd immunity') serve the collective need and that coverage should be viewed as a public good.[40]

This position blunts accusations that major public health tools like vaccination and its companions 'surveillance and containment' are assaults on individual rights, a stance brought into prominence by AIDS activists in the 1980s;[41] these civil liberties concerns have reappeared in the face of counter-terror measures like 'preparedness'.[42] Although public health ethics is a limited area of research, it suggests that once public trust in the state is lost, there will be a 'reframing' of vaccination programmes to label them as, in effect, assaults on individuals' rights.[43]

Historians have documented many times the resistance evoked when state authorities enforce vaccination too energetically. Since the earliest state-led vaccination of infants in mid-nineteenth-century Britain, there was opposition, ranging from simple household-level non-compliance, to parents with cudgels chasing away health officers, to nationwide anti-vaccination campaigns fuelling parliamentary wrangles.[44] Compulsion, which took the form of repeatedly fining non-compliant parents, inflamed class feeling and sowed antagonism between religious groups. Opposition to vaccination, and to intrusive health measures more generally, eventually caused officials to give ground – for example, when confronted by massed conscientious objectors – and to listen more carefully and speak more cautiously – or more cunningly – to affected publics.[45] Arguably, sustained opposition to Victorian public health programmes re-shaped the state's administration. Some of the UK's experience was repeated elsewhere, and many a European, American and colonial medical official was forced to back down from the Jennerian vision of smallpox's 'annihilation'. Some degree of resistance was a constant feature in UK and US immunisation campaigns through the 1940s.[46] Determined scepticism, non-compliance, rejection (whether of vaccinations in general or of specific vaccines) and insistence on the right to choose have become widespread in the late twentieth to early twenty-first centuries.[47]

Vaccination and national identity

In Part I of this book the authors explore how vaccination campaigns and new vaccine technologies have wittingly or unwittingly shaped national identity at different times and places. Paul Greenough's chapter foregrounds difficulties the US Communicable Disease Center (CDC) faced in 1958 in transferring its epidemiological expertise into Cold War Pakistan as a host of political groups, private citizens and other non-state actors vied to rescue the neglected eastern province from raging epidemics of smallpox and cholera. Though the US government saw an opportunity to intervene with vaccines and new methods of surveillance, civil society in East Bengal had already appropriated vaccination and succeeded in reshaping it as a popular project that contributed to the region's emerging anti-Pakistani identity. Chapter 2, by Niels

Brimnes, plumbs discursive resistance to vaccination in India beginning in the late colonial period and continuing well into the early decades of Independence; while there were at least four oppositional positions, elite authors (including Mahatma Gandhi) concurred that a free and self-reliant India would be damaged rather than strengthened by public health immunisation.

The two final chapters in Part I bring to light hitherto 'hidden' vaccination histories by narrating the 'uniting' effects of vaccines on opposed Cold War entities like 'the free world' and 'occupied Europe'. In Dora Vargha's chapter one discerns how a western fantasy of an authoritarian 'communist' top-down approach to vaccination became the model for successful vaccination campaigns in the West. As in the case of East Pakistan in the late 1950s, Cold War tropes played a role in shaping and developing vaccines and vaccination campaigns.

Finally, Eun Kyung Choi and Young-Gyung Paik's chapter brings to light a fascinating story of the four-way contention from the early 1950s through the 1980s among foreign and domestic medical researchers, agents of the government and the pharmaceutical industry and popular perceptions that together helped to shape and re-shape the modern South Korean nation. The chapters in this section thus reflect the mixed record of both top-down and bottom-up enthusiasms for and antagonisms toward vaccines and vaccination, thereby deepening recognition that immunising technologies are growth media that can both foster and erode national and transnational solidarity.

Nationality, vaccine production and the end of sovereign manufacture

In Part II the authors focus on vaccine production, which began around the start of the twentieth century, typically in municipal or state-run public health laboratories. The chapters follow a chronological timeline starting with sovereign state production and ending with diminished (if not privatised) production; this arc parallels significant changes in the organisation of contemporary society and the emergence of a global commoditisation of pharmaceuticals. The case studies of Mexico told by Ana Maria Carrillo and of the Netherlands by Stuart Blume narrate the on and off successes of national (centralised) vaccine production over the last century, showing how decisions were taken by state actors to manufacture vaccines against particular diseases and how questions of safety and efficacy were handled in vaccine production.

Yet both chapters conclude with a downward spiral and loss of public-sector manufacturing capacity as autonomous production gave way in the face of free market ideology and the resources of the global pharmaceutical industry. In marked contrast, as Jaime Benchimol relates in his account of invention and production in Brazil, the narrative arc of sovereign vaccines and vaccination rose rather than fell as various mid-twentieth century regimes determined to continue making yellow fever and other vaccines; indigenous Brazilian research and production organisations succeeded in acquiring and then innovating on the most advanced vaccine technologies. Brazil thus sets itself apart from the other stories of loss of national capacity under conditions of globalisation; instead it built on the country's earlier capacity for adoption and innovation and underwent a regeneration that is uncommon elsewhere. Julia Yongue tells another unique story of vaccine production in Japan, in which a sense of Japanese uniqueness is traced to the pre-war history of uncoordinated decisions by non-state firms to manufacture vaccines and sera.

Reading these four chapters together clarifies the signal importance of particular individuals and their networks and highlights how closely vaccine production and vaccination campaigns are tied. Above all, this section shows how institutional actors like state agencies, industrial houses, supranational health organisations, local and global philanthropic organisations, have determined distinctive national trajectories of vaccination.

Vaccination, the individual and society

In Part III the authors take up the storms and stresses of bottom-up versus top-down approaches to vaccination in various countries. Andrea Stöckl and Anna Smajdor's chapter analyses the MMR (measles, mumps, rubella) vaccine debate in the UK, 1998–2003, through the lens of Prime Minister Tony Blair's failure to disclose his own son's vaccination status. This chapter links the role of public figures and ideas of 'anti-vaccination' to the erosion of trust within, and between, strata of the British class system. In modern Sweden, with its rather different social system, and which began to vaccinate early, vaccination has tended to adhere to the idea of Swedish national 'solidarity'. Britta Lundgren and Martin Holmberg's chapter shows this ideal eroded by a scandal that surrounded the last influenza pandemic in which global (WHO) criteria for administering a national campaign were substituted for the usual Swedish ones; subsequently serious side-effects were found in some vaccinated Swedish children.

Elisha Renne's case study of polio vaccination in Nigeria shifts the focus to current politics of vaccination campaigns that focus on global eradication, and which are strongly backed by supranational and philanthropic organisations that sideline regional and national concerns. The proponents of such campaigns take it for granted that governments lack the resources and the competences – and some would say the right – to determine their own vaccine needs and to meet them through production or procurement. States like Nigeria have no choice but to rely on donors' largesse and the policy directives that accompanies it. This is of course still more true of smaller countries, where independent vaccine production is wholly infeasible, and where health systems are largely dependent on donor funds.

To summarise, Part III reveals that vaccination technologies, which once flourished as a means by which nation-states demonstrated their power to protect their citizens and keep them immune in times of epidemics, have now become another medium by which weakened states in the north (or states in the south with weak governing capacity) exemplify the loss of an older index of health sovereignty to market globalisation. As noted, Brazil is a striking exception to this generalisation.

Part III also invokes the figure of the individual, whose rights, choices and health security under epidemic conditions are all conditioned by a looming, anxious state. These chapters nicely demonstrate the collective tropes and implicit understandings according to which a healthy 'society' functions, and how choice-bearing 'individuals' are conceptualised, idealised and historically situated as members in coherent national 'societies'. In the afterword William Muraskin demonstrates how illusory these scripted notions of rights-bearing individuals who are protected by their state can be.

Muraskin unravels the astonishing circumstances in which a few (white male western) individuals, acting in concert with global institutions that they either control or can steer, have been able to turn global vaccination policy toward their favoured practice of disease eradication.

Notes

1 Following common usage, 'vaccination' and 'immunisation' are used interchangeably throughout. Similarly, the terms 'immunisation programme' and 'vaccination campaign' are equivalent.
2 H. J. Larson, C. Jarrett, E. Eckersberger, D. M. D. Smith and P. Paterson, 'Understanding Vaccine Hesitancy Around Vaccines and Vaccination from a Global Perspective: A Systematic Review of Published Literature, 2007–2012', *Vaccine*, 32:19 (2014), pp. 2150–9; L. A. Jana and J. E. Osborn, 'The History of Vaccine Challenges: Conquering Diseases, Plagued by Controversy', in A. Chatterjee (ed.), *Vaccinophobia and Vaccine Controversies of the 21st Century* (New York, Dordrecht, Heidelberg and London: Springer, 2013), pp. 1–13.
3 S. Blume (Chapter 6); B. Lundgren and C. Holmberg (Chapter 10); W. Muraskin (Afterword) ; E. Renne (Chapter 11); A. Stöckl and A. Smajdor (Chapter 9).
4 S. Blume (Chapter 6); J. Benchimol (Chapter 7); A. Carrillo (Chapter 5); and J. Yongue (Chapter 8).
5 Muraskin, 'Afterword'.
6 P. Baldwin, *Contagion and the State in Europe, 1830–1930* (Cambridge: Cambridge University Press, 1999).
7 D. Brunton, *The Politics of Vaccination: Practice and Policy in England, Wales, Ireland and Scotland, 1800–1874* (Rochester: University of Rochester Press, 2008).
8 C. Gradmann and V. Hess (eds), 'Vaccines as Medical, Industrial, and Administrative Objects', Special issue of *Science in Context*, 21:2 (2008).
9 *Ibid.*; K. Kroker, J. Keelan and P. M. H. Mazumdar (eds), *Crafting Immunity: Working Histories of Clinical Immunology* (Ashgate: Aldershot, 2008).
10 L. Galambos with Jane Eliot Sewell, *Networks of Innovation. Vaccine Development at Merck, Sharp & Dohme, and Mulford, 1895–1995* (Cambridge: Cambridge University Press 1997).
11 J. Colgrove, *State of Immunity: the Politics of Vaccination in Twentieth Century America* (Berkeley, Los Angeles and London: California University Press, 2006); J. Liebenau, *Medical Science and Medical Industry: The Formation of the American Pharmaceutical Industry* (Basingstoke: Macmillan, 1986).

12 For example, R. MacLeod and M. Lewis (eds), *Disease, Medicine and Empire. Perspectives on Western Medicine and the Experience of European Expansion* (London: Routledge, 1988); Margaret Vaughan, *Curing their Ills: Colonial Power and African Illness* (Cambridge: Polity Press, 1991); D. Arnold, *Colonizing the Body: State Medicine and Epidemic Disease in 19th Century India* (University of California Press, 1993); M. Harrison, *Public Health in British India: Anglo-Indian Preventive Medicine, 1859–1914* (Cambridge University Press, 1994); L. Manderson, *Sickness and the State: Health and Illness in Colonial Malaya, 1870–1940* (Cambridge: Cambridge University Press, 1996); Michael Worboys, 'Colonial Medicine', in R. Cooter and J. Pickstone (eds), *Companion Encyclopedia of Medicine in the Twentieth Century* (New York: Routledge, 2002), pp. 67–80; S. Bhattacharya, *Expunging Variola: The Control and Eradication of Smallpox in India, 1947–1977* (Hyderabad: Orient Longman, 2006); A. Janetta, *The Vaccinators: Smallpox, Medical Knowledge, and the 'Opening' of Japan* (Palo Alto, CA: Stanford University Press, 2007).

13 For example, P. J. Weindling (ed.), *International Health Organisations and Movements 1918–1939* (Cambridge: Cambridge University Press, 1995).

14 M. Echenberg, *Plague Ports: The Global Urban Impact of Bubonic Plague, 1894–1901* (New York: New York University Press, 2007).

15 Ilana Löwy 'Producing a Trustworthy Knowledge: Early Field Trials of Anticholera Vaccines in India', in S. A. Plotkin and B. Fantini (eds), *Vaccinia, Vaccination, Vaccinology: Jenner, Pasteur and their Successors* (Paris: Elsevier, 1996), pp. 121–6; P. Chakrabarti, *Bacteriology in British India: Laboratory Medicine and the Tropics* (Rochester: University of Rochester Press, 2012).

16 A. Kumar (ed.), *Medicine and the Raj: British Medical Policy in India, 1835–1911* (New Delhi: Sage Books, 1998).

17 J. Farley, *To Cast Out Disease: A History of the International Health Division of Rockefeller Foundation, 1913–1951* (New York: Oxford University Press, 2003).

18 A. M. Moulin, *L'Aventure de la vaccination* (Paris: Fayard, 1996); A. M. Moulin, 'The International Network of the Pasteur Institute: Scientific Innovations and French Tropisms', in C. Charle, J. Schriewer and P. Wagner (eds), *The Emergence of Transnational Intellectual Networks and the Cultural Logic of Nations* (New York: Campus Verlag, 2004), pp. 135–62. See also K. Pelis, *Charles Nicolle, Pasteur's Imperial Missionary: Typhus and Tunisia* (New York: Rochester University Press, 2006).

19 M. Cueto (ed.), *Missionaries of Science: The Rockefeller Foundation and Latin America* (Bloomington: Indiana University Press, 1994). See also C. Abel, 'External Philanthropy and Domestic Change in Colombian Health Care,

the Role of the Rockefeller Foundation, *c.*1920–1950', *Hispanic American Historical Review*, 75 (1995), pp. 339–76.

20 I. Löwy, 'Yellow Fever in Rio de Janeiro and the Pasteur Institute Mission (1901–1905): the Transfer of Science to the Periphery', *Medical History*, 34 (1990), pp. 144–63. Though see also M. Cueto, 'Sanitation from Above: Yellow Fever and Foreign Intervention in Peru, 1919–1922' *Hispanic American Historical Review*, 72 (1992), pp. 1–22.

21 M. Servín Massieu, *Microbiología, vacunas y el rezago científico de México a partir del siglo XIX* (México City: Plaza y Valdés, 2000); A. C. Rodríguez de Romo, 'La ciencia pasteuriana a través de la vacuna antirrábica: el caso mexicano', *Dynamis*, XVI (1996), pp. 291–316; A.M.Carrillo, 'La patología del siglo XIX y los institutos nacionales de investigación médica en México', *Laborat-ACTA*, XIII:1 (2001), pp. 23–31.

22 M. Espinosa, *Epidemic Invasions: Yellow Fever and the Limits of Cuban Independence, 1878–1930* (Chicago: University of Chicago, 2009).

23 But see S. A. Amrith, *Decolonizing International Health: India and Southeast Asia, 1930–65* (London: Palgrave 2006).

24 Colgrove, *State of Immunity*; T. J. Keefe and M. W. Zacher, *The Politics of Global Health Governance: United by Contagion* (New York: Palgrave Macmillan, 2008); R. Packard, 'Post-colonial Medicine', Cooter and Pickstone (eds), *Companion Encyclopedia of Medicine in the Twentieth Century*, pp. 97–112.

25 World Health Organization (WHO), *Expert Committee on Biological Standardization, Report on the Third Session, London 2–7 May 1949* (Geneva: WHO, 1950); W. C. Cockburn, B. Hobson, J. W. Lightbown, J. Lyng, D. Magrath, 'The International Contribution to the Standardization of Biological Substances. II. Biological Standards and the World Health Organization 1947–1990. General Considerations', *Biologicals*, 19:4 (1991), pp. 257–64.

26 F. Fenner, D. A. Henderson, Isao Arita, Zdenek Jezek and Ivan D. Ladnyi, *Smallpox and its Eradication* (Geneva: WHO, 1988).

27 L. Brilliant, *The Management of Smallpox Eradication in India: A Case Study and Analysis* (Ann Arbor: University of Michigan, 1985); Bhattacharya, *Expunging Variola*; D. A. Henderson, *Smallpox: The Death of a Disease – The Inside Story of Eradicating a Worldwide Killer* (Amherst, NY: Prometheus, 2009); I. Arita, *The Smallpox Eradication Saga: An Insider's View* (Hyderabad: Orient BlackSwan 2010); W. Foege, *House on Fire: The Fight to Eradicate Smallpox* (Berkeley, Los Angeles, London: University of California Press, 2011).

28 S. Bhattacharya, 'Uncertain Advances: a Review of the Final Phases of the Smallpox Eradication Program in India, 1960–1980', *American Journal of Public Health* 94:11 (2004), pp. 1875–83.

29 P. Greenough, 'Intimidation, Coercion and Resistance in the Final Stages of the South Asian Smallpox Eradication Campaign, 1973–1975', *Social Science & Medicine*, 41:5 (1995), pp. 633–45; Foege, *House on Fire* (2011).

30 J. Okwo-Bele and T. Cherian, 'The Expanded Programme on Immunization: A Lasting Legacy of Smallpox Eradication', *Vaccine*, 29, suppl. 4 (2011), pp. D74–D79. For the close link between the SEP and polio eradication, see Muraskin, 'Afterword.'

31 S. Blume, 'Anti-vaccination Movements and their Interpretations', *Social Science & Medicine*, 62:3 (February 2006), pp. 628–42.

32 A. M. Moulin, 'The Vaccinal Hypothesis: Towards a Critical Anthropological Approach on a Historical Phenomenon', *História, Ciências, Saúde -Manguinhos*, 10, suplemento 2 (2003), pp. 499–517.

33 D. P. Fidler, *SARS, Governance, and the Globalization of Disease* (London: Palgrave 2004).

34 N. B. King, 'Security, Disease, Commerce: Ideologies of Postcolonial Global Health', *Social Studies of Science*, 32 (2002), pp. 763–89.

35 T. M. Brown, M. Cueto and E. Fee, 'The World Health Organization and the Transition from International to Global Public Health', *American Journal of Public Health*, 96 (2006), pp. 62–72.

36 W. Muraskin, 'The Global Alliance for Vaccines and Immunisation: Is it a New Model for Effective Public–Private Cooperation in International Public Health?', *American Journal of Public Health*, 94:11 (2004), pp. 1922–5; W. Muraskin, *Polio Eradication and its Discontents* (Delhi: Orient BlackSwan, 2012).

37 H. Potts and P. Hunt, *Accountability and the Right to The Highest Attainable Standard of Health* (Colchester: University of Essex, Human Rights Centre, 2008).

38 R. G. Bernheim, J. F. Childress, A. Melnick and R. J. Bonnie, *Essentials of Public Health Ethics* (Burlington MA: Jones & Bartlett, 2015).

39 R. Bayer and A. L. Fairchild, 'The Genesis of Public Health Ethics', *Bioethics*, 18 (2004), pp. 473–92.

40 A. Dawson, 'Herd Protection as A Public Good: Vaccination and Our Obligations to Others', in A. Dawson and M. Verwei (eds), *Ethics, Prevention and Public Health* (Oxford: Oxford University Press, 2007), pp. 160–78; L. Ortmann and J. I. Iskander, 'The Role of Public Health Ethics in Vaccine Decision Making: Insights from the Centers for Disease Control and Prevention', in Chatterjee (ed.), *Vaccinophobia and Vaccine Controversies of the 21st Century*. Note 2 above.

41 P. Treichler, *How To Have Theory in an Epidemic: Cultural Chronicles of AIDS* (Durham, NC: Duke University Press, 1999); D. Gould, *Moving Politics: Emotion and ACT UP's Fight Against AIDS* (University of Chicago Press, 2009).

42 Institute of Medicine (IOM), *The Smallpox Vaccination Program: Public Health in the Age of Terrorism* (Washington, DC: National Academies Press, 2005); Stephen S. Morse, 'Global Preparedness for Public Health Emergencies', *Journal of Public Health Policy*, 28:2 (2007), pp. 196–200; A. Richmond, L. Hostler, G. Leeman and W. King, 'A Brief History and Overview of CDC's Centers for Public Health Preparedness Cooperative Agreement Program', *Public Health Reports*, 125, suppl. 5 (2010), pp. 8–14.

43 E. Obadare, 'A Crisis of Trust: History, Politics, Religion and the Polio Controversy in Northern Nigeria', *Patterns of Prejudice*, 39 (2005), pp. 265–84.

44 N. Durbach, *Bodily Matters: The Anti-vaccination Movement in England 1853–1907* (Duke University Press 2004).

45 *Ibid.*; Brunton, *The Politics of Vaccination*.

46 R. D. Johnston, *The Radical Middle Class: Populist Democracy and the Question of Capitalism in Progressive Era Portland, Oregon* (Princeton: Princeton University Press, 2003); E. Conis, *Vaccine Nation: America's changing relationship with immunization* (Chicago: University of Chicago Press, 2013); C. Welch, 'New Approaches to Resistance in Brazil and Mexico', *Hispanic American Historical Review*, 93:3 (2013), p. 539.

47 Colgrove, *State of Immunity*; L. O. Gostin (ed.), *Public Health Law and Ethics: A Reader*, 2nd edn (Berkeley and Los Angeles: University of California Press, 2010); Chatterjee (ed.), *Vaccinophobia and Vaccine Controversies*.

I
Vaccination and national identity

1

The uneasy politics of epidemic aid: the CDC's mission to Cold War East Pakistan, 1958

Paul Greenough

Epidemic outbreaks, political struggle, civil society response

Historians warn against narratives in which actors are spared the dilemmas of chance and choice. No doubt prolepsis, anachronism and teleology should be avoided, but I find it difficult to tell a story about East Pakistani politics and disease control in 1958 without underlining two facts that emerged later – that East Pakistanis would win a bitter struggle for independence from West Pakistan in 1971, and that smallpox would be eradicated from Asia in 1975, when the very last case was traced to a child in a remote village of the new nation of Bangladesh.

While my story does not directly engage the Bangladesh civil war or the final push for smallpox eradication, it narrates some of the prehistory of both. Put differently, the unity of Pakistan and the survival of the *Variola* (smallpox) virus were both threatened by developments in 1958. Further, an exotic institutional actor, the US Communicable Disease Center (CDC, later renamed the Centers for Disease Control and Prevention), played a leading role in these developments.[1] Little note was taken of CDC's involvement at the time, because not only was its future global leadership unsuspected, but the diplomatic significance of foreign assistance in humanitarian crises was still being established.[2] Most observers at the time assumed that the long-established Red Cross and Red Crescent societies and the newly founded World Health Organization (WHO) would be the key international players. However, an opening for CDC came when smallpox and cholera broke out everywhere in East Pakistan in the spring of 1958.[3]

Cholera and smallpox were endemic to both East and West Bengal.[4] The diseases were historically embedded in regional culture, and Hindu and Muslim devotees were known to worship disease deities in village shrines and temples.[5] Indeed, the bacteria that cause cholera (*Vibrio cholerae*) are thought to have evolved in the waters at the face of the Ganges-Meghna-Brahmaputra delta, and local variants of cholera have emerged seven times since 1817 to encompass the world.[6] Smallpox was just as deeply entrenched as cholera; it had a multi-year epidemic cycle, the severity in any given year depending on the number of susceptible infants and children. By mid-April of 1958, according to official sources, at least 700 Bengalis were dying of cholera weekly and another 1,500 of smallpox.[7] While these numbers are large, they had been larger in previous years. However, public anxiety was greater than usual in spring of 1958, because political and technical troubles had crippled the East Pakistan (EP) Department of Public Health. The department was small and poorly funded; it had twenty-five district health officers to serve 43 million people.[8] Vaccination was performed by badly paid vaccinators supervised by a handful of sanitary inspectors.[9] An Institute of Public Health in Dacca produced 48 million doses of smallpox lymph each month, enough for every East Pakistani. But in April 1958, at the very moment when smallpox mortality was rising, production fell to 14 million doses, because a province-wide outbreak of rinderpest had caused a shortage of calves needed to make vaccine.[10] The supply of cholera vaccine, considerably less immunogenic than smallpox vaccine, was less of an issue, but it too was limited.[11]

In addition to epidemics, political crises continuously agitated EP public life in the spring of 1958. There were three chief points of contention. First, provincial autonomy: many Bengalis asked, why should the elected government in Dacca be unable to appoint its own officials and commit provincial resources without waiting on orders from distant ministers and bureaucrats in the West? Second, official language: why should the Bangla language, spoken by 43 million East Pakistanis, not receive the same official recognition in public life and education as Urdu, a language spoken by millions fewer West Pakistanis? Third, ideology: why should Pakistan be bound to military alliances with USA and the UK instead of forging closer ties with more obvious allies in communist China and the Soviet Union?[12] Party and personal power struggles along these lines led to affrays in the legislative chamber, and there was frequent churning of ministerial leaders in Dacca.[13] As a result public services, including education and public health, were often paralysed.

In January 1958 newspapers in Dacca began to report outbreaks of smallpox and cholera in peripheral districts, giving a few lines to each on inside pages (Figure 1.1). Because smallpox and cholera were familiar seasonal diseases, these initial reports produced little public response.

NEWS FROM DISTRICTS

DACCA

10 Pox Deaths

MUNSHIGANJ. Feb. 24:— Cases of smallpox are reported from the villages of ,Hashail Union of the Tangibari Police Station. So far 10 persons died of small-pox. Dearth of pure drinking water is reported to be sesponsible for the spread of smallpox.—UPP.

School Managing Body

MUNSHIGANJ. Feb. 24:— The District Magistrate, Dacca has dissolved the existing Managing Committee of the Sholghar A. K. S. High English School of Sreenagar Police Station. An ad-hoc Committee has been appointed with Mr. U. C Sarkar, Circle Office, Lohaganj as Secretary, it is learnt. UPP.

Govt. Grant

MUNSHIGANJ. Feb. 24:— The Government of East Pakistan has allotted a sum of Rs. 13,000 for the re-excavation of Taltala-Lohajang Canal, it was learnt here.—UPP.

Bengali Drama

BARISAL

Ex-Servicemen Assocn.

FROM OUR CORRESPONDENT

BARISAL. Feb. 22:—Local Ex-Servicemen at a meeting, held recently in the Zilla School ground have formed an association under the name of Barisal Exservicemen Association. The association will be non-political and non-communal in character and aims at working for the social and economical upliftment of the ex-servicemen of the district.

An eleven-member Executive Committee was formed with Capt. M. Ahmed, M.B. as the president and Messrs S. M. Dutta Chowdhury and B B. Chowdhury as the Joint Secretaries.

Office-Bearers Of Bar Assocn.

FROM OUR CORRESPONDENT

BARISAL, Feb. 22:—The office-bearers of the local Bar Association for the year 1958 have been elected at an annual general meeting held here recently, Mr. Abani Nath Kush sitting President and Mr Mohd Yunus have been elected as President and Secretary respectively of

RAJSHAHI

Scarcity Of Cigarettes

FROM OUR CORRESPONDENT

RAJSHAHI, Feb. 23:—Acute Scarcity of cigarettes is prevailing in the local town since long and Scissors is selling @ 10 annas and Capstan @ Ropee one and annas four per packet.

It may be mentioned here that army officials have arrested one person for selling cigarettes at higher rates. They have also raided the shop of local cigarette agents but found nothing, it is further learnt.

Outbreak Of Pox

FROM A CORRESPONDENT

NATORE, Feb. 22:—Outbreak of smallpox and other epidemic diseases have been reported from whole Natore Sub-division dhe to tee want of pure drinking water.

The Government of East Pakistan have been urged to pay immediate attention in this regard.

Figure 1.1 Fragmentary news reports of smallpox outbreaks from EP districts of smallpox, *Pakistan Observer*, 23 February 1958. News reports were a source of outbreak intelligence that travelled faster than the EP Health Department's passive surveillance.

As the spring advanced, however, the capital itself was threatened, and alarmed letters to the editor and editorials appeared on the front and inside pages.[14] By April cholera and smallpox concerned readers in West Pakistan as well.[15] On 9 April the Chief Minister in Dacca, Ataur Rahman Khan (Awami League), acceded to pressure and called a public meeting to review the epidemic situation.[16] On this occasion the provincial Health Minister, D. N. Datta, announced mortality estimates and the extent of his department's vaccine problems.[17] After hours of discussion, the Chief Minister proclaimed the formation of a Citizens Provincial Epidemic Control Committee (CPECC) to manage the epidemics through civil society means. The Citizens Committee included physicians, medical college professors, a few provincial assembly members, a few Health Department officials and representatives from social, political, student and welfare organisations.[18] 'In effect, this replaced the Health Department by a voluntary organisation', noted a foreign observer, T. A. Cockburn.[19] A smaller 'Operational Committee' was responsible for day-to-day activities and met frequently for several months.

While the CPECC urged an increase in the Health Department budget, its chief proposal was to recruit and train volunteers who would first vaccinate in Dacca and then fan out across the province. The requirements for success were, first, to mobilise a huge number of enthusiastic students and, second, to secure copious vaccine supplies from abroad. The same foreign observer inferred that the Chief Minister's motive was 'to shift responsibility for the epidemic disaster from his own Government to the Committee' – it was to be, in effect, a 'vigilante' organisation.[20] This is an exaggeration – the CPECC was never wholly out of control – but it quickly developed an agenda that drove out dissenters. For example, it endorsed casual vaccination methods that riled the few committee members who were public health professionals. Dacca newspapers, delighted by the CPECC's energy and novelty, mostly supported its efforts; they also urged their readers, 'Get yourself inoculated. Cholera and smallpox are spreading in the city.'[21]

Arrival of international aid, March–April 1958

The Government of Pakistan (GOP), facing criticism for unacceptably high mortality in EP, and already anxious about the success of the

Communists in the 1954 provincial legislative elections, made an effort to relieve the epidemics.[22] In early April it turned to the International Federation of the Red Cross and Red Crescent Societies and the WHO for help. The WHO took the lead and broadcast a global call for vaccines and other supplies. Although there was then no mechanism to stockpile and dispatch relief aid, twenty-five countries sent Pakistan more than 22 million doses of smallpox vaccine between April and June 1958. The first country to respond was the USA, specifically a specialised agency within the State Department, the International Cooperation Administration (ICA, antecedent to the Agency for International Development), which had staff in the Karachi embassy and Dacca consulate.

Some US vaccine arrived in Dacca within two weeks of the GOP/WHO request, and by the end of June the USA had supplied more than half of the total imports.[23] Other major donors included Republican China, France, Canada, the Soviet Union and the WHO itself (Table 1.1). While most smallpox vaccine arrived as liquid lymph under

Table 1.1 Major donors of smallpox vaccine to East Pakistan, spring 1958[a]

Doses of lymph (wet) or freeze-dried vaccine (dry)
USA and US Red Cross Society 11.81 million, wet
Chinese Red Cross Society (Taiwan) 2.88 million, wet and dry
Soviet Union 2.25 (3.0) million, dry[b]
World Health Organization 1.72 million, dry
Canadian Red Cross Society 1.4 million, wet
French Catholic Relief Society 1.1 million, dry
India 0.43 million, wet
Turkish Red Crescent Society 0.10 million, wet
Germany and German Red Cross Society 0.69 million, wet and dry

[a] Cockburn, 'Epidemic Crisis in EP', p. 3, CDC-RG 442. There was a great profusion of vaccines arriving from different countries in variously sized vials, bottles, ampoules, and so on, with different labels and instructions.
[b] The larger figure for Soviet dry vaccine was noted by the American consul in Dacca. Gene Caprio to Department of State, Foreign Service Despatch no. 362, Dacca, 17 June 1958, CDC-RG 442.

refrigeration, the vaccine furnished by the Soviet Union (USSR) came freeze-dried – a promising new mode unaffected by ambient temperatures.[24] Smaller amounts of cholera vaccine were also sent, including one million doses from the People's Republic of China.[25]

The swift and generous response from the USA to the call for vaccine was no mystery. South Asia was a Cold War theatre in 1958, and Pakistan belonged to two US military alliances – CENTO (the Baghdad Pact) and SEATO.[26] US security doctrine in this period held that grinding poverty, unchecked epidemics and other such features predisposed underdeveloped countries to turn toward Communism; further, the USSR was suspected of playing on 'local aspirations, resentments and fears' to advance an anti-American agenda.[27]

Since the mid-1950s US diplomats had been monitoring the rise of the leftist National Awami Party (NAP) in East Pakistan, which they believed to be intent on exploiting epidemics and food shortages to disparage Pakistan's pro-western policies. Hence in early April of 1958, ICA staff assembled an emergency aid package that, in addition to scouring the earth for vaccine, also brought in a US Naval Medical Research Unit (NAMRU 2) from Taiwan to Dacca to work on the cholera threat.[28] Furthermore, the ICA set in motion the appointment of a Chief Public Health Adviser to the Government of East Pakistan, Dr Aidan T. Cockburn, MBBS, DPH.[29] Cockburn, a 46-year-old British epidemiologist who had previously served as WHO adviser to the government of Ceylon, arrived with his family in Dacca on 20 April. Cockburn was being paid by ICA and was seconded to the Pakistan government. He quickly gained the trust of the Pakistan central Minister of Health and the EP provincial Minister of Health; the latter named him director of the Institute of Public Health in Dacca.[30] US Information Service (USIS) units in Dacca and Karachi arranged for these developments to be covered favourably in local newspapers and their own Bangla-language newsletter, *Markin Parikrama* (American Survey).

CDC epidemiologists and active surveillance

News of the US aid package for Pakistan caught the attention of Dr Alexander D. Langmuir, MD, MPH, chief epidemiologist of the US Communicable Disease Center in Atlanta.[31] Langmuir, a 48-year-old public health physician, was a graduate of Harvard College and Cornell

Medical School and had been a professor of epidemiology at Johns Hopkins University School of Hygiene and Public Health before joining CDC in Atlanta in 1949. He was the US Government's top investigative or field epidemiologist.[32] Since 1951 he had built up a field epidemiology training programme at CDC, rather colourfully named the Epidemic Intelligence Service (EIS), which enjoyed a reputation for coping with difficult outbreaks and other health crises in the US.[33] By 1958 Langmuir was chafing to test his EIS officers – most of whom were conscripted physicians trained in field epidemiology by being directly planted in state and local health departments – in deeper waters abroad. He was openly scouting opportunities in third-world settings where he knew 'active surveillance' methods would prove valuable (Figure 1.2).[34]

Tipped off by Cockburn about developments in Pakistan, Langmuir cabled the US Embassy in Karachi on 22 April, offering a team of

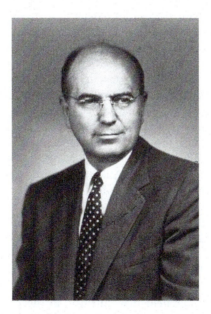

Figure 1.2 Dr Alexander D. Langmuir, Chief Epidemiologist, Communicable Disease Center, Atlanta GA, c.1955. Source: National Library of Medicine.

epidemiologists for service in EP.[35] He and Cockburn were of the same generation; both had been army epidemiologists during the Second World War, and Cockburn had been a CDC Chief of Encephalitis Branch from 1948 to 1954 before moving to the WHO. The two of them had co-authored a paper a year earlier.[36] ICA administrators in Karachi, reasoning that two senior epidemiologists might be better than one, agreed to fund the CDC team's expenses. The ensuing effort in EP was CDC's first group aid mission abroad.[37]

Langmuir's reputation as a giant of epidemiology was due to his successful practice of an investigative method he called 'active surveillance', by which he meant 'continued watchfulness over the distribution and trends of [disease] incidence through the systematic collection, consolidation and evaluation of morbidity and mortality reports and other relevant data.'[38] 'Continued watchfulness' required the collection and interpretation of data that revealed the velocity and route of a pathogen's movement through a defined population. Active surveillance was to be contrasted with 'passive surveillance' such as was practised in EP, which involved the slow peregrination of an uncertain diagnosis from an illiterate village watchman to the Health Ministry via intermediaries and an unreliable postal system.[39] Active surveillance, in contrast, took place in real-time as an outbreak occurred. If a disease could be quickly profiled – whether in a school, temple or mosque, barrack, factory, city or state – then a rapid, precise response would be launched.

Of course, it helped to know the infective agent's identity – was it influenza, salmonella or polio? – and its means of transmission – mayonnaise or mosquitos? But when a pathogen was unknown, CDC microbiologists stood ready in Atlanta to identify it. The investigative goal was not deep thoroughness but elegant sufficiency: collect just enough data to see a pattern, then work out where and how to halt the outbreak. EIS officers received their training on the job and learned how to make their own inquiries, going from hospital to hospital, clinic to clinic, and even patient to patient. They stood ready to travel when stressed-out city or state officials summoned, and glossy magazine journalists in the USA took to calling them 'disease detectives'.[40]

Further, Langmuir held that 'intrinsic in the concept [of surveillance] is the regular dissemination of the basic data to all who have contributed and to all others who need to know.'[41] Not only must field epidemiologist share their data, they must also renounce credit for any success in favour of the agency that had summoned them; it was politic to give away the glory. Following these principles, Langmuir and CDC had made allies in state and local health departments; over several decades, active surveillance became an essential tool of US and then international public health practice.[42]

Cockburn, who arrived in Dacca three weeks before the EIS contingent, met with strong objection on being appointed to the CPECC by the Pakistan Minister of Health. He was the only foreigner on an all-Bengali Committee pursuing a left-populist agenda. His role – 'Public Health Adviser to East Pakistan' – had been invented by ICA, and it seemed plausible to many that he was a US agent. In any case, he knew precious little about the Bengalis, their culture and their homeland. As a consequence, he noted later, the CPECC Operational Committee was 'extremely vicious to me', and he faced several weeks of 'bitter fighting and arguing'.[43] Once accepted on to the Committee, he found it to be often dysfunctional. Here is his account of a CPECC meeting in May:

> The Committee set to work with the avowed intention of destroying the Public Health Department. The Committee originally had many civil servants on it, but the unofficial members insulted these civil servants so much that they stopped attending the meetings. By the date of my arrival on May 20 [*sic*; his actual arrival was 20 April], the effective committee now consisted of about eight members who had complete control of all matters dealing with smallpox and cholera. This committee consisted of a veteran newspaper reporter, a private practitioner, a medical student, and the remainder were very junior doctors in government employ. Not only was the whole [Health] Department afraid of this group, but the Minister himself dared not oppose it. At one of the meetings that I attended they demanded more money for their work, and when the Minister stated he did not have any more, they rose to their feet shouting at the Minister and insulting him. One young doctor harangued the Minister for nearly ten minutes, his voice rising higher and higher to a thin scream, until finally it cracked and he burst into tears. The Secretary and the Director of Public Health both sat silent and the Minister kept his head bowed in an abject posture, even though this particular doctor was only a junior member of the health department. The Committee got the money they demanded.[44]

Bowing to the Committee's will, Cockburn agreed to support a mass campaign based on volunteers rather than on trained public health staff. He then threw himself into the recruitment of university students. This shift, dictated initially by political necessity and later defended as an effective strategy, preceded the arrival of Langmuir and his EIS team and marked a professional divide that would never be overcome (Figure 1.3).

After briefings in Karachi, Langmuir and his eight-man team flew to Dacca on 12 May and were met by consular, ICA and USIS officers.[45]

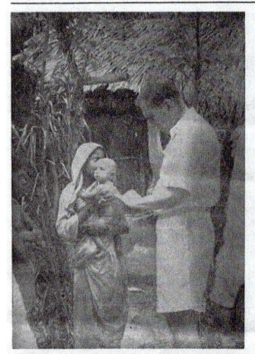

Figure 1.3 Dr T. Aidan Cockburn, East Pakistan Provincial Health Adviser, vaccinating an infant in Barisal district. Source: *Markin Parikrama* ('American Survey'), May 1958.

The week of their arrival coincided with peak smallpox mortality. Accompanying Langmuir as his deputy were Glenn Usher, an unflappable CDC physician-epidemiologist, and seven EIS physician-trainees.[46] Their plane was loaded with vaccine on ice, and USIS staff had planned a publicity blitz around the arrival of experts and supplies.

While the Dacca papers took note of the Americans' arrival, their enthusiasm was restrained; some journalists were openly anti-American, others were at best lukewarm; the US team had arrived under the auspices of the Karachi government at a time of elevated anti-central government sentiment. When a Russian team of bacteriologists landed a few days later, also bearing large quantities of vaccine, the Dacca press was much more welcoming. Langmuir, following Cockburn's advice, established cordial relations with the Soviet team, which was given workspace next to the Americans in the Institute of Public Health. It soon became clear that the Russians were mainly interested in cholera research.[47] While the Russian scientists researched, Soviet diplomats tried to funnel the two million doses of freeze-dried vaccine to the pro-communist National Awami Party for the party's own team of volunteer vaccinators. Cockburn intervened to ensure that all vaccine was stored together in the Institute of Public Health for allocation through the CPECC.[48]

Langmuir quickly discovered that the CPECC would not tolerate the US direction of the campaign and that the CDC's role would be to support, not to command.[49] On 18 May – just six days after the US team arrived – the Chief Minister, Atur Rahman Khan, called a press conference to announce that, given abundant epidemiological expertise and copious supplies of foreign vaccine, the CPECC had decided to ramp up what had been a smallpox control campaign to an *eradication* campaign. The CPECC, the Chief Minister promised, would raise a volunteer force of 20,000 students that would stamp out both smallpox and cholera in East Bengal in four months.[50] A pamphlet stating these aims was distributed to the press.[51] Cockburn approved of the pamphlet, and it is likely that he was its author.[52] The projected eradication campaign rested on three premises: first, that vaccination was a simple procedure and could be easily taught to volunteers; second, that vaccine was abundant and possessed immunological potency; and third, that volunteers would come forward in large numbers. Smallpox eradication would thus become a people's movement, because, in Cockburn's sympathetic view, 'the citizens of the country had started a vast spontaneous, unplanned, uncoordinated effort to vaccinate themselves.'[53] Cockburn fully endorsed the premise that motivated volunteers could accomplish great tasks in public health.[54]

While the three premises proved to be more or less correct, success did not, in fact, come as easily and swiftly as had been promised. This did not escape the Chief Minister who, one month after the campaign began, reconsidered the unbridled authority he had made over to the CPECC. At a meeting on 25 May he announced to members that henceforth Cockburn would be in control of the campaign. Thereafter Cockburn directed, to the chagrin of many. However, the Chief Minister also insisted that a Bengali doctor would serve as the committee's figurehead chair. Now in charge, Cockburn made no dramatic changes in CPECC's volunteer methods, rather he laboured to make them work smoothly and to ensure that public health personnel supported rather than opposed the volunteer campaign.[55]

Langmuir's men were enraged by Cockburn's abandonment of standard public health methods, but they kept quiet. They had no doubt that the Chief Minister had announced the eradication campaign in mid-May because he had learned from Cockburn that the WHO would be debating global eradication at the World Health Assembly (WHA) in June.[56] By proclaiming an EP eradication plan, his government was stealing a march on domestic opponents and the rest of the world. Langmuir, who thought eradication unlikely under the best of circumstances, was flushed out by Bengali reporters and said diplomatically: '[if] the basic organisation [were] there, there was no reason why the East Pakistan government should not be able to eradicate smallpox.'[57] But of course he knew that 'the basic organisation' – meaning a health department of trained professionals backstopped by a well-equipped infrastructure – was not there at all.

The popular vaccination campaign, April–July 1958

Within a few weeks of the CPECC's creation in April, several hundred volunteers were recruited, beginning with students from the Medical College on the campus of Dacca University.[58] Most university students were patriotic supporters of regional autonomy, having waged a protracted, sometimes violent but successful campaign to secure full recognition for the Bengali language in Pakistan's public life a few years before.[59] The call for a people's vaccination campaign was another opportunity to aid fellow Bengalis and serve their province. Cockburn is still remembered for an address he made to 1,000 university students in May 1958; he spoke animatedly about vaccination, but his medical terminology required translation. Thereupon many students volunteered.[60]

Within a few weeks students had vaccinated nearly 300,000 inhabitants of Dacca.[61] They then set off for district towns. The CPECC provided them with four rupees a day for food, and they had permission to travel free on the state railways.[62] By late May, citizens' subcommittees had been established in most district and sub-divisional towns, where they organised evening health spectacles to galvanise the public and attract volunteers. With the assistance of magistrates, army officers and other notables, they staged parades, organised lectures, held concerts and screened short films about health and sanitation. New volunteers were trained, given lists of targeted wards or villages, and sent off with boxed vials of vaccine. In some places schoolteachers taught their students to vaccinate, and it was noticed that schoolgirls could freely enter homes to vaccinate women in purdah. In other places local officials called on *Ansars*, a part-time force of police auxiliaries, usually farmers, urging them to volunteer. The volunteers' efforts, where backstopped by district officers and available public health staff, resulted in widespread acceptance of vaccination, which was understood to be a project by Bengalis for Bengalis. There were no reports of resistance or opposition. Yet in districts where official support was lacking or where there was inter-party competition, the coverage was distinctly spotty.[63]

Significantly, the vaccination methods taught to volunteers were streamlined until only the bare essentials of standard Health Department inoculation protocols were retained. First, the vaccine cold chain was ignored, apparently without ill effects.[64] Second, alcohol swabbing before vaccinating was given up, as was bandaging vaccinees' slight wounds. Third, in lieu of medically purposed needles or rotary vaccination lancets, ordinary needles were widely used (the ICA sourced 11 million sewing-machine needles, which were distributed like prizes). Fourth, there was no common method of inoculation: 'all vaccinators

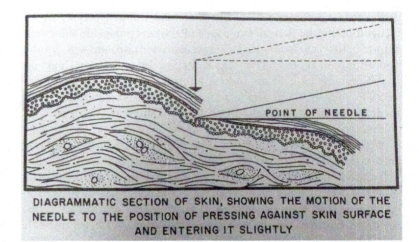

POINT OF NEEDLE

DIAGRAMMATIC SECTION OF SKIN, SHOWING THE MOTION OF THE
NEEDLE TO THE POSITION OF PRESSING AGAINST SKIN SURFACE
AND ENTERING IT SLIGHTLY

Figure 1.4 Professional methods of vaccination. WHO, *Handbook for
Smallpox Eradication Programmes in Endemic Areas* WHO/SE/67.5 (Geneva
1967), pp. III–10.

soon went their own ways, some making punctures, others making
long scratches, while some did elaborate cross hatchings'. Fifth, record-
keeping was minimised, and volunteers kept track only of the number
of doses administered without taking down names or other information.[65] These modifications, made in the interest of speed and simplic-
ity, were suited to an amateur force whose energy and enthusiasm were
key ingredients in the campaign (Figure 1.4).

Admittedly, enthusiasm could flag, and unopened boxes of vaccine
were sometimes found abandoned.[66] An EIS observer who shadowed
volunteers in the Brahmanbaria subdivision of Tippera district noted
that they were primarily

> local students of upper school and lower college levels ... The students
> have no field or family commitments to worry about; yet they work in
> their own union so they can return to their home or a friend's home each
> night after work. Their morale and sense of public service is far higher
> than the *ansars'* [i.e. home-guards]. They have been granted an extended

vacation so that they are free to do their work ... They work in small teams, each with a supervising teacher, village by village. They are far more literate and reliable as reporters of their activities than *ansars* ... There are problems, however. Morale is declining as the volunteers enter their third week ... The ASDO [Assistant Sub-divisional Officer] admits that the students are missing a good number of persons due to unwillingness to be vaccinated or absence in the field.[67]

The observer estimated that 30,000 Bengalis were vaccinated daily by these unorthodox means at the height of the campaign.[68] The cholera and smallpox epidemics both subsided spontaneously, as was normal, with the monsoon's arrival in late June.

CDC field epidemiologists go into the districts

In EP the most basic data for understanding disease trends, such as hospital admissions, lab-confirmed diagnoses, and morbidity and mortality statistics, were often non-existent. It was estimated that only one in ten cases of smallpox was officially reported.[69] Thus a principal mechanism for finding outbreaks was via the several daily newspapers to which stringers in outlying areas sent brief reports by telegraph. These reports came to notice more swiftly than the Health Department's chain of reporting, but were not always accurate. Langmuir and his team were eager to analyse health data, but they lacked the ability to generate the numbers themselves – they could neither read, nor speak nor count in Bengali and were ignorant of the cultural and political terrain. Under these circumstances, what could they do that would be of real significance? After discussions with Cockburn, the health ministers and the CPECC committee, the CDC team agreed to become 'the "eyes and ears" of the smallpox control programme' by visiting all seventeen districts and preparing reports that would 'evaluate the current control campaigns in the districts and identify areas of success and failure ... [and other] epidemiological factors of importance to the smallpox control programme'.[70] In short, Langmuir's team took on an evaluation task; they had no authority over vaccination policy nor over volunteer vaccinators.[71] Langmuir promised the reports would be completed by late June, when monsoon floods always put an end to most rural travel. He and Usher would stay behind in Dacca to attend to logistics.[72]

From 19 May until 15 June the seven EIS officers fanned out into the districts, each with a volunteer Bengali physician-guide. They traced vaccine supply chains, observed volunteers in training and action, and counted the frequency of scars from previous vaccinations. They tested the Soviet freeze-dried vaccine and determined it was just as effective as liquid lymph. They found that prior vaccination did not always confer long-term immunity. They discovered great unevenness in coverage and determined that the campaign would not reach its goal of 80 per cent coverage. They estimated that hundreds of thousands of infants and children were being missed.[73] In Comilla district, which was considered the most successful in the province, EIS officer Fred Dunn found that 'a sizable and particularly vulnerable segment of the population [children] will still remain unprotected'.[74]

In Brahmanberia sub-division of Comilla, '12 percent of children under four years of age and 27 percent of infants under 1 year of age remained unvaccinated after the campaign had completed in those areas'.[75] Coverage was even less complete in the other districts. At the end of their tours, the EIS officers prepared reports containing mostly negative accounts of volunteer-based smallpox control. The gist of these, but not the reports themselves, were shared with EP health officials and district magistrates in late June meetings.

During this four-week period – late May until late June – relations between Cockburn and CDC team members came to the brink of collapse. They despised him for failing to stand up to Bengali politicians. They repeated a rumour that he enjoyed ministerial favour, and especially his appointment as Director of the Institute of Public Health, because he had promised millions of dollars from the Americans to furnish and equip the near-empty building.[76] They loathed his encouragement of volunteerism and referred to the eradication programme as 'Aidan's circus' and 'Operation Cockburn Fantastique'. Their criticisms went beyond his 'wandering minstrel' show to the man himself, whom they mocked as a bumbler, a 'madman' who 'hopped up and down' when agitated, and who impulsively 'ran out of the room'. As physicians, they decided he needed tranquillising.[77] In these and other ways they undercut his authority as Chief Public Health Adviser and threw cold water on the volunteer campaign. The most likely cause of this venomous criticism was that they felt vulnerable for being so closely associated with an unprofessional and wasteful campaign they expected to fail.[78] Usher wrote to Langmuir,

> I've been uneasy all along about the position of our team in relation to this situation, and I'm still uneasy. We are all thoroughly convinced that Aidan's whoop-de-doo campaign is going to fall far short of vaccinating 80% or 90% of the population in four months. But he has announced loudly that *he* will accomplish this, and in so doing he has antagonised a lot of people, including the entire membership of the Committee ... When the campaign fails to achieve its goal in the allotted time, they will hit him hard and I'm afraid we'll get splattered with some of the mud.[79]

Yet, despite their unhappiness, the appearance of civility was maintained. Meanwhile, EP political life became ever more confused. On 22 June the appointed Governor suddenly dismissed the elected EP government and took over administration of the province. Langmuir suggested to Usher that 'all in all it would seem very wise for the epidemiological team to withdraw as fast as possible; that is, as fast as can be achieved without rocking the boat or blowing off more booby traps'. Yet despite his feeling that the aid mission to EP had been a 'rollercoaster', a 'wild and wondrous ride', he called it a 'complete success' – for the ironic reason that it could have been so much worse.[80]

When an elected EP ministry returned in August, political struggle among the major parties only intensified, leading to physical violence on the floor of the Legislative Assembly in October. Cockburn was somehow able to ride this roller-coaster while still attending to his duties.

Absorbing the lessons of the 1958 East Pakistan epidemics

After the EIS team returned to the USA in June, Langmuir and Usher prepared trip reports and sent detailed proposals to ICA and the EP Ministry of Health for strengthening anti-smallpox and anti-cholera measures.[81] There was considerable back and forth of draft documents between Atlanta and Dacca, where Cockburn continued to be the EP point-person for public health. However, Cockburn and CDC epidemiologists were often at loggerheads about these proposed projects. A scathing note on a manuscript by an EIS officer reads: 'I'm getting

sick & tired of Cockburn's brief ridiculous letters – we probably should
end all correspondence with the idiot – there seems no point in continuing these nonsensical arguments.'[82] Eventually, Cockburn realised
his views were unwelcome to CDC, and he vented his bitterness in a
note to his employers in ICA:

> I regret that I was not consulted in the production of any of the CDC
> reports ... Reading through [them] one has the impression the CDC
> came, saw and conquered the epidemic single-handed, and that any
> achievements of the Pakistani government (which are hardly men-
> tioned) or other teams were negligible ... One wonders what would
> have happened if [the CDC team] had not come here. Twenty million
> [sic] people would still have been vaccinated, and the programme would
> have gone on much the same ... In all the reports the CDC seems to be
> looking at the situation through American rather than Asian eyes.[83]

While Langmuir and Cockburn were fundamentally on the same side
– the side of scientific medicine, effective public health and American
aid – their rapport had ended. Cockburn wrote to Langmuir to say rue-
fully: 'You once said that our basic philosophies were different. That is
very true. You like to assemble facts in a selected order and build a kind
of pyramid that is solid. I take a few facts and arrange them until I see
a kind of general outline and then attempt to fill in the gaps. To you
things are much more static than to me. To me, everything moves.'[84]

In May 1959 the Twelfth World Health Assembly, meeting in
Geneva, adopted smallpox eradication as an official WHO programme.[85] There was now considerable interest in what had occurred
in EP the previous year. Langmuir and Cockburn were the obvious
ones to give a public account, but their long-mooted, jointly authored
article documenting the campaign was a casualty of their falling out.
Instead, Langmuir and Usher decided to prepare an article presenting
the aid mission's results from CDC's perspective, while Cockburn
drafted his own article, defending volunteer methods and CPECC's
record. Unusually, and perhaps uncomfortably for the authors, the
articles appeared side by side without editorial comment in the January
1960 *Public Health Reports*, official journal of the US Public Health
Service.[86]

Langmuir and Usher agreed to focus on a single question: What light
did the 1958 EP campaign shed on the problems of eradicating a

disease in a high-density setting? When faced with the need to commit himself to paper, however, Langmuir bowed out, writing to Usher, as follows:

> We have read and been rather disenchanted with Dr. T. A. Cockburn's efforts at producing a publishable manuscript ... Reluctantly we have come to the firm conclusion that we do not have good enough epidemiological data to warrant a published paper ... we realize that we have a fine adventure story to tell, but not much of a scientific contribution to make ... If you wish to prepare some sort of manuscript ... you should feel perfectly free to do so.[87]

Usher, who had some definite ideas about the EP campaign, accordingly prepared an article for publication. The article, entitled 'The Feasibility of Smallpox Eradication', ignored cholera to focus on smallpox. In a several tables and graphs it laid out the 1958 epidemic's total mortality, the rates of mortality, and age- and sex-specific mortality rates and presented similar data from past epidemics for comparison. Predictably, he painted a negative picture of volunteerism as a model for WHO eradication work. A discussion section then addressed the reasons that made smallpox eradication in East Pakistan such a challenge. One reason was that smallpox was deeply entrenched; despite demonstrably high rates of vaccination – between 80 and 90 per cent – the epidemiologists had been 'unable to find a correlation between the proportion of the population that had been vaccinated and either the time of onset or the intensity of the epidemic in various districts'.[88] In other words, mass vaccination in EP had not generated the 'herd immunity' that in other places favoured eradication.[89] Usher concluded that 'the time of epidemic onset and the intensity of the epidemic were more closely related to population density than to vaccination status'.[90]

Such matters of fact – mortality, immunity, population density, endemicity – are the regular concerns of field epidemiology, and Usher's article put these features of the EP epidemic on a firm numerical basis. However, when he turned to answer a burning policy question – how to tackle entrenched smallpox in poor, densely settled countries – he departed from numerical evidence and entered the terrain of judgement. His key recommendation was that eradicators must be prepared to use constraint against 'groups that [respond] poorly to vaccination campaigns and [experience] high attack rates.'[91] To quote him at some length:

> In the surveillance or 'firefighting' phase of an eradication programme selective vaccinating of exposed persons (sometimes referred to as 'ring containment') is, of course, desirable, but it is not considered advisable to rely entirely upon this for the emergency containment of outbreaks. This is especially true in a country like East Pakistan where health services are not fully developed, and there is a shortage of qualified personnel for the performance of contact investigations. In such circumstances it seems essential to rely on 'area containment,' that is, an immediate, very intensive campaign to raise to the highest possible level the vaccination status of a community where an outbreak has occurred. The successful execution of the 'firefighting' phase of the eradication programme where the problem is as difficult as it is in East Pakistan may require rather drastic measures, such as area quarantine, during the time required to vaccinate a community in which an outbreak has occurred. Enforcement of emergency measures will need to be determined and persistent.[92]

Why did Usher recommend 'drastic', 'determined' and 'persistent' measures? What had he and other EIS epidemiologists seen in EP that made 'emergency' or 'firefighting' measures like area containment – meaning that whole villages would be corralled and no one could exit without vaccination, whatever their prior immune status – necessary? From their unpublished exchanges it is evident the CDC team had been appalled by the circus-like atmosphere whipped up during the 1958 'citizens' campaign. Such popular methods, with their admittedly casual inoculation technique, uneven coverage, neglect of small children and thinly disguised political purpose, must never be repeated. Only trained health staff that possessed the will to take 'drastic measures' would succeed. Voluntary methods that wasted vaccine and depended on 'herd immunity' would never be able to enforce necessary discipline. To be sure, Usher's views were consonant with post-war assumptions everywhere, which held that public health immunisation requires military rigour and organisation.[93]

Cockburn's article, 'Epidemic Crisis in East Pakistan, April–July, 1958', could not have been more different. While acknowledging the value of the CDC's work collecting information from rural districts, he underlined the success of the volunteer-based approach and recommended it as a model for the coming global eradication campaign. In a key passage he observed that:

> Smallpox is easy to prevent; vaccination is simple and can be done by illiterate people. The vaccine is cheap and can be mass-produced. It should be possible for each country in Southeast Asia to vaccinate 90 percent of its people within a year and to repeat the operation every 3 to 5 years. The resulting level of immunity would probably cause the disease to disappear completely ... mass vaccination is not basically a medical undertaking but a layman's job of organisation, propaganda and logistics.[94]

Indeed, Cockburn's position was that vaccination was a simple matter, even for children: 'The children easily picked up the vaccination technique from their teachers, who were trained by the sanitary inspectors. The teams of children, supervised by their teachers, worked in the villages around the schools.'[95] While unsterile technique, breaks in cold chain integrity, and poor record-keeping were admitted defects, Cockburn found them tolerable – his key finding was that eradication was attainable with sufficiently large numbers of motivated volunteers, abundant freeze-dried vaccine and 'herd immunity'. There was no need for careful training or even for exacting supervision. These were the very ideas that had driven Usher and his colleagues to distraction.

Conclusion

From a local perspective it was Bengali middle-class anxiety, conjoined with political opportunism and student enthusiasm, that briefly linked East Pakistanis to each other through the shared experience of vaccination; to that extent, the 'citizens' campaign' can be said to have strengthened a growing realisation among the educated middle class that Bengalis could act together to avert common dangers. This realisation, strengthened in later years by a series of natural and political disasters, ultimately led to Bangladeshi separatism and civil war. Yet, whatever the eventual nationalist benefits, a coup by the Pakistan Army on 24 October 1958 destroyed EP's tattered democracy and civil-society experiments.[96] From a global perspective the 1958 epidemics allowed a military-industrial behemoth, the USA, to project humanitarian aid and technical assistance into a contested region, cementing a strategic alliance with Pakistan. Yet CDC epidemiologists, aiming to save lives and spread the doctrine of active surveillance, found themselves hampered by other actors with different agendas. At stake was whether CDC, authorised for the first time to operate abroad, could demonstrate its prowess in an international health crisis. While Langmuir considered the 1958 mission a failure, the State Department did not. US diplomats measured success mainly in terms of favourable Pakistani opinion of US assistance.[97] The CDC clearly reaped intangible benefits: cementing ties with ICA, USIS and NAMRU; negotiating with Pakistani ministers; laying the groundwork for a cholera research centre in Dacca; and debating virology with eminent Russian scientists – all matters that enhanced CDC's reputation and justified a further global role.

In time even Langmuir took a longer view of the EP mission. He wrote to Usher, 'Someday I have hopes of developing a truly adequate smallpox programme that can lead, both in this country and in the world eradication programme. The Dacca episode … will constitute a major first step, premature, wild and wondrous as it was.'[98] He was right – 1958 *had* been premature; the vaccination campaign in EP was an experiment in the pre-history of global eradication. Fourteen years later CDC epidemiologists returned to Bangladesh and guided the final push in 1974–75 that halted smallpox transmission in Asia; active surveillance proved to be powerfully effective.[99] But, true to Usher's preferences, CDC's successful method of 'surveillance and containment' excluded the public and required the occasional use of force that would never have been tolerated in the USA.[100] In short, 'drastic, determined and persistent firefighting' was effective but hardly popular.

Cockburn would be pleased to learn that at present 'best practices' for immunisation campaigns include, as a matter of course, soliciting volunteers and forging collaborations with local leaders, activists and celebrities; present-day immunisation campaigns are communications-rich and share responsibility with parents, NGOs, political parties and other stakeholders.[101] While he was no doubt erratic and impulsive, Cockburn was also visionary in seeing that disease control is as much a matter of social and political mobilisation, and a recognition that rights must be respected, as of strictly applying almost veterinary methods of restraint. This is especially true in settings of 'complex emergencies', where health crises are compounded by political instability, excess mortality and a meltdown of markets and administration.[102] At the same time, modern disease control campaigns rely heavily on CDC's tried and tested methods of intense surveillance and field investigation; at the time of writing there is a global network of field epidemiology training programmes in fifty countries, all based on Langmuir's training principles of quick responses, modesty in claiming credit and 'learning by doing'.[103] Hence, Usher and Cockburn were both right in their advocacy of essential elements for successful disease control programmes.

Acknowledgements

I thank Mrs Ameena Akbar and Assistant Professor Bilal Hossein, both residents of Dhaka, for finding and compiling print sources from 1958 EP. I am grateful to Sanjoy Bhattacharya, Jaime Benchimol, Stuart Blume, Niels Brimnes, Michaela Hoenicke-Moore, Elisha Renne and Anne Wallis who made helpful suggestions on earlier drafts. Special thanks go to Robert B. Wallace (EIS 1969–70) who first interested me in field epidemiology.

Notes

1 The Communicable Disease Center (CDC) was established in Atlanta in 1946. For several decades the CDC was a small agency in a federal system that resisted centralisation of public health and firmly reserved disease control to the individual states. For a brief account see Bindu Tharian, 'Centers for Disease Control and Prevention', in *New Georgia Encyclopedia for Educators*, www.georgiaencyclopedia.org/articles/science-medicine/centers-disease-control-and-prevention (accessed 24 November 2016). For a full history, see E. W. Etheridge, *Sentinel for Health: A History of the Centers for Disease Control* (Berkeley: University of California Press, 1992).

2 Connections between epidemic threats and global diplomacy date from the mid-nineteenth century and a series of international sanitary conferences mostly concerned with the spread of cholera; see Valeska Huber, 'The Unification of the Globe by Disease? The International Sanitary Conferences on Cholera, 1851–1894', *The Historical Journal*, 49:2 (June 2006), pp. 453–76.

3 Key publications and documents for this episode are: A. D. Langmuir to
   Director, USOM/P Karachi, 'Epidemic Aid – Smallpox and Cholera, EP,
   First Progress Report' (June? 1958), in National Archives and Records
   Administration (NARA), Communicable Disease Center, Public Health
   Service (NARA, CDC Record Group 442.2.3, hereafter CDC-RG 442);
   US Epidemic Aid Team to EP, 'Smallpox in EP' (June? 1958), pp. 1–17
   with appendixes, CDC-RG 442; G. S. Usher, 'Terminal Report: Epidemic
   Aid Mission to EP. May to July 1958', typescript (mid-November 1958),
   pp. 1–19, Records of the US Foreign Assistance Agencies, 1948–61/, ICA,
   Office of the Deputy Director for Ops, Office of Public Health, Near East,
   South Asia, Far East Division, Country Files, Pakistan 1954–60 (NARA,
   ICA-Record Group 469, hereafter ICA-RG 469); Glenn S. Usher. 'The
   Feasibility of Smallpox Eradication', *Public Health Reports*, 75:4 (1960),
   pp. 37–42; Thomas A. Cockburn, 'Epidemic Crisis in EP, April–July,
   1958', *Public Health Reports*, 75:1 (1960), pp. 26–36. A more detailed draft
   version of Cockburn's article is 'Epidemic Crisis in EP, April–June, 1958',
   MS, 32 pages (CDC-RG-442). The author also maintains a personal
   archive of documents received from former EIS officers.
4 In August 1947 the British colony of India was partitioned at independence between Pakistan and India; simultaneously, the colonial province
   of Bengal was also partitioned between (Indian) West Bengal, with its
   capital at Calcutta (present-day Kolkata), and (Pakistani) EP, with its
   capital at Dacca (present-day Dhaka).
5 In the active delta – 40,000 square miles of low-lying alluvial plain criss-
   crossed by large and small rivers and subject to annual monsoon flooding
   – dense waterways allowed Bengalis to move about in small skiffs from
   paddy-growing and fishing villages to marketplaces and mosques, which
   favoured the steady transmission of pathogens.
6 D. A. Sack, R. B. Nair and A. K. Siddique, 'Cholera', *Lancet*, 363:9404 (17
   January 2004), pp. 223–33. The International Center for Diarrheal
   Disease Research (IDDR-B), commonly called 'The Cholera Lab', was
   founded in Dacca in 1962 on the premise that the Bengal delta was cholera's primordial home.
7 While EP's disease reporting system was unable to determine exact morbidity and mortality, the reported prevalence of cholera in 1958 was
   10,438 cases of which 6,684 died (CFR = 64 per cent); the corresponding
   reported figure for smallpox was 44,736 cases, of which 20,444 died (CFR
   = 46 per cent), Usher, 'The Feasibility of Smallpox Eradication', pp. 37–42,
   figures 1 and 2. See also Cockburn, 'Epidemic Crisis in EP', pp. 27–30.
8 Each of EP's 17 districts had a District Health Officer, a Sanitary Inspector
   with two assistants and a single vaccinator; two additional vaccinators

and three additional Sub-divisional Health Officers were temporarily appointed for three months in each district in 1958; Usher, 'Terminal Report', p. 6.

9 F. Fenner, D. A. Henderson, I. Arita, Z. Jezek and I. D. Ladnyi, *Smallpox and Its Eradication* (Geneva: World Health Organization, 1988), p. 811.

10 Vaccine was prepared from lymph harvested from calves' infected bellies. At least 600 calves were required each month. Usher gives monthly totals of smallpox vaccine manufactured in Dacca and imported from elsewhere during January–June 1958. Apparently up to 85 per cent of this amount was wasted because of the scarcity of refrigeration. See Usher, 'Smallpox in EP', p. 12, table 9.

11 No cholera vaccine was manufactured in EP in this period; all supplies were imported.

12 An overview of EP politics in this period is given in Willem Van Schendel, *A History of Bangladesh* (Cambridge University Press, 2009), pp. 107–20. The Pakistan National Assembly met in session twice a year, alternating between Karachi and Dacca.

13 The four leading EP political parties were the Muslim League (pro-Pakistan, anti-communist), the Awami League (pro-Bengal autonomy, anti-communist), the Krishak Praja Party (pro-Bengal autonomy, anti-communist) and the National Awami Party (pro-Bengal autonomy, pro-communist). A good political summary is G. W. Chowdhury, 'The EP Political Scene, 1955–1957', *Pacific Affairs*, 30:4 (1957), pp. 312–20. A fuller account is Salahuddin Ahmed, *Bangladesh Past and Present* (Dhaka: APH Publishers, 2004), pp. 138–51.

14 For example, 'Four more small-pox [sic] cases were admitted to the Mitford Hospital [Dacca] yesterday. It will be recalled here that almost daily four to six smallpox patients were being admitted to the hospital according to ... authorities', *Pakistan Observer* (6 April 1958).

15 For example, 'Distressing reports continue to be received about the havoc caused by the serious epidemics of smallpox and cholera raging in EP ... proof of the shocking – one could even say criminal – failure of the provincial health authorities to control the epidemic?', *Dawn* (Karachi), editorial (13 April 1958), p. 1.

16 'No Concrete Plan to Combat Epidemic', *Pakistan Observer* (Dacca, 10 April 1958), p. 1. Ataur Rahman Khan or ATA (1907–91) became Chief Minister of EP in September 1956 and held the position (with brief interregnums) until martial law was declared and democracy suspended in mid-October 1958.

17 'No Concrete Plan to Combat Epidemic'.

18 Aidan Cockburn to Assistant Director, USOM/Dacca, Confidential Memorandum of Conversation (23 July 1958), p. 2, ICA-RG 286. In time, CPECC grew to include sixty members, but operational control of the vaccination campaign was in the hands of a sub-committee of six or so persons.

19 Cockburn, 'Epidemic Crisis in EP', MS, p. 2.

20 Ibid.

21 For example, Pakistan Observer (13 April 1958).

22 In the March 1954 EP legislative elections, the Communist Party of Pakistan (CPP) entered the Assembly and deepened its influence by forming a united front with other parties. CPP candidates directly and indirectly won a total of 26 seats, making it an important legislative force. See Tariq Ali, The Clash of Fundamentalism. (London: New Left Books, 2002), p. 395.

23 See, for a narrative of the sequence of events leading to significant US aid to Pakistan in 1958, CDC, Epi Aid Memo 58–37–1 (7 May 1958). 'Epidemic Aid-Smallpox – Cholera', CDC-RG 442.

24 Cockburn, 'Epidemic Crisis in EP', pp. 27–30. The EP epidemic was an important trial for freeze-dried vaccine in semi-tropical conditions. There was commercial interest among US drug manufacturers to learn as much as possible about its continued potency at temperatures of more than 40 C (104 F). Foreign Service Despatch no. 362, Dacca (no date), CDC-RG 442.

25 Ibid.

26 CENTO = Central Treaty Organization (also known as the Baghdad Pact) and SEATO = Southeast Asia Treaty Organization. See Lubna Saif, 'Pakistan and SEATO', Pakistan Journal of History and Culture, XXVIII:2 (2007), pp. 77–90.

27 US, National Security Council, Record of Actions Taken, Acting Executive Secretary, to the National Security Council, 13 February 1956. DDRS Document Number: CK3100395518, www.archives.gov/research/search/ (accessed 1 June 2014). See also R. W. Benjamin and J. H. Kautsky, 'Communism and Economic Development', in American Political Science Review, 62:1 (March 1968), pp. 110–23.

28 The 1958 mission to Dacca by the NAMRU-2 team led to the establishment in 1960 of the Pakistan-SEATO Cholera Research Laboratory (the antecedent to the International Centre for Diarrheal Disease Research, Bangladesh ICDDR, B) in June 1979. See Cockburn, 'Epidemic Crisis in EP', p. 3.

29 Cockburn remained in Dacca through the mid-1960s and published a weekly column on public health issues for The Morning News. Foreign Service Despatch no. 42, Dacca, 18 December 1958, CDC-RG 442.

30 Cockburn (1912–81) obtained his medical degree from Durham and a doctorate in Public Health from the Royal Institute of Hygiene and Public Health, London, in 1940. Like Langmuir, he was a trained wartime epidemiologist whose skills became valuable in the post-war world. He worked at CDC from 1948 to 1954 and took US citizenship. He then made a career shift into international health and held WHO assignments in Egypt, Canada and Ceylon before arriving in Dacca. See J. L. Angel and M. R. Zimmerman, 'T. Aidan Cockburn, 1912–1981: A Memorial', *American Journal of Physical Anthropology*, 58:121 (1982): pp. 121–2.

31 The Communicable Disease Center was renamed the Centers for Disease Control and Prevention in 1992 but has retained the CDC acronym.

32 Langmuir's title at CDC was Chief of Epidemiology Branch and Director of the Epidemic Intelligence Service, a position he held from 1951 to 1970. See 'Alexander D. Langmuir – A Brief Biographical Sketch with Emphasis on his Professional Activities', *American Journal of Epidemiology*, 144:8, Supplement (October 1996), pp. S1–S10.

33 See S. B. Thacker, A. L. Dannenberg and D. H. Hamilton, 'Epidemic Intelligence Service of the Centers for Disease Control and Prevention: 50 years of Training and Service in Applied Epidemiology', *American Journal of Epidemiology*, 154:11 (2001), pp. 985–92; W. Schaffner and F. M. LaForce, 'Training Field Epidemiologists: Alexander D. Langmuir and the Epidemic Intelligence Service', *American Journal of Epidemiology*, 144:8 Supplement (1996), pp. S16–22; and A. D. Langmuir, 'The Epidemic Intelligence Service of the Center for Disease Control', *Public Health Reports*, 95:5 (September–October 1980), pp. 470–7.

34 At its creation in 1946 the CDC's scope was entirely domestic; however, with the support of the ICA/AID the CDC gained regular authorisation to send EIS officers and aid teams abroad.

35 A. D. Langmuir, 'CDC, Epi Aid Memo 58–37–1, 7 May 1958, Epidemic Aid-Smallpox – Cholera' and A. D. Langmuir, 'CDC, no date, 'Epidemic Aid-Smallpox – Cholera, First Progress Report', CDC-RG 442.

36 T. A. Cockburn, C. A. Sooter and A. D. Langmuir, 'Ecology of Western Equine and St. Louis Encephalitis Viruses. A Summary of Field Investigations in Weld County, Colorado, 1949 to 1953', *American Journal of Hygiene*, 65 (1957), pp. 130–46.

37 Individual CDC personnel had gone abroad before 1958, and CDC officers occasionally accompanied foreign delegations.

38 A. D. Langmuir, 'The Surveillance of Communicable Diseases of National Importance', *New England Journal of Medicine*, 268:4 (24 January 1963), pp. 182–3; A. D. Langmuir, 'Newer Surveillance Methods in the Control of Communicable Diseases; Developing Concepts in Surveillance', *Milbank Memorial Fund*, Q 43:2, pt. 2 (1965), pp. 369–72; and A. D.

Langmuir, 'Evolution of The Concept of Surveillance in the United States', *Proceedings of the Royal Society of Medicine*, 64 (June 1971), pp. 9–12.

39 As described in Fenner *et al.*, *Smallpox and Its Eradication* (Geneva: World Health Organization, 1988), p. 817.

40 *Time, Newsweek* and other mass magazines fostered the disease detective image. From the 1960s through the 1980s Langmuir maintained a working relationship with a staff writer at the *New Yorker*, who published striking articles about EIS sleuthing in a recurring column, 'The Annals of Epidemiology'.

41 Langmuir, 'The Surveillance of Communicable Diseases of National Importance', p. 183.

42 S. B. Thacker and M. B. Gregg, 'Implementing the Concepts of William Farr: the Contributions of Alexander D. Langmuir to Public Health Surveillance and Communications', *American Journal of Epidemiology*, 144:8, Supplement (1996), pp. S24–5. The official history of the World Health Organization recognises that 'active epidemiological surveillance' was a powerful mid-century public health advance but fails to acknowledge CDC's role in refining it. See WHO, *The Second Ten Years of the World Health Organization, 1958–1967* (Geneva: WHO, 1968), pp. 94–6.

43 A. Cockburn to Assistant Director, USOM/Dacca, Confidential Memorandum of Conversation, 23 July 1958, page 2, ICA-RG 286.

44 *Ibid.*

45 Langmuir earlier spent several weeks in Dacca during August–September of 1954 when the State Department sent him to assist with threatened epidemics during a major flood. No epidemics developed, and he considered the trip a waste of time. A. D. Langmuir to Sally Langmuir, 2 September 1954 (aerogramme), Alan Mason Medical Archives, Johns University, Alexander Langmuir papers (hereafter Langmuir Papers).

46 Besides Langmuir and Usher the CDC team included Drs Frederick Dunn, James Mosley, Yates Trotter, Jacob Brody, Bruce Dull, Chandler Dawson and Malcolm Page. Teams from other agencies and countries arrived in Dacca in the same month to assist with epidemic control – a nine-man American military team from NAMRU-2, as noted, a six-member delegation of microbiologists from the USSR, 20 experienced vaccinators from Afghanistan, and a single French researcher. Cockburn, 'Epidemic Crisis in EP', p. 5, table 2.

47 'USSR Medical Team in Karachi', *Pakistan Observer* (12 May 1958) and 'Russia Medical Aid Lauded' *Pakistan Observer* (13 May 1958). For

the Russian account, see B. N. Pastukhov, 'Visit of Soviet Doctors to Pakistan to Assist in the Campaign Against Cholera and Smallpox' (English translation from Russian), *Journal of Microbiology, Epidemiology and Immunobiology*, 30:2 (1959), pp. 148–51.

48 Consul General's dispatch no. 317, Dacca, 'Political Aspects of Epidemic and Food Shortage in EP' (15 May 1958), p. 3, ICA-RG-469.

49 'It soon became apparent that we could not function in the manner that had been specified in the cable requesting our services, namely to "principally organize control [of] mass vaccination throughout EP". In order to perform in this way it would have been necessary to confer administrative authority upon our team members. This was manifestly not feasible.' Usher, 'Terminal Report', p. 8.

50 'Four-Stage Plan to Eradicate Epidemics', *Pakistan Observer* (19 May 1958). After this date there is less evident concern about cholera in the press record, and smallpox becomes the chief preoccupation.

51 Government of EP and Provincial Epidemic Control Committee. Director of Public Relations, *Eradication of Smallpox and Cholera: A Plan for EP* (Dacca, May 1958), 3 pages. A million copies were printed in Bengali and English, CDC-RG 442.

52 According to Cockburn, it was he who conceived the eradication campaign, but the decision to launch was taken by the Pakistan health minister with the concurrence of the EP Chief Minister. Though they belonged to different parties, both could share in the glory of eradication, which Cockburn assured them was feasible. In Cockburn's words, 'I suggested that something Churchillian was needed – "we shall vaccinate them in the towns, we shall vaccinate them in the paddy fields, etc. etc." I left Mr Huq and the Chief Minister discussing what I said.' Cockburn to Assistant Director, USOM/Dacca, Confidential Memorandum of Conversation (23 July 1958), p. 3, CDC-RG 286.

53 Cockburn, 'Epidemic Crisis in EP', p. 16.

54 It is unclear whether Cockburn knew about contemporary mainland Chinese methods of mass mobilisation for disease control. As a WHO physician he was better informed than most about new developments in public health, and communist politicians in Bengal were in direct contact with Chinese diplomats.

55 A. Cockburn to Assistant Director, USOM/Dacca, Confidential Memorandum of Conversation (23 July 1958), enclosed on p. 4, ICA-RG 286.

56 The USSR's representatives proposed smallpox eradication to the WHA in June 1958. The Assembly decided on one year of further study, and the eradication programme was not adopted by the WHA until 1959. See Fenner *et al.*, *Smallpox and Its Eradication*, pp. 366–71.

57 'Eradicating epidemics from E. Pakistan; Dr. Langmuir Hopeful', *Pakistan Observer* (16 May 1958); 'East Wing Will Be Able to Eradicate Smallpox – US Expert', *Dawn* (Karachi, 25 May 1958).

58 There were competing, party-political efforts to recruit students as vaccinators. For example, the Krishak Sramik Party's Youth League set up an Epidemic Control and Famine Relief Committee that sent students to villages, *Pakistan Observer* (14 April 1958), p. 1 and *Pakistan Observer* (15 May 1958), p. 1.

59 Students had spearheaded the Language Movement (1952–56). In an infamous clash with police, three students were killed on the Dacca University campus on 21 February 1952, an event that is memorialised every 21 February as a Bangladesh national holiday. See 'Language Movement', *Banglapedia, National Encyclopedia of Bangladesh,* revised 2nd edn (2012), www.banglapedia.org/HT/L_0066.htm (accessed 12 June 2014). http://en.banglapedia.org/index.php?title=Language_Movement (accessed 24 November 2016).

60 Interviews in Dacca with Professor K. M. Mohsin (20 February 2013) and Professor Abdul Momin Chowdhury (23 February 2013), who were recruited as vaccinators by Cockburn in May 1958.

61 Despite this campaign in Dacca, smallpox continued at a low level in the city throughout 1958; an August 1958 survey found that 5 per cent of the population in municipal Dacca and 16 per cent of the population in non-municipal Dacca had not been vaccinated. T. A. Cockburn to A. D. Langmuir (10 September 1958) enclosing 'Survey to Determine the Vaccination Status of the Population of Dacca August 2–7, 1958', 3 pages. CDC-RG 442.

62 Cockburn, 'Epidemic Crisis in EP', p. 46. Four rupees would buy approximately 1 lb of raw rice. 'Government to Raise Rice Prices', *Pakistan Observer* (11 May 1958), p. 1.

63 The vaccination campaign coincided with intense factional conflicts in the Awami League as well as fights between it and other parties; hence 'leaders of the Government parties as well as the Opposition are literally stumping the province ... to give the people their version of the food problem and the epidemics'. US Consul General, dispatch no. 317, Dacca, 'Political Aspects of Epidemic and Food Shortage in EP' (15 May 1958), 'Comment', p. 4, ICA-RG-469.

64 The 'cold-chain' refers to efforts made to ensure appropriate low-temperature storage and transportation so that vaccines arrive in field settings without spoilage or loss of potency.

65 Cockburn, 'Epidemic Crisis in Bengal', pp. 17–19.

66 *Ibid.,* pp. 9–13. Government vaccinators also sometimes pitched their vaccine supplies.

67 F. Dunn (?), 'Administrative Confidential Report, Progress of Volunteer Smallpox Vaccination Program in Tippera District', mimeograph enclosure to letter, T. A. Cockburn to R. C. Kriegel (24 June 1958), CDC-RG 442.

68 *Ibid.*

69 Fenner *et al.*, *Smallpox and Its Eradication*, p. 811.

70 Usher, 'The Feasibility of Smallpox Eradication', p. 37.

71 Usher,' Terminal Report', pp. 8–9.

72 *Ibid.*, pp. 2, 9–11. When Langmuir returned to the USA at the end of May, Usher was left in charge.

73 'It is impossible with volunteers to concentrate activities upon the segments of the population that are in greatest need of vaccinating', Usher, 'Terminal Report', *Ibid.* p. 11, ICA-RG- 469.

74 'Supplementary Report to USOM/EP, Epidemic Aid Mission to EP, July 19, 1959', mimeograph document, RG 469, p. 11.

75 US Epidemic Aid Team to EP, 'Smallpox in EP' (June? 1958), pp. 1–17 with appendixes, CDC-RG 442; US Epidemic Aid Mission to EP, 'Supplementary Report to USOM/EP, July 19, 1959', ICA-RG 469; Usher, 'Terminal Report', p. 11, ICA-RG-469.

76 G. Usher to A. Langmuir, aerogramme (22 June 1958). CDC-RG 442.

77 Usher prevailed on Cockburn to take Miltown, noting in a letter to Langmuir that, 'I am opposed to the promiscuous use of tranquilizers but think in Aidan's case it is fully justified and its regular use will have a remarkable effect', Usher to Langmuir, aerogramme (20 June 1958). CDC-RG 442.

78 G. Usher to A. Langmuir, aerogramme (12 June 1958), CDC-RG 442.

79 *Ibid.*

80 A. Langmuir to G. Usher, personal letter, 27 June 1958, p. 2, CDC-RG-442.

81 CDC, Epidemic Aid Mission to EP, *Supplementary Report to USOM/EP*, Public Health Service, US Department of Health, Education and Welfare on Loan to US Operations Mission to EP, 12 July 1958, 14 pages, CDC-RG 442.

82 CDC, loose sheet, no date (1959?), CDC-RG 442.

83 A. T. Cockburn to D. Harwood, ICA Assistant Director, Dacca, Confidential letter on 'Supplementary Report of the CDC Epidemiologists' (15 July 1958), CDC-RG 442.

84 A. T. Cockburn to A. D. Langmuir (1 June 1959), CDC-RG 442.

85 See note 56.

86 Cockburn, 'Epidemic Crisis in EP', and Usher, 'The Feasibility of Smallpox Eradication'.

87 A. D. Langmuir to G. S. Usher, personal letter (1 June 1959), CDC-RG 442.

88 Usher, 'The Feasibility of Smallpox Eradication', pp. 38–9.
89 P. E. M. Fine, 'Herd Immunity: History, Theory, Practice', *Epidemiologic Reviews*, 15:2 (1993), pp. 265–302.
90 Usher, 'The Feasibility of Smallpox Eradication', pp. 38–9.
91 *Ibid.*, p. 40.
92 *Ibid.*, p. 41.
93 As noted in D. Vargha's chapter in this volume, 'Vaccination and the Communist State: Polio in Eastern Europe'.
94 Cockburn, 'Epidemic Crisis in EP', p. 32.
95 *Ibid.*
96 K. B. Sayeed, 'The Collapse of Parliamentary Democracy in Pakistan', *Middle East Journal*, 13:4 (1959), pp. 389–406; Van Schendel, *History of Bangladesh*, pp. 121–30.
97 Diplomatic opinion in Dacca, Karachi and Washington deemed the CDC mission and associated publicity a success and resolved to increase US aid. Consul, Foreign Service Dispatch 55, Dacca, 'Smallpox in EP and US Assistance' (6 August 1958), ICA-RG 469, pp. 1–7.
98 A. D. Langmuir to G. S. Usher, CDC, Washington (10 December 1959). CDC-RG 442.
99 Fenner *et al.*, *Smallpox and Its Eradication*, chapters 15–16; Sanjoy Bhattacharya, *Expunging Variola: The Control and Eradication of Smallpox in India, 1947–1977* (Hyderabad: Orient Longman, 2006); W. Foege, *House on Fire: The Fight to Eradicate Smallpox* (Berkeley and Los Angeles: University of California Press, reprint edn 2012), chapter 5.
100 P. Greenough, 'Intimidation, Coercion, and Resistance in the Final Stages of the South Asian Smallpox Eradication Campaign, 1973–1975', *Social Science and Medicine*, 41:5 (1995), pp. 633–45.
101 S. E. Findley, 'Effective Strategies for Integrating Immunization Promotion into Community Programs', *Health Promotion Practices*, 10:2 supplement (2009), pp. 128S–137S; US Agency for International Development, 'Working with Communities to Strengthen Immunization', *Immunization Snap Shots*, 9 (June 2009), www.immunizationbasics.jsi.com/Newsletter/Archives/snapshots_volume9.htm (accessed 15 October 2014).
102 M. H. Merson, E. E. Black and A. J. Mills, *Global Health: Diseases, Programs, Systems and Policies*, 3rd edn (Burlington, MA: Jones & Bartlett, 2012), pp. 539–613.
103 CDC, Global Health, 'Field Epidemiology Training Program, www.cdc.gov/globalhealth/fetp/about.html (accessed 14 June 2014); D. M. Schneider, M. Evering-Watley, H. Walke and P. B. Bloland, 'Training the Global Public Health Workforce Through Applied Epidemiology Training Programs: CDC's Experience, 1951–2011', *Public Health Reviews*, 33 (2011), pp. 190–203.

2

Fallacy, sacrilege, betrayal and conspiracy: the cultural construction of opposition to immunisation in India

Niels Brimnes

Immunisation in India – an outline

In January 1819 the *Madras Courier* published an interesting note by Calvi Virumbon, in which it was claimed that vaccination against smallpox was known in India before Jenner's famous discovery in 1796. Virumbon wrote that he had discovered an ancient text in Sanskrit describing a way to avoid smallpox, which was indistinguishable from vaccination.[1] Together with other more or less convincing references to the existence of pre-Jennerian vaccination in India, Virumbon's claim caused significant interest over the next century. Today, however, there seems to be agreement that the claim was a 'pious fraud' made by a British civil servant in an attempt to inscribe vaccination into the Indian medical tradition, which already included the practice of variolation – inoculation of real smallpox matter – as a preventive against smallpox.[2] This fraud is nevertheless interesting as an attempt to 'indigenise' a foreign medical practice, which the British expected to be well received by the Hindus due its connection with the sacred cow.

The cowpox vaccine reached India via Persia in 1802, and the colonial medical authorities immediately began to promote it. In many areas they had to convince Indians to shift from variolation to vaccination, either because the former was an established indigenous practice or because it had been actively promoted by the colonial authorities.[3] It was in this context that the colonial authorities expected to capitalise on the connection between vaccination and the cow. In the Asiatic Annual Register from 1803 it was, for instance, noted that: 'From the veneration in which the animal is held by Hindus it requires only an intimation that such a blessing was within their reach, to ensure its earliest dissemination throughout this division or class of the inhabitants of Bombay.[4]

The hopes that vaccination was particularly well attuned to Indian cultural sensibilities were, however, soon dashed, as Indians turned out to be no less reluctant than other populations across the world in accepting an unknown practice performed directly on their – or their infants'– bodies. By contrast, to the extent that religious and moral considerations had any impact on the dissemination of vaccination in India, they tended to work against it.

Vaccination against smallpox made only slow and uneven progress in colonial India. Throughout the nineteenth century vaccination was a crude and unreliable operation, and it was not obvious that it was superior to variolation in preventing smallpox.[5] However, the introduction of lymph derived from calves towards the end of the century and the establishment of large vaccine-producing units from the first decades of the twentieth century secured a constant supply of more reliable vaccine.[6] Together with the gradual introduction of revaccination these developments meant that vaccination made more progress, and it was one of the few public health interventions in British India that is believed to have had an impact on mortality figures in the first part of the twentieth century.[7] Through most of the nineteenth century the term vaccination invariably meant vaccination against smallpox, but from the 1890s other types of immunisation were introduced and also referred to as 'vaccination'. Most notably, the Russian bacteriologist Waldemar Haffkine was based in India from 1893, where he tested vaccines against cholera and plague.[8]

Indians often reacted to vaccination with indifference or resistance. Some might have rejected it, because it was foreign and unknown or because it was seen as secular rival to the religiously inscribed practice of variolation. In such instances, vaccination might have served as 'a site of conflict between malevolent British intent and something Indian, something sacred, that was under threat of violation and destruction.'[9] Many more might have avoided vaccination for more practical reasons: because it was difficult to access, harmful, unpleasant and in many cases without effect.[10] Immunisation against plague caused significant opposition, as did most of the other draconian measures introduced by the colonial state during the plague emergency around 1900.[11] In the twentieth century a more articulate and organised opposition emerged, which often drew on the activities and arguments of the strong anti-vaccination movement in Britain. They did, however, never form a united front against vaccination in India.[12]

By 1947 immunisation was an established and integrated part of the public health service in India. In 1946 a committee under the chairmanship of Sir Joseph Bhore published a report with suggestions for the development of the health services in post-war – and presumably post-colonial – India. The report was widely referred to in the decades after 1947, even if actual politics often differed from its recommendations. It advocated the doctrine of 'social medicine', which favoured broad sanitary interventions over narrow, technology-driven advances against specific diseases. However, if the report warned against believing that proper health could 'be achieved through a bottle of medicine or a surgical operation'; it nevertheless strongly supported vaccination.[13] Noting that India had the highest incidence of smallpox among all countries featuring in League of Nations statistics, it declared vaccination to be 'the quickest and the most effective means of controlling the disease' and deemed it to be 'essential that primary vaccination should be made compulsory throughout the country without delay'.[14] The report also favoured immunisation against cholera and plague.[15]

In the first decade after independence diseases other than smallpox, cholera and plague took centre stage in India. Top priority was now given to malaria and tuberculosis, and to some extent vaccination against smallpox suffered from this development.[16] The new focus brought, on the other hand, the controversial BCG vaccine against tuberculosis to India. In late 1948 the Government of India secured international assistance in introducing mass BCG vaccination. The Indian BCG campaign developed into the largest immunisation campaign the world had seen, and the goal was to reach all Indians below the age of 25 (estimated at 170 million people) by the end of the second five-year plan period in 1961. It was, however, difficult to overcome logistical challenges and to keep pace with population growth, and the campaign continued until BCG was incorporated into the general immunisation programme in 1978.[17] On top of this, the campaign also encountered a well-articulated opposition, which is analysed here.

From the late 1950s the interest in smallpox returned as WHO began to promote the goal of global eradication. A resolution made by the

Twelfth World Health Assembly in 1959 marked the official beginning of the eradication effort, and also led to increasing activities in India.[18] A National Smallpox Eradication Programme (NSEP) was launched in 1962, which aimed to reach 80 per cent coverage in three years.[19] Despite access to international assistance the programme was a disappointment. With only 44.9 per cent of the population vaccinated, it was – in Sanjoy Bhattacharya's assessment – obvious to all involved that 'the NSEP timetable had gone completely awry and, even more worryingly, it was very apparent that no one was completely sure when – or if – smallpox would ever be expunged from India'.[20] Marked progress did not come until after the launching of an 'Intensified Campaign' (INSEP) in 1973. INSEP meant more national and international funding, a shift to the 'containment and surveillance' strategy and enhanced focus on the four major endemic states Bihar, Madhya Pradesh, Uttar Pradesh and West Bengal.[21] In May 1975 the last indigenous case of smallpox was reported from Bihar and two years later India was certified free from smallpox.[22] Vaccination had achieved its greatest triumph in India.

In 1974 – while India was still struggling to eradicate smallpox – WHO launched its 'Expanded Programme of Immunization', which included vaccines against six childhood diseases: diphtheria, tetanus, whooping cough, polio, measles and tuberculosis (BCG). This programme was adopted in India from 1978. In 1985 the programme was renamed the Universal Immunisation Programme (UIP) and an attempt made to extent it to the entire country.[23] One recent account has described UIP as the largest immunisation programme in the world, catering annually to 27 million infants and 30 million pregnant women. The same account also notes, however, that after twenty-five years the coverage of UIP is still poor in many areas and that millions of infants are not immunised according to schedule.[24] In 1994, following another call from the WHO for a single-disease eradication programme, India intensified its efforts to eradicate polio. The means to reach this goal was another mass immunisation campaign, known as the Pulse Polio Programme. While the polio programme was met with criticism from some professional quarters, India has succeeded in eliminating polio from its territory and is at the time of writing expecting to be officially certified as polio free.[25] From the controversial attempt to control tuberculosis with the BCG vaccine to the removal of polio from Indian soil, independent India's immunisation record is, therefore, largely one of acceptance and implementation of the international agenda set by WHO. The responses to immunisation in post-colonial India did not deviate much from those seen in colonial India. The majority of Indians accepted immunisation and reluctance to accept vaccines was often due to indifference or vague fears about imperfectly understood practices.[26]

In the official WHO account of the eradication of smallpox this type of response has been conveniently couched as 'cultural and religious' resistance stemming from 'traditions and folklore', but in an analysis of resistance to vaccination in the final stages of smallpox eradication, Paul Greenough has linked such opposition to the coercive measures employed by campaign officials.[27] Organised political or ideological opposition was, however, rare. The cases analysed by Greenough were spontaneous and local, and while Bhattacharya does identify more politically motivated opposition to the smallpox eradication drive in the 1970s, he also notes that it was 'relatively easy to isolate'.[28] Organised, political or ideological opposition to immunisation was exceptional, and the following sections analyse four instances of this type of opposition, in order to understand how immunisation was constructed in relation to ideas about being Indian, the features of Indian society and India's place in the world.

Immunisation as fallacy

In 1921 N. F. Billimoria of the Bombay Humanitarian League – an animal welfare organisation – published a pamphlet against vaccination entitled *Vaccination and Small-pox*. The pamphlet consisted of three parts: a piece written by Billimoria himself, a piece written by the Secretary to the National Anti-Vaccination League in Britain, Ms Lily Loat, and a compilation of authoritative opinions by influential men (and a single woman). Billimoria's own contribution 'Vaccination: A Fallacy' attacked the practice on several fronts. He duly began with the pain caused to the calves used in the production of vaccine lymph, but soon turned to the more 'utilitarian' argument that vaccination had no effect. Referring to official statistics he claimed that there were as many deaths from vaccination as from smallpox itself in Britain in 1914–15; he saw a correlation between a falling vaccination coverage and fewer cases of smallpox in England and Wales between 1912 and 1917; and he asked why Germany and Japan with their strict regimes of compulsory vaccination still had a considerable number of smallpox cases. In a short digression to Indian conditions Billimoria mentioned that despite the efforts to vaccinate Indians, there were several hundred deaths from smallpox in Bombay city every month. He also claimed that vaccination made 'men more susceptible to other diseases', and questioned the 'craze' for giving sera and vaccines against any possible ailment.[29]

This led to a more general argument about medical strategy. Referring to the well-known example of Leicester, where smallpox was quite successfully combatted without vaccination, he juxtaposed *sanitation* to *vaccination*. He quoted a British professor to the effect that in the English city of Leicester, which was famous for rejecting vaccination: 'we have *real* immunity, *real* protection; and it is obtained by attending to sanitation and isolation, coupled with the almost total neglect of vaccination'. Applying this opposition to the Bombay slums, he asked: 'Now if vaccination has nothing whatever to do with sanitary measures, why vaccination could not prevent the epidemics in the overcrowded and filthy areas? And yet we are taught by our medical friends that small-pox has nothing to do with sanitary measures.'[30] Billimoria also drew on moral arguments about the right to intervene in the order of nature and he invoked the purity and vitality of the nation's youth: 'We want to bring our children into such a splendid condition of health by means of pure milk, pure diet, pure air and pure living generally; we want to bring the nation generally into such a condition of health as will resist any onslaught of such poisons as small-pox &c.'[31] Vaccination was not only cruel to animals, it was also useless, a violation of the relation between man and nature and it harmed the strength of the nation.

Lily Loat's contribution 'Vaccination and Small-pox in India', argued along the same lines. She fielded three objections to vaccination: the cruelty committed towards lymph-producing animals, the pain and risk suffered by children taking the vaccine, and a lack of measurable effects. In relation to the latter argument and after going through official statistics, she concluded that vaccination had 'not had the slightest effect in diminishing small-pox in India'. To the contrary, she found that death rates in India had gone up with the increase of vaccination.[32] Loat was also worried about purity, albeit in a more direct way. Vaccines were, she argued, 'swarming with micro-organisms' and the ultimate origin of material used in vaccination remained obscure.[33] If Billimoria was concerned about the purity of the national body, Loat warned against pollution of individual bodies. Finally, Loat saw herself as the spokesperson for 'the vast mass of inarticulate poverty-stricken Indians', who could not speak for themselves. Yet, the conventional colonial rhetoric was turned upside down, when she declared that the Indian masses were ready to throw off the superstitious belief in vaccination; the problem rested with the educated classes, which had 'imbibed Western ideas'.[34] There was no reason why India should follow the false path taken by a superstitious Britain.

Perhaps the most salient feature of pamphlet was the predominance of the British experience. Most of the figures came from Britain, and most of the references were to British Government reports and information appearing in the organ of the Anti-Vaccination League in Britain, *The Vaccination Inquirer*. This impression is reinforced by the compilation of authoritative opinions in the third and last part of the pamphlet. These were overwhelmingly British, with Florence Nightingale being the sole woman. It would seem that Billimoria's and Loat's opposition to vaccination was inspired by, and imported from, Britain. If vaccination was inappropriate in Britain, it would be inappropriate in India for the same reasons. There was no specifically Indian element in the reservations raised in Billimoria's pamphlet, and I would characterise this type of opposition to immunisation as cosmopolitan.

Vaccination as sacrilege

A notable – and available – Indian voice absent from Billimoria's collection of opinions against vaccination was Gandhi. Through the early *satyagrahas* and the non-cooperation campaign Gandhi had by 1921 taken the position as the key figure in the nationalist movement, and he had also articulated views on health issues. From the publication of the well-known pamphlet *Hind Swaraj* in 1909 Gandhi emerged as a vocal opponent to western medicine. In 1913 he published a series of articles in *Indian Opinion* under the title 'General Knowledge About Health', which were modified and republished in 1921 as *A Guide to Health*.[35] Throughout his life he continued to comment on issues of health and medicine and vaccination was among the practices he most fervently criticised. Gandhi had two reservations against vaccination. First it hindered discipline over the body and control over the mind. In *Hind Swaraj* Gandhi argued that if the doctor did not intervene in the body – with drugs or vaccines – 'nature' would do its work 'and I would have acquired mastery over myself'.[36] This resembled Billimoria's objection to interfere in the order of nature; and it is noteworthy that Billimoria referred to Spencer rather than Gandhi on this issue.[37]

It also violated his religious instincts, his vegetarianism and his notion of purity. Many medical remedies contained alcohol or animal substances, and in one of the articles published in 1913 he was very clear about his views:

> Vaccination seems to be a savage custom. It is one of the poisonous superstitions of our times the equal of which is not to be found even among so called primitive societies ... Vaccination is a filthy remedy. Vaccine from an infected cow is introduced into our bodies; more, even vaccine from an infected human being is used ... I personally feel that in taking this vaccine we are guilty of a sacrilege.[38]

By 1929 Gandhi held the same views. In a comment on F. L. Brayne's book *Village Uplift in India* Gandhi commented that various forms of immunisation were 'soul destroying remedies making man a weakling dying many times before his natural death'.[39] Gandhi was ready to admit that vaccination gave 'a sort of temporary immunity from smallpox', but he also affirmed his religious objections to the practice.[40] In the weekly newspaper *Navajivan* he wondered how 'vegetarians can ever take such vaccine' and in a private letter he described vaccination as 'tantamount to partaking of beef'.[41] In this way vaccination became emblematic of all that was wrong with western medicine.

It would not, however, do justice to Gandhi to see him as simply rejecting western medicine. Although he identified doctors in *Hind Swaraj* as one of the great evils of western civilisation, and in the same year in a private letter for the first – but not the last – time described western medicine as 'the essence of black magic', he did acknowledge and approve the scientific approach of the discipline. The problem was the way it was used.[42] When Gandhi opened the 'Tibbia' medical college in Delhi in 1921 he first reiterated his statement that western medicine was 'black magic', but immediately continued: 'Having said that much

I would like to pay my humble tribute to the spirit of research that fires the modern scientists. My quarrel is not against that spirit. My complaint is against the direction that the spirit has taken.'[43] To a German interviewer, in 1937, Gandhi explained that he did not despise all medical treatment that came from the West and emphasised safe maternity and the care of infants as fields where India could learn from the West.[44] It would be more accurate to say that Gandhi's criticism focused on a number of specific practices, which he found particularly objectionable, and that various forms of immunisation were prominent among them.

Instead, he found the virtues of science in two other fields related to health: nutrition and sanitation. In Gandhi's universe they seem to have been complementary; the first dealing with inward and personal purity, the latter with outward corporate cleanliness. Both Joseph Alter and Sunil Amrith have noted how Gandhi turned to the emerging science of nutrition and the authority of the League of Nations Health Organization to substantiate his claim for the importance of a balanced diet.[45] But personal cleanliness and a proper diet were not enough. As he wrote in *Young India* in 1929, Indians had a reputation for being a personally clean people, but that cleanliness was bought 'at the expense of our neighbours ... We are clean as individuals but not as members of the society or the nation of which the individual is but a tiny part.'[46] In order to achieve cleanliness at the corporate level Gandhi turned to sanitation.

As early as 1913 Gandhi discovered that 'hygiene' was a science distinct from, and superior to, medicine because it was preventive rather than curative.[47] In 1921, he stated this even more clearly: 'The science of sanitation is infinitely more ennobling, though more difficult of execution, than the science of healing.'[48] The issue of sanitation surfaced more prominently in Gandhi's writings as he became engaged in village reconstruction work from the 1920s and featured in his 'constructive programme' from the 1940s.[49]

Like Billimoria, Gandhi opposed vaccination and sanitation. In 1929 he advised that 'those who do not get themselves vaccinated ought to know and follow the rules of sanitation', thereby suggesting – as in Billimoria's reference to Leicester – that sanitation was an alternative to vaccination.[50] Referring to the Bombay slums Billimoria had also suggested that insanitary surroundings would cancel out any potentially positive effects of vaccination; but this was not a central part of Gandhi's opposition. His was not an argument about the relative efficacy of vaccination; it was about substituting morally sound sanitary behaviour for an immoral practice.

Gandhi was a genuinely cosmopolitan thinker, who drew inspiration from both Indian and non-Indian sources. He was no great admirer of India's own medical traditions and inspiration for his cherished strategy of village sanitation came from the West. In 1927 he declared that Indians 'have yet got to learn much from the Britisher in the matter of sanitation' and a decade later he told an interviewer that he had 'copied' his ideas about sanitation from the British doctor, George Vivian Poore.[51] In his specific opposition to vaccination he also looked abroad and referred to the anti-vaccination movement in Britain and its arguments with approval.[52] A close examination of Gandhi's writings might, therefore, lead one to conclude that his opposition to vaccination was every bit as cosmopolitan as the opposition manifested in Billimoria's pamphlet.

Yet, Gandhi's anti-vaccination rhetoric did assume a particularistic touch. His appearance as the main figure of the Indian nationalist movement and his explicit exploitation of specifically Indian idioms made this inevitable. Identifying western doctors as one of the major evils of western civilisation in the widely circulated *Hind Swaraj* only reinforced this reading. If European doctors were 'the worst of all', if they violated '*our* religious instinct', and if studying European medicine was 'to deepen our slavery', it was indeed obvious to think of vaccination as immoral *because* it was European.[53] Later, Gandhi dampened his anti-western rhetoric on medical issues, but the notion that western medicine was unsuited to Indian conditions persisted. In 1939 he told a medical missionary: 'if I were asked to advise missionaries or Mission Boards, I would ask them not to try to transplant the entire system of Western medicine into India. We could not afford it. There is ever so much to be gleaned and had from the study of indigenous drugs and medicines.'[54] Similarly, in 1947, Gandhi urged Indian doctors and scientists to remain in India, instead of going abroad to pick up the latest curative technologies. He encouraged them to turn their attention to India's numerous villages: 'They will find that all medical men and women can find work to do there. Not in the Western fashion, of course, but in our own fashion in the villages.'[55]

From the aggressive rhetoric in *Hind Swaraj* to the milder insistence on a medical approach suited to the conditions of the Indian villages, Gandhi's position always implied a notion of Indian difference. Despite cosmopolitan inspiration his religiously informed opposition to any kind of immunisation was bound to be understood as an insistence on Indian distinctiveness.

Immunisation as an act of betrayal[56]

When the Government of India in 1948 invited the Scandinavian 'International Tuberculosis Campaign' (ITC) to assist in the introduction of the BCG vaccine against tuberculosis, it was a manifestation of the modernist aspirations of the new state and its belief in modern technology. The reservations of Gandhi and like-minded people were sidelined as the Government authorities promised that 'BCG constitutes a potent and speedy method of bringing under control the high incidence of tuberculosis which has been spreading rapidly through the country'.[57] Those who cared to look would find claims that BCG provided 80 per cent protection and could reduce the tuberculosis problem in India to a fifth over 15–20 years of intensive vaccination.[58] They would also find, however, that both the safety and the efficacy of BCG were questioned. The effort to control tuberculosis through vaccination triggered, therefore, the largest and best articulated anti-immunisation campaign in post-colonial India – and possibly in the post-colonial world.

The opposition radiated from Madras in South India, but was noted throughout India and even beyond. It began before the first expert from ITC had set foot in India. In November 1948 the former sanitary engineer of the Government of Madras, A. V. Raman, wrote a critical editorial in *People's Health*; a monthly publication edited and run, it seems, mainly by Raman himself.[59] As the Indian authorities and Scandinavian experts in February 1949 prepared to inaugurate the BCG vaccination campaign in Madras, Raman raised his voice again. And his opposition to BCG began to appear in newspapers throughout India. On 14 February – just two days before the official inauguration of the campaign – he published a lengthy piece in the most prominent newspaper in the Madras area, *The Hindu*.[60] Raman succeeded in putting the Indian authorities on the defensive, and in his opening address P. V. Benjamin – the adviser on tuberculosis to the Government of India – conceded that the Government had opted for BCG because it had limited resources and BCG promised to be an affordable solution to an extensive and costly health problem.[61] Raman collected the contributions to the heated dispute over BCG and published it in the February issue of *People's Health*, adding an extensive editorial entitled 'BCG What about it?'[62] Until 1951 Raman succeeded in temporarily putting the implementation of BCG vaccination to a halt in Madras, but in other regions his opposition did not have a similar impact.[63]

In July 1951 ITC withdrew from India leaving the field and the challenge to expand mass vaccination to the Indian authorities, WHO and UNICEF. In 1954 Halfdan Mahler, the WHO senior medical officer, believed that it was time to reinvigorate the BCG campaign in Madras State, where it had suffered since Raman's opposition. One reason for this was the resignation of the Chief Minister in the state, Chakravarti Rajagopalachari. Simply known as C. R. or 'Rajaji' among Tamils, he was the prime figure in the nationalist movement in southern India. A close associate of Gandhi and part of the Congress leadership, he had been Chief Minister in the Congress Government of Madras from 1937 to 1939 and held several high offices after 1947. In April 1952 he became once again Chief Minister of Madras, a position he resigned in 1954 after falling out with the dominant faction of the Congress Party in Madras.[64] Rajagopalachari was also a close friend of Raman and shared his scepticism towards BCG vaccination. From 1952 he communicated his views on BCG in letters to the Union Minister of Health and ardent supporter of BCG, Rajkumari Amrit Kaur.[65] With his resignation the Indian authorities and their UN supporters were given the opportunity to restart the campaign in Madras, but the former Chief Minister was also free to voice his scepticism in public.

Rajagopalachari first openly challenged BCG in a public speech on 7 May 1955. Benjamin answered Rajagopalachari's criticism in *The Hindu* only to find a long reply two days later.[66] The controversy was up and running and surfaced regularly over the next two years. The controversy culminated in the summer of 1955 when Rajagopalachari published a pamphlet entitled *BCG – Why I Oppose It*. As a response to Rajagopalachari's pamphlet the Government of Madras published a counter-pamphlet entitled *Truth about BCG. Why Government Have Launched a Mass Campaign*, which attempted to address both the scientific debate and the popular concerns about the vaccine.

Rajagopalachari's opposition resonated throughout India and caused a dramatic, if relatively short-lived, drop in the number of people reached by the BCG teams over the summer of 1955. It made the biggest impact in South India – particularly in Madras State – where it seems to have adversely affected campaign figures until 1957.[67]

The opposition to BCG was complex and although Raman and Rajagopalachari agreed on many things, they also differed in important aspects of their opposition. I therefore analyse the opposition to BCG through the identification of four overlapping and interdependent 'strains'. First, specific criticism was directed against the BCG vaccine. This 'strain' featured prominently because – in contrast to the vaccine against smallpox – the value of BCG was contested among scientists.[68] BCG was the first vaccine based on attenuated live bacteria, and it had been connected with the death of seventy-six infants in the German city of Lübeck in 1930. By 1948 medical experts agreed that BCG was safe, but suspicion lingered on and was also employed by its Indian opponents. Raman explicitly referred to the tragedy in Lübeck, while Rajagopalachari indirectly utilised the safety issue by declaring: 'What one cannot, however, agree to is the injection into tens of thousands of our children, of live bacilli when we have no authority to claim certainty of harmlessness on the basis of the attenuation of those bacilli.'[69]

If experts considered BCG safe by 1948, they continued to disagree on its protective value. Many held that the vaccine did not provide significant protection, and its Indian opponents noted that it was not used in the USA and that the British medical authorities were only slowly adopting it. In a letter to *The Hindu* on 17 May 1955 Rajagopalachari formulated his criticism in two questions, combining the quite different reservations against the vaccine: '(1) Is there no danger in mass inoculation by live BCG? (2) Does the attenuated Bovine tubercle bacillus create an immunity against the normal human infection?'[70] In this way the BCG vaccine was simultaneously portrayed as both dangerously virulent and hopelessly ineffective. These shortcomings together with the fact that BCG was not used on a mass scale in the countries assisting the Indian campaign obviously opened the guinea-pig issue. In 1949 newspapers quoted Raman's exclamation: 'I strongly protest in the name of India … against our boys and girls being made a sort of cannon-fodder and treated like guinea-pigs for the sake of experimentation.'[71]

The specific uncertainties connected to BCG provided, however, also a platform for a discussion of more general issues. For Raman this was the flawed, techno-centric strategy behind a narrow, single-disease campaign. What India needed, Raman argued, was 'environmental engineering': broad health programmes concentrating on improving the basic living conditions of the Indian poor. This was the second strain of opposition, and it was introduced in Raman's first editorial against BCG from November 1948:

> Of what earthly use is BCG in the present living condition of the Indian masses; every moment of their lives, they take a dose of infection; they continue to take in heroic doses of it day in and day out ... The Minister of Health can just as well pass a resolution that every home should be a BCG factory and every hospital a tuberculosis hospital.[72]

Raman later repeated his criticism of the narrow vaccination strategy; and he did so by invoking two interesting authorities in the debate over public health in independent India:

> We would give the first and foremost priority to the improvement of nutritional and environmental conditions. The Bhore Committee has said so. Long before the Bhore Committee, Mahatmaji said so. The fact, however, is that there is hardly a single Health Minister in any province today, who is troubled by the disparity between official policies and the Mahatmaji's teachings.[73]

The reference to the authoritative Bhore Committee was not surprising. The report had been published only three years earlier, and Raman shared a belief in the doctrine of 'social medicine' with the committee. He wanted the Indian state to intervene in public health through comprehensive programmes of environmental engineering that addressed basic health issues such as village sanitation and clean drinking water. The reference to Gandhi was less straightforward, but perhaps more powerful. Raman employed Gandhi's famous remark about western medicine as 'the essence of black magic', although he did not share this view. When Raman invoked Gandhi's name, it was not as the critic of western medicine but as the ardent supporter of nutrition and sanitation. To Raman BCG was a dubious and untested 'technological fix'. By adopting it the young Indian state had betrayed the hopes held for a new departure in public health as well as the ideals of the Mahatma.

Rajagopalachari did not join Raman on this issue. If Raman felt the state intervened too little and too superficially in public health, Rajagopalachari felt it intervened too much. After stepping down as Chief Minister in 1954, he increasingly fell out with the Nehruvian version of socialism and the omnipotent role of the state, and in 1959 he became the leading figure in the establishment of the conservative anti-statist Swatantra Party.[74] This suggests that we understand his opposition to BCG vaccination as part of this transformation and consequently that it was directed as much against the policies pursued in Nehru's India, as against the controversial vaccine itself. A conservative uneasiness with the increasing role of the Indian state was, therefore, a third 'strain' underpinning the opposition to BCG.

A final and obvious 'strain' was nationalism. Inevitably, the adoption of a disputed and possibly second-rate vaccine provoked nationalist sentiments in the newly independent state. India had finally emerged as a nation in its own right and on a par with western countries; it now demanded the same standard of public health remedies. The guinea-pig issue turned up again; this time accompanied by concerns about India's status as a nation in relation to other communities. Raman remarked that experiments with BCG had been conducted 'on guinea-pigs, calves and American Indians ... I am driven by the irresistible conclusion that the authorities are exposing the people of this country to be utilised by research workers for their benefit.'[75] Rajagopalachari joined him by claiming that, 'Indian children are being offered for mass expectation on the same plan as was put in operation among the people in war-ravaged areas and uncivilised dependent communities'.[76] As members of a new and sovereign nation, neither Raman nor Rajagopalachari could accept being treated like American Indians or 'dependent communities'! One of Rajagopalachari's many correspondents made the point even clearer: 'The Britishers would never have done it, not even in Kenya.'[77] BCG was again seen as an act of betrayal, this time against the newly won nationhood.

Immunisation as neo-colonial conspiracy

After the BCG controversy died down towards the end of the 1950s, the following three decades seems to have witnessed little visible and vocal opposition to immunisation. Towards the end of the 1980s, however, a new sceptical voice made itself heard, at least among academics and bureaucrats. This voice belonged to Debabar Banerji. Having graduated from Calcutta Medical College in 1953, Banerji's career took an unusual turn, when he was employed as a sociologist attached to the National Tuberculosis Institute in Bangalore in 1961. He joined Jawaharlal Nehru University (JNU) in Delhi in 1972 where he became Professor at the Centre of Social Medicine and Community Health.

Banerji's criticism of immunisation in India targeted the UIP. In two near identical articles from 1990 Banerji disputed the Indian government's claim that vaccination was one of the most cost-effective health interventions and accused it of launching 'a massive, expensive and very complicated programme ... without even finding out what the problem was'.[78] Banerji raised a range of issues: the programme lacked, 'the baseline epidemiological data' on the six diseases that it was supposed to cover, internal evaluation was flawed, the 'cold chain' supposed to keep vaccines potent in the field was not sufficiently monitored, and attempts were made to 'cover up' the dismal performance, which – according to Banerji – did not reach the target of 85 per cent coverage in any of the Indian states.[79] The UIP was therefore grouped with other 'ill-conceived and ill-designed, techno-centric, target oriented and time bound programmes'.[80]

In 2004 Banerji applied a similar criticism to the Global Programme for Polio Immunisation (GPPI), and its Indian avatar, the Pulse Polio Programme. This time he was backed by several other critics, many of them based at his former workplace, The Centre for Social Medicine and Community Health at JNU. According to William Muraskin's instructive account of the global effort to eradicate polio, India gave rise to 'the most powerfully argued and cogent' protest against this enterprise. It was the existence of a sufficiently large, critical mass of highly educated medical men in India that enabled the formation of a group labelled the 'Indian dissenters' by Muraskin.[81] As a central voice among these dissenters, Banerji pointed out that, seen from non-western regions, polio was not a sufficiently important health problem to merit a costly eradication effort. By following the lead taken by western countries, the Indian authorities failed 'to attend to far more important health problems'.[82] Immunisation against polio continued on the flawed strategy of the UIP and the GPPI was, he concluded, an expensive, epidemiologically unsound disaster: 'It should never have been attempted. It has diverted attention from some of the most pressing problems of child mortality and morbidity among the poor in the world. It has turned out to be highly expensive. It presents unsurmountable problems of implementation.'[83]

While the other members of 'Indian dissenters' group continued to criticise the campaign against polio based on clinical and epidemiological considerations,[84] Banerji's position had always included elements far beyond epidemiology. In one of his articles, he situated his specific criticism of immunisation in the larger context of asymmetrical, neo-colonial relations of power:

> In the existing immoral and unethical North–South divide, which is based on unequal terms of exchange, by imposing such programmes on the South the North seems to come back to the South with a tiny fraction of what it has plundered from it and, adding insult to injury, seems to be telling the South condescendingly: 'Here we come with our technological magics. We have a magical wand to remove your health problems. What does it matter if you are forced to live under degrading conditions of poverty, illiteracy, exploitation, and social injustice? After all, you and your children are alive! Look how we have raised your life expectancy'.[85]

This echoed both the prose of the Bhore Committee and of Raman's arguments that immunisation was a 'cheap' technological fix offered to post-colonial countries as a poor substitute for real progress in public health. Like Raman, Banerji was an ardent advocate of primary health care, and – unlike Raman – he was able persistently to refer to the most powerful international manifestation of that approach: WHO's 1978 Alma-Ata Declaration. To Banerji the Declaration was a 'watershed' in the history of public health and a 'major victory for the masses of people in the world'.[86]

In 2004 Banerji published an interesting article, in which he developed these views into a historical narrative of the development of public health in India. The article set out by describing the introduction of western medicine as one of the adverse effects of colonial rule in India. The priority given to western medicine had an adverse effect on the already stagnant indigenous traditions of medicine. Out of this misery grew, however, 'a number of internally generated – "endogenous" – movements for developing alternative approaches to improving people's health'.[87] Banerji identified three such 'home-grown' alternatives: Gandhi's promotion of naturopathy, hygiene and environmental sanitation;

the distinguished Indian physician and nationalist politician, B. C. Roy, who advocated integration of western medicine and indigenous traditions; and the sub-committee on health of the National Planning Committee established in 1938 by the Indian National Congress. According to Banerji the latter had 'made an attempt to bring together the ideas for an alternative health service for the country'.[88] Invoking these 'internally generated' alternatives to colonial, western style medicine, Banerji introduced the issue of an Indian distinctiveness that called for a particular, nationally appropriate health strategy.

In his treatment of the health services in independent India, Banerji applauded the priorities and visions of the Bhore Committee and regarded its report as an authoritative document. Although the early years of independence were tough, the new regime was – Banerji argued – compelled to listen to the people in the planning of public health and 'India could develop an endogenous, alternative body of knowledge that was more suited to its prevailing social, cultural, economic, and epidemiological conditions'.[89]

In a rare endorsement of the achievement of public health policies in India between 1947 and 1977, Banerji narrated how primary health centres were set up (as advised by the Bhore Committee) and how programmes such as the National Tuberculosis Programme (to which Banerji was associated in his early career) received world-wide attention because they resisted the imposition of a western 'pre-fabricated technological package'.[90] Banerji even vouched for the problematic DDT-based National Malaria Eradication Programme; often viewed as the prototype of a techno-centric, vertical disease control programme.[91] By 1977, 'India thus came quite close to the Alma-Ata Declaration on Primary Health Care', which clearly epitomised Banerji's favoured medical strategy. In Banerji's narrative, a new approach to the study of public health was developed, which was 'specially tailored for a country such as India'.[92]

Soon after, however, the 'fall from grace' occurred. Before the ink on the Alma-Ata declaration had dried, western countries backed down from the promises made in Kazakhstan. Primary health care was turned into *selective* primary health care, which focused more narrowly on the specific fields of growth monitoring, oral rehydration, breastfeeding, and – notably – childhood immunisation. To Banerji this amounted to a 'retreat from the commitments made at Alma-Ata'.[93] The Indian government's launch of the UIP was – both in Banerji's specific criticism of the programme and in his larger narrative – presented as a result of this retreat from and counter-attack on the principles of primary health care. Implementation of Pulse Polio in India simply added insult to injury.

Two things should be emphasised in Banerji's views on immunisation. First, he never rejected the practice of immunisation as such; his criticism was always about the way in which it was conducted. Although the Oral Polio Vaccine was controversial and had many flaws, Banerji did not – by contrast to the critics of BCG – delve extensively into this issue.[94] Similarly, he ended his criticism of the UIP on the note that: 'The question is not of rejecting *all* technology; the question is to see through the dangers of the market forces in both the North and the South.'[95] Second, while his attacks on the IUP and polio eradication programmes were 'universal', in the sense that he positioned himself as speaking on behalf of the poor throughout the developing world,[96] his later and more historically informed reflections introduced the notion of a specifically Indian, 'endogenous' tradition of public health that was able to devise strategies particularly suited to the demographic, social and cultural characteristics of Indian society. These strategies excluded the wholesale acceptance of immunisation programmes designed by rich, western countries and their adherents in international organisations. While Banerji's aggressive rhetoric might have had a limited impact on the actual public health policy in India, it does illustrate the persistence of the notion that something in Indian society makes immunisation particularly problematic there.

Conclusion

The history of immunisation in India is mainly about some of the world's most extensive programmes and about millions of people accepting the introduction of micro-organisms into their bodies for preventive purposes. This chapter has, by contrast, focused on four instances of opposition to immunisation. While articulate opposition represents the exception and has largely been an elite phenomenon, it points to a least two important tensions in modern Indian society: between universal science and cultural distinctiveness and between international intervention and national integrity.

The four cases analysed each provide a distinctive illustration of how immunisation and the opposition to it was culturally constructed and linked to an imagined Indian nation. The opposition to vaccination against smallpox in Billimoria's pamphlet was as imported as the practice of vaccination itself: even if vaccination harmed the national body, the pamphlet looked to Britain both for arguments and evidence. While Gandhi was in agreement with many of the arguments employed by anti-vaccinationists in Britain, his emergence as the leading representative of the Indian nation, and his general anti-modernist rhetoric meant that his reservations against immunisation were bound to be read as a culturally embedded rejection of a medical practice that was both immoral and unsuited to Indian conditions. With reference to Gandhi, Indians could display their 'Indianness' by rejecting immunisation, and later both Raman and Banerji did indeed invoke his name as they discarded externally designed immunisation programmes.

While independent India readily embraced immunisation and largely followed the stance taken by WHO and other international organisations, opposition continued to be articulated. BCG vaccination was countered by a complex set of arguments in the first decade after independence. In the present context the most salient feature was that mass vaccination with BCG was constructed as a betrayal of both Indians' expectations to be offered public health interventions that matched those in the West, and of their newly won nationhood. The theme of betrayal also featured in the last of the cases analysed, this time of the principles of primary health care enshrined in the Alma-Ata declaration. Debabar Banerji saw the way in which immunisation was implemented as a manifestation of continued unequal neo-colonial relations of power. Moreover, he developed a historical narrative in which global immunisation programmes were opposed to a specifically 'endogenous', Indian way of approaching public health challenges.

From these examples it is clear that Paul Greenough was correct when he remarked that 'encounters with government vaccinators are never about immunization alone.'[97] Three of the cases analysed feature the notion of a distinctive 'Indianness' that made imported ways of conducting immunisation particularly problematic. This suggests that David Arnold's contention that vaccination in the nineteenth century was constructed as a site of conflict between malevolent British intent and something 'Indian' is also relevant for the twentieth century; not so much for the ordinary Indian, but for the Indian elite that was concerned with the formulation and preservation of a distinctive national identity. To the voices analysed in this chapter immunisation was not building the nation, but threatened to destroy it.

Acknowledgements

I am particularly grateful to Rajib Dasgupta for comments on a first draft of this chapter. The responsibility for any errors or misjudgements remains with me.

Notes

1 D. Wujastyk, ' "A Pious Fraud": The Indian Claims for Pre-Jennerian Smallpox Vaccination', in G. J. Meulenbed and D. Wujastyk (eds), *Studies on Indian Medical History* (Groningen: Egbert Forsten, 1987), pp. 131–67, on p. 134.

2 *Ibid.*, pp. 164–7.

3 N. Brimnes, 'Variolation, Vaccination and Popular Resistance in Early Colonial South India', *Medical History*, 48:2 (2004), pp. 199–228.

4 Quoted in Wujastyk, 'A Pious Fraud', p. 151. See also D. Arnold, *Colonizing the Body. State Medicine and Epidemic disease in Nineteenth-Century India* (Berkeley: University of California Press, 1993), p. 136.

5 P. R. Greenough, 'Variolation and Vaccination in South Asia *c.*1700–1865: A Preliminary Note', *Social Science and Medicine*, 14D (1980), pp. 345–47; Arnold, *Colonizing the Body*, p. 139; S. Bhattacharya, M. Harrison and M. Worboys, *Fractured States: Smallpox, Public Health and Vaccination Policy in British India 1800–1947* (Hyderabad: Orient Longman, 2005), p. 59.

6 Arnold, *Colonizing the Body*, pp. 140–1; Bhattacharya *et al.*, *Fractured States*, pp. 178–203.

7 R. Jeffery, *The Politics of Health in India* (Berkeley: University of California Press, 1988), p. 96.

8 Arnold, *Colonizing the Body*, pp. 197–8, 221–3.

9 *Ibid.*, pp. 143–4.

10 Bhattacharya *et al.*, *Fractured States*, pp. 66–9, 72.

11 Arnold, *Colonizing the Body*, pp. 221–3.

12 Bhattacharya *et al.*, *Fractured States*, pp. 203–17.

13 *Report of the Health Survey and Development Committee* 2 (Calcutta: Government of India Press, 1946), pp. 1–4.

14 *Ibid.*, quoted from pp. 169 and 171.

15 *Ibid.*, pp. 179, 185

16 Sanjoy Bhattacharya, *Expunging Variola. The Control and Eradication of Smallpox in India 1947–77* (Hyderabad: Orient Longman 2006), pp. 50, 99

17 Government of India, 'Second Five Year Plan', chapter 25 Health, para 37, at http://planningcommission.nic.in/plans/planrel/fiveyr/welcome.html (accessed 5 June 2013). N. Brimnes, 'Another Vaccine, Another Story: BCG Vaccination Against Tuberculosis in India, 1948 to 1960', *Ciência & Saúde Coletiva*, 16:2 (2011), pp. 397–407.

18 F. Fenner *et al.*, *Smallpox and its Eradication* (Geneva: WHO 1988), pp. 366–71.

19 R. N. Basu, Z. Jezek and N. A. Ward, *The Eradication of Smallpox from India* (New Delhi: WHO, 1979), pp. 21–8.

20 Bhattacharya, *Expunging Variola*, p. 133. For the 44.9% figure, see p. 126. See also Basu, *The Eradication of Smallpox*, p. 28.

21 Bhattacharya, *Expunging Variola*, pp. 176–210; Basu, *The Eradication of Smallpox*, pp. 29–32.

22 Bhattacharya, *Expunging Variola*, pp. 215, 230; Basu, *The Eradication of Smallpox*, pp. 32–4.

23 WHO/UNICEF, *State of World's Vaccines and Immunization* (Geneva: WHO, 1996), pp. 11–14; S. K. Pradhan, 'Time to Revamp the Universal Immunization Program in India', *Indian Journal of Public Health*, 54 (2010), pp. 71–4, www.ijph.in/text.asp?2010/54/2/71/73273 (accessed 7 June 2013); Ministry of Health and Family Welfare, *National Vaccine Policy* (Delhi: Government of India, 2011); V. M. Vashishtha and P. Kumar, '50 Years of Immunization in India: Progress and Future', *Indian Pediatrics*, 50:1 (2013), pp. 11–118, on p. 112.

24 Pradhan, 'Time to Revamp'.

25 Vashishtha and Kumar, '50 Years of Immunization', p. 112; S. K. Mittal, 'Pulse Polio Program – A National Perspective, *Indian Journal of Pediatrics*, 63:1 (1996), pp. 1–8; P. Chatterjee, 'How India Managed to Defeat Polio', *BBC News India*, 13 January 2014, www.bbc.co.uk/news/world-asia-india-25709362 (accessed 18 February 2014).

26 M. Nichter, 'Vaccinations in South Asia: False Expectations and Commanding Metaphors', in M. Nichter (ed.), *Anthropology and International Health: South Asian Case Studies* (Dordrecht, Boston: Kluwer Academic Publishers, 1989), pp. 200–11; M. Nichter, 'Vaccinations in the Third World: A Consideration of Community Demand', *Social Science and Medicine*, 41:5 (1995), pp. 617–32.

27 Basu, *The Eradication of Smallpox*, pp. 112–14; P. R. Greenough, 'Intimidation, Coercion and Resistance in the Final Stages of the South Asian

Smallpox Eradication Campaign, 1973–1975', *Social Science and Medicine*, 41:5 (1995), pp. 633–45.

28 Bhattacharya, *Expunging Variola*, pp. 237–8.

29 N. F. Billimoria, 'Vaccination: A Fallacy', in *Vaccination and Small-pox* (Bombay: Bombay Humanitarian League, 1921), pp. 9–10, 20–6.

30 *Ibid.*, pp. 29, 33.

31 *Ibid.*, p. 18.

32 L. Loat, 'Vaccination and Small-Pox in India', in *Vaccination and Small-pox* (Bombay: Bombay Humanitarian League, 1921), p. 46.

33 *Ibid.*, pp. 39–41.

34 *Ibid.*, pp. 42, 46.

35 Sometimes also referred to as *The Health Guide*. See M. K. Gandhi, *A Guide to Health* (Madras: S. Ganesan, 1921).

36 'Hind Swaraj', in *Collected Works of Mahatma Gandhi* (hereafter CWMG) (New Delhi: Government of India, 1959–84), X, pp. 6–64, on p. 35.

37 Billimoria, 'Vaccination: A Fallacy', p. 11.

38 'General Knowledge About Health – XXIV', *Indian Opinion* (14 June 1913), in CWMG, XII, p. 111.

39 'Village Improvement', *Young India* (14 November 1929), in CWMG, XLII, pp. 146–7.

40 'Notes', *Young India* (18 July 1929), in CWMG, XLI, p. 192.

41 'Smallpox and Cholera', *Navajivan* (30 June 1929), in CWMG, XLI, p. 141; 'Letter to Manilal and Sushila Gandhi' (30 June 1929), in CWMG, XLI, p. 146.

42 'Hind Swaraj', in CWMG, X, pp. 35–6. Letter to Henry S. L. Polak, 14. October 1909, in CWMG, IX, p. 479.

43 'Speech at opening of Tibbi College, Delhi, *Bombay Chronicle* (15 February 1921), in CWMG, XIX, p. 358.

44 'Interview to Capt. Strunk', *Harijan* (3 July 1937), in CWMG, LXV, p. 361.

45 J. S. Alter, *Gandhi's Body. Sex, Diet and the Politics of Nationalism* (Philadelphia: University of Pennsylvania Press, 2000), p. 20. S. S. Amrith, *Decolonizing International Health. India and Southeast Asia 1930–65* (Basingstoke: Palgrave Macmillan, 2006), p. 33.

46 'A National Defect', *Young India* (25 April 1925), in CWMG, XL, p. 283.

47 'General Knowledge about Health – I', *Indian Opinion* (4 January 1913), in CWMG, XI, p. 428.

48 'Speech at opening of Tibbi College, Delhi, *Bombay Chronicle* (15 February 1921), in CWMG, XIX, p. 357.

49 See, for instance, 'Implications of Constructive Programme', *Harijan* (18 August 1940), in CWMG, LXXII, pp. 378–81.

50 'Smallpox and Cholera', *Navajivan* (30 June 1929), in CWMG, XLI, p. 141.
    Gandhi did refer implicitly to the experience of Leicester. 'General Knowl-
    edge About Health – XXV', *Indian Opinion* (21 June 1913), in CWMG, XII,
    p. 116.
51 'Speech at Mayavaram', *The Hindu* (15 September 1927), in CWMG,
    XXXIV, p. 529; 'Interview to Capt. Strunk', *Harijan* (3 July 1937), in
    CWMG, LXV, p. 361. For examples of Gandhi's scepticism towards the
    ayurvedic tradition of medicine, see CWMG, LXXVI, pp. 45, 161–2, 201–2,
    257.
52 'General Knowledge about Health – XXV', in CWMG, XII, pp. 115–17.
53 'Hind Swaraj', in CWMG, X, p. 36. Emphasis added.
54 'Discussion with Dr Chesterman', *Harijan* (25 February 1939), in CWMG,
    LXVIII, p. 420.
55 'Speech at Prayer Meeting', Delhi (2 June 1947), in CWMG, LXXXVIII,
    p. 62.
56 This section is adapted from the more detailed treatment of the opposition
    to BCG vaccination in C. W. McMillen and N. Brimnes, 'Medical Mod-
    ernization and Medical Nationalism: Resistance to Mass Tuberculosis Vac-
    cination in Postcolonial India, 1948–1955', *Comparative Studies in Society
    and History*, 52:1 (2010), pp. 180–209. For a later and further-developed
    version of this analysis, see also Niels Brimnes, *Languished Hopes: Tuber-
    culosis. The State and International Assistance in Twentieth-century India*,
    (Hyderabad: Orient BlackSwan, 2016), pp. 148–82.
57 'Press Note', printed in *Indian Medical Gazette* (January 1948), pp. 50–1.
58 'First Five Year Plan', chapter 32 Health, para. 37; 'Second five Year Plan,
    chapter 25 Health, para. 37, both at http://planningcommission.nic.in/
    plans/planrel/fiveyr/welcome.html (accessed 5 June 2013).
59 *People's Health*, 3:2, p. 53.
60 *Indian Express* (5 February 1949); *The Hindu* (14 February 1949). Articles
    that referred to Raman's critique of BCG from *Indian Express*, *Nagpur
    Times* and *Sunday Times* were all reproduced in *People's Health*, 3:5, pp.
    206–8.
61 *People's Health*, 3:5, p. 222.
62 I assume Raman is the author of the editorial, which has no signature.
63 Raman stopped publishing *People's Health* in 1951, most likely for financial
    reasons.
64 A. Copley, *The Political Career of C. Rajagopalachari 1937–1954. A Moralist
    in Politics* (Madras: Macmillan, 1978), p. 246.
65 Tamil Nadu State Archive, Chennai, Health Department, 1216, 1953;
    Nehru Memorial Library, New Delhi, C. Rajagopalachari Papers, Instal-
    ment VI–XI, Subject files no. 28.

66 *The Hindu* (15 and 17 May 1955).
67 P. Larsen (UNICEF, New Delhi) to T.G. Davies (UNICEF, New York) 17 September 1955. UN Archives (UNICEF), Box CF/RA/BX/PD/1962/T008, folder A124. See also the numbers given in Amrith, *Decolonizing International Health*, pp. 141–2.
68 For the controversial history of BCG and the official WHO position on its use, see N. Brimnes, 'BCG Vaccination and WHO's Global Strategy for Tuberculosis Control 1948–1983', *Social Science and Medicine*, 67 (2008), pp. 863–73.
69 *The Hindu* (17 May 1955). For Raman's reference to Lübeck, see *The Hindu* (14 February 1949). Also reproduced in *People's Health*, 3, p. 204.
70 *The Hindu* (17 May 1955).
71 *Indian Express* (5 February 1949). See also *The Hindu* (5 February 1949). Both reproduced in *People's Health*, 3:5, p. 198.
72 *People's Health*, 3:2, p. 53.
73 *People's Health*, 3:5, p. 188.
74 Copley, *The Political Career*, pp. 14, 161, 236; H. L. Erdman, *The Swatantra Party and Indian Conservatism* (Cambridge: Cambridge University Press, 1967), p. 65.
75 *The Hindu* (14 February 1949). Important trials with BCG had been carried out on American Indians from the 1930s. See, Christian W. McMillen, ' "The Red Man and the White Plague": Rethinking Race, Tuberculosis, and American Indians, ca.1890–1950', *Bulletin of the History of Medicine*, 82:3 (2008), pp. 608–45.
76 C. Rajagopalachari, *B.C.G. – Why I Oppose It*, n.p. [1955], p. 1.
77 S. Soundararajan (Madras) to C. Rajagopalachari (Madras), 3 August 1955. Nehru Memorial Library, Delhi, C.Rajagopalachari Papers, instalment V, Subject file no. 135.
78 D. Banerji, 'Politics of Immunisation Programme', *Economic and Political Weekly*, 25:14 (1990), p. 715; D. Banerji, 'Crash of the Immunization Programme: Consequences of a Totalitarian Approach', *International Journal of Health Services*, 20:3 (1990), pp. 501–10.
79 Banerji, 'Crash', pp. 505–6.
80 Banerji, 'Politics', p. 717.
81 W. Muraskin, *Polio Eradication and its Discontents. A Historian's Journey Through an International Health (un)Civil War* (Hyderabad: Orient BlackSwan, 2012), pp. 94–128. Quoted from p. 94.
82 D. Banerji, 'Global Programme of Polio Eradication in India', pp. 1–26, quoted from p. 8. This document is dated 12 April 2004 and posted, though without the references, at the website of the International Association of Health Policy. See: wwwhealthp.org/node/17 (accessed 13 May 2013).

83　*Ibid.*, p. 19.
84　C. Sathyamala *et al.*, 'Polio Eradication Initiative in India: Deconstructing the GPEI', *International Journal of Health Services*, 35:2 (2005), pp. 361–83.
85　Banerji, 'Crash', p. 507.
86　D. Banerji, 'Technocentric Approach to Health. Western Responses to Alma-Ata', *Economic and Political Weekly*, 31:28 (1986), pp. 1233–4; Banerji, 'Politics', p. 715; Banerji, 'Crash', p. 501.
87　D. Banerji, 'The People and Health Service Development in India: A Brief Overview', *International Journal of Health Services*, 34:1 (2004), pp. 123–42. Quoted from p. 126.
88　Banerji, 'The People', p. 127.
89　*Ibid.*, p. 130.
90　*Ibid.*, p. 131. See also Banerji, 'Global Programme', p. 2.
91　Banerji, 'Global Programme', p. 20.
92　Banerji, 'The People', p. 132.
93　Banerji, 'Crash', p. 502; Banerji, 'Technocentric Approach', p. 1233.
94　On the problems with the Oral Polio Vaccine (OPV), see Muraskin, *Polio Eradication*, pp. 12–18.
95　Banerji, 'Crash', p. 507; Banerji, 'Politics', p. 717. Muraskin, *Polio Eradication*, p. 124, note 42.
96　Muraskin, *Polio Eradication*, p. 94.
97　Greenough, 'Intimidation', p. 633.

3

Vaccination and the communist state: polio in Eastern Europe

Dora Vargha

In December 1959, Hungary introduced into its national immunisation programme the Sabin vaccine, the live poliovirus vaccine that has been the tool of the Global Polio Eradication Initiative since 1988. This campaign put Hungary in the front line of polio vaccination with live virus vaccines along with the Soviet Union and Czechoslovakia, where the Sabin vaccine was tested. Czechoslovakia became the first country in the world to practically eradicate polio in 1960[1] and the Hungarian model of annual intensive mass vaccination campaigns became one of the bases on which the WHO built its global strategy of polio eradication.[2]

How did Eastern Europe come to play such an important role in laying the foundations of polio eradication during the early Cold War? Was there something particular about Eastern European states that made this region especially fitting or receptive to mass trials and vaccination campaigns that then had a global effect?

This chapter aims to get to the heart of this matter by examining Eastern European experiences with polio in the 1950s and early 1960s. Two states played a particularly important part in the history of the Sabin vaccine, and thus stand in the focus of this analysis: Hungary and Czechoslovakia. The vaccine trials and prevention efforts with the Sabin vaccine in the late 1950s and early 1960s are placed in the broader context of experiences with polio in Eastern Europe with the caveat that the description of regional vaccination policies is far from complete. The political diversity of Eastern Europe, paired with the linguistic and cultural differences in the region make the accessibility of an overall Eastern European experience very challenging. Moreover, the critical history of vaccination programmes and public health organisation have been – until recently – largely unexplored, leaving historians of Eastern European medicine with a Herculean task when attempting to piece an overall narrative together.

In what follows, I argue that Eastern European states saw themselves, as they were seen by the West, to be particularly well suited to test and apply polio prevention with live virus vaccine on a mass scale. State paternalism and disease prevention as the cornerstone of communist public health dogmas on the one hand, and the particular organisation of public health practices and society more broadly on the other, contributed to the region becoming a reference point in scientific debates on the use of the Sabin vaccine and on polio eradication. Although these ideas and concepts rooted in ideology and a Cold War view of Eastern European states were often divorced from realities, such internal and external perceptions of Eastern European states had significant practical consequences not only in polio prevention, but also in building bridges between East and West.

Polio in Eastern Europe

To understand the significance of polio in Cold War Eastern Europe, we must consider the social, economic and political history of the era. In a wider context, the looming threat of a nuclear war overshadowed the Cold War. Military and strategic considerations contributed to the formation of Big Science and affected research funding structures and research practices all over the world.[3]

While the potential threat of destruction was pervasive, other results arising from the Second World War were equally important: the impact on the economy, on concepts of what citizens' roles are, on beliefs in progress in medicine and science, and on concerns over ethical issues in medicine. Moreover, this time saw the advent of new international agencies, such as the WHO; an era of decolonisation; the establishment of new regimes; and the emergence of particular ideas about what modern societies should be. One of the key sites of new regimes that worked with particular ideas of modernity was Eastern Europe, where, in accordance with the Soviet Union, communist governments emerged to gain exclusive political control between 1945 and 1952.

One would not expect polio to play a central role in such a setting – especially since, in terms of number of people affected, it was not a major health threat. Even at the climax of an epidemic, the increased incidence numbers were not particularly high when compared to the morbidity and mortality of other diseases of the era. However, as in many post-war societies, population politics became increasingly important in Eastern Europe in the wake of long years of devastating and bloody battles, deportations, genocide and starvation. Moreover, an intensive concentration on heavy industry and material output in the 1950s, and an ideology that placed robust physical workers at the heart of communism's success furthered interest in the reproduction of healthy and productive bodies.

Faced with the after-effects of the Second World War and the economic goals and ideals of the new era, several states enforced a strict pro-natalist policy in the early 1950s, most prominently abortion bans,[4] in the hope of increasing live births and thereby the number of productive workers. The general idea and goal undergirding pro-natalist policies was a shared attribute in the Eastern Bloc. As historian Gail Kligman put it, 'Mobilization and control of the population were of critical strategic importance for the maximization of development potential, and attention to demographic phenomena was essential to securing long-term interests. In order to meet the relatively high labor needs of such economies, reproduction of the labor force became a priority planning item.'[5]

In all countries of the Eastern Bloc, with the exception of Albania, the bans were lifted after abortion was made possible on request in the Soviet Union in 1955.[6] The short increase during the years of the abortion ban was soon followed by the decrease in live births. In Hungary, the 1956 Revolution, followed by a massive emigration of dissidents further added to the decrease in the current and future workforce.[7]

The epidemic waves of polio came to Eastern Europe at the time of this demographic shock and challenged the process of social, political and economic reorganisation. The relatively new communist governments that positioned themselves as the answer to a bright and productive future, had to deal with the traumatic effects of polio epidemics, which threatened communist ideals.

A disease that targeted the youngest of the population, leaving them physically disabled and removing them from the potential workforce was an effect that could not be taken lightly, on either sides of the Iron Curtain. From the communist state's point of view, this effect was aggravated when the visibly disabled bodies of polio victims were pitted against the robust bodies of workers and peasants omnipresent in murals, statues, magazines and schoolbooks. Polio simply did not fit the communist utopia.

Severe polio epidemics started to appear in Eastern Europe around the early 1950s. In Romania, epidemics began in 1949 and peaked in 1957 with an incidence rate of a stunning 42.5 cases per 100,000.[8] In Poland the most severe year was the first, 1951, with an incidence rate of 12.7,[9] while in Hungary, where epidemics began raising concern in 1952, the worst epidemic year of 1957 produced a relatively high incidence rate in the region: 23.8 per 100,000.[10] In Bulgaria, apart from the epidemic year of 1941, polio began taking its toll every three years from 1951 onwards, reaching a peak in 1957 with a morbidity rate of 13.8 per 100,000 inhabitants.[11] An exception to the rule was Czechoslovakia, where 1939 marked the beginning of the polio era.[12] However, in the early 1950s the incidence rate reached its highest peak, rising from 1.52 in the 1930s to 10.03 per 100,000.[13]

Polio, primarily a disease of children, raised the stakes for the state's provider role in public health. While health care was consistently low among spending priorities, and always took a backseat to the development of heavy industry in rebuilding the country after the war, it was also one of the key elements of the communist state that set the East apart from the West.

The ideological stance in public health objectives, which framed theories of health and disease on dialectical-materialist ideas, was based on the post-war Soviet model of public health and was adopted in several Eastern European countries following the communist takeover around 1948.[14] As historian of medicine Bradley Moore points out, preventive and prophylactic interventions against external threats to the health of the body were key in this Eastern European thinking about public health.[15] Moreover, free access to health care for workers provided by the paternalistic state was a fundamental idea in how the system worked, or at least was supposed to work. Polio, with its debilitating effects and its patients' need for long-term treatment, visibly challenged the provider role that the state set up for itself through policies and communication. More importantly, the fact that polio affected children made it imperative to meet its challenge successfully.

State paternalism and socialised medicine were not unique to the Eastern part of Europe. In the post-war era, national health care schemes and states' strong intervention in health matters were on the rise in countries such as Great Britain, France and Sweden. As Lundberg and Holmberg show (Chapter 10 in this book), it is a historical heritage that countries, like Sweden, still grapple with today.

However, not only was public health in general, and prevention in particular, a cornerstone of the communist ideal, but mass public health programmes, such as prevention of infectious diseases by vaccination were ideal terrains in which the communist state could demonstrate its power and legitimate its authority. If vaccination worked, the result would be immediate and visible. If not, factors unconnected to the state, like science could be blamed.[16]

Salk vaccine behind the Iron Curtain

Polio vaccination in Eastern Europe became such an enterprise with vaccines that appeared in the West in the second half of the 1950s. As the incidence of the disease appeared with more frequency and with higher and higher rates around the world, vaccine development became especially pressing and therefore gained priority in securing research funds. The first vaccine to be widely produced and distributed was the Salk vaccine in 1955, developed by Jonas Salk in the USA, which induced immunity to the disease with the help of inactivated or killed poliovirus.

Developing the vaccine was one important step. Establishing its efficiency was quite another. American authorities moved quickly when it came to approving and licensing the Salk vaccine;[17] it took them merely two hours after Thomas Francis, director of the University of Michigan Poliomyelitis Vaccine Evaluation Center, officially announced the results of the field trial involving 1.8 million schoolchildren on 12 April 1954.[18]

On 25 April 1955 in California, a child previously inoculated with the Salk vaccine was admitted to the hospital with signs of polio. The following day, five similar cases were reported. All of these patients received vaccine produced by the Cutter Laboratories, and on 27 April the Surgeon General requested that Cutter recall all its vaccines. In the course of the next two months, 94 vaccinated patients, 126 family contacts and 40 community contacts were diagnosed with poliomyelitis[19] in what would be termed the Cutter incident. This situation had tremendous impact: it shook public trust in the vaccine, changed vaccine regulation and control in the USA and ultimately affected the story of another, live-polio vaccine developed by Albert Sabin.[20] While American and worldwide confidence was soon restored in the only available vaccine, in the following years, based on varying experience with its application around the world, the efficacy of the Salk vaccine would be debated at international conferences and on the pages of medical journals well into the 1960s.

These debates did not seem to appear in the decision-making of Eastern European polio vaccine use. In the wake of the threat against the bodies of their citizens and their modernist projects, with a particular, ideological and practical emphasis on disease prevention, most Eastern European countries introduced the Salk vaccine without much public or professional deliberation. This set them apart from many of their western counterparts, where, despite intense state involvement in polio prevention, extensive professional debates surrounded and informed governments' decisions in choosing and implementing vaccination strategies.[21]

The timing of the introduction of polio vaccines in Eastern Europe, however, did follow the same pattern as in the West: governments generally took action only when the imminent threat of a severe epidemic was unfolding. One of the explanations for this is that polio was not an omnipresent threat. It usually caused outbreaks in the summer months, and did not come every year. Another important aspect was the financial commitment vaccination required: importing vaccines was a costly enterprise and setting up domestic vaccine production required significant investment, like building new laboratories, training staff and importing and keeping expensive lab animals.[22] This latter, economic aspect was especially important in Eastern Europe, since both vaccine import and the establishment of domestic production required hard currency that was not easy to come by.[23]

Czechoslovakia was among the first in the region to introduce inactivated Salk vaccine. While preparations for local polio vaccine production began in 1956, an atypical epidemic wave in that same year urged the government to change its original plans to start polio vaccination with domestic vaccine at the end of 1957. Instead, Czechoslovakia acquired vaccine from the Canadian Connaught Laboratories and started immunisation in the spring of 1957, before the onset of the epidemic season. Paediatricians and Red Cross volunteers aided the vaccination process. They followed the so-called 'Danish method' of injecting a low vaccine dose intradermally, using 0.1 and 0.15 ml vaccine in two doses.[24] The Czechoslovak hygienists were upfront about choosing this method 'to inoculate the maximum number of children with the limited amount of vaccine available'.[25] A year later the Czech health authorities calculated the effectiveness of the initial vaccination campaign to be 66 per cent in the Czech regions and 72 per cent in Slovakia for children under the age of 7. They found the results to be promising and decided to continue vaccinations with domestically produced Salk vaccine in 1958.[26] However, state hygienists soon became interested in another vaccine developed by Sabin, turning a significant part of the country into a field-testing site.

Like their Czechoslovak counterpart, the Hungarian government chose to import Canadian and American vaccine to begin the immunisation of the population in 1957. Although preparations were also made for domestic vaccine production, the process was significantly delayed, mostly due to the revolution that broke out in the autumn of 1956, while an evaluation study was being prepared. However, there was no time to lose, since the most severe polio epidemic in the history of Hungary was unfolding in the summer of 1957. Thus, mass vaccination began with the imported Salk vaccine, mostly produced by the Canadian Connaught Laboratories, and American manufacturers Eli Lilly and Co. and Parke-Davis and Co.,[27] along with shipments from the WHO and smaller contributions from religious organisations.[28] In an effort to stretch vaccine supplies as far as possible, the Hungarian Health Ministry also chose the Danish method to administer the vaccine. This method, which used close to 1/10th of the conventional, intramuscular vaccination method came under scrutiny[29] when, despite the widespread vaccination campaigns, a new, severe epidemic occurred in 1959, with an incidence rate of 18.3 per 100,000.[30] This new epidemic also marked the end of domestic Salk vaccine production in Hungary, which had begun earlier that year.[31] Instead, the government decided to rapidly test and then introduce Sabin's new, live vaccine by the end of 1959.

Other Eastern European countries followed similar patterns with the Salk vaccine. Poland began domestic production in 1957 on a small scale[32] and started mass production in the second half of 1958. The vaccination was to be covered partially by domestic, and partially by imported, Salk vaccine.[33] As in many countries, an epidemic served as motive for the Bulgarian government to introduce mass vaccination in September 1957. Bulgaria used imported vaccine until 1959 (from the American Merck and Connaught Laboratories), when it switched to the inactivated vaccine produced in the Soviet Union.[34] The East German government began vaccination with the inactivated vaccine in 1958, using the so-called 'Berna' vaccine, produced by the Swiss Serum and Vaccine Institute in Bern. In order to spare vaccine, the East German method of choice was also intradermal injection. This method changed with the arrival of Salk vaccine prepared in Moscow – with the availability of larger quantities of more affordable vaccine, East Germany changed to the intramuscular injection of 1 ml vaccine for the first dose.[35] Instead of using Salk's polio vaccine, Romania began immunisation with a different inactivated vaccine: the recently released Lépine vaccine, developed in France by Pierre Lépine, physician and biologist, and manufactured by the Pasteur Institute of Paris.[36]

As the story of Eastern European Salk vaccination shows, the Iron Curtain did not stand in the way of polio prevention. Moreover, it was not only the vaccines that crossed over the firm border dividing West from East. Eastern European scientists were regular participants in the international (European and global) conferences on poliomyelitis, exchanging experiences with vaccination and research on the polio vaccine. In addition, since Salk vaccine production required a particular and strict procedure, along with elaborate laboratory equipments and the keeping of live monkeys, Eastern European virologists and public health specialists crossed to western countries like Denmark and Sweden to gain experience in inactivating the virus and producing the vaccine.[37]

Sabin vaccine and the Eastern European trials

The scientific interaction across the Iron Curtain continued with the development, testing and implementation of the Sabin vaccine. The novelty of the new vaccine was that instead of containing killed virus, it aimed to achieve immunity with the presence of live, attenuated virus – that is, poliovirus that had been sufficiently weakened so as not to cause illness, but potent enough to elicit an immune response. Like wild poliovirus strains, the attenuated strains were also excreted by the vaccinees, creating the possibility of indirectly immunising people who had not been vaccinated. The live virus vaccine was also different from the Salk in another important way: it could be administered orally, instead of by injection.

Live poliovirus vaccine was never tested on a mass scale in the USA, for several reasons. First, with the widespread use of the Salk vaccine, the main funding body of polio prevention and care, the National Foundation for Infantile Paralysis, along with US authorities, lost interest in investing greatly in yet another vaccine. Moreover, after the Cutter incident, they were wary of embarking on a potentially risky polio vaccine trial.[38] Therefore, live poliovirus trials were, for the most part, conducted outside the USA.

The history of live poliovirus vaccines has been mostly explored through the Cold War cooperation between the American Albert Sabin and the Russian Mikhail Chumakov.[39] The common pursuit of these two scientists led to the largest field trial in the history of polio vaccination, involving almost 17 million people in the Soviet Union.[40] As soon as Sabin finished selecting the most optimal strain for creating the vaccine, he sent samples to Anatol Smorodintsev, Chumakov's colleague in Leningrad. Field trials with the strain started in 1957 on a very small scale with the vaccination of 67 children. This number gradually grew to 150, then to 2,010, and finally to 20,000 in 1958.[41] Parallel to Smorodintsev's trials, another field trial, initiated by Chumakov, then director of the Poliomyelitis Research Institute in Moscow, took off in greater proportions. Chumakov asked Sabin to send him 'the greatest possible amount' of vaccine for testing and producing. Sabin sent enough to vaccinate 300,000 children.[42] Chumakov started the trial with 20,000 and, following its initial success, was able to conduct the largest field trial to date in the history of polio vaccines.

By the end of 1959, over 15 million people spanning fourteen republics of the Soviet Union were vaccinated in the trial. Smorodintsev and his team immunised more than 1.5 million of the subjects; the rest received vaccine from Chumakov's lab in the Institute for Poliomyelitis

Research in Moscow. The Soviet Union's Minister of Health issued an order on 16 December 1959 for the mass immunisation of the whole population between the ages of two months and 20 years by July 1960. This meant vaccinating 77 million people in a matter of months.[43] The *British Medical Journal* deemed this campaign a 'Blitzkrieg against poliomyelitis'.[44]

However, the story of further Eastern European trials, equally important to their Soviet counterparts, remains largely unexplored. Live vaccines fared even worse than the Salk vaccine in creating consensus in vaccine efficiency, and more importantly, safety. Fears that vaccines made with attenuated live viruses could cause or spread disease instead of curbing epidemics were persistent throughout the development of the live vaccines in the 1950s and the early 1960s. Trials in Eastern Europe became important reference points in vaccine efficiency and safety considerations both in scientific debates and in governments' decision-making processes on the introduction of the vaccine.

The Hygiene and Epidemiological Service of Czechoslovakia organised relatively large field trials in 1958 and 1959 with vaccines prepared from the Sabin strains by the Institute of Sera and Vaccines in Prague, with additional batches of vaccines acquired from Chumakov in the Soviet Union.[45]

Sabin, whose help the Czechoslovak scientists requested through the WHO,[46] personally aided the bureaucratic process of shipping the strains from Cincinatti to Prague in the spring of 1958 and kept a close eye on the trials.[47] The trials were conducted in four regions (Ústi nad Labem, Liberec, Juhlava and Ostrava)[48] and in total 140,000 children between the ages of 2 and 6 were vaccinated.[49]

Finding the serological results favourable, and based on studies by mostly Soviet scientists,[50] the vaccination programme was extended nationwide in 1960. Using domestically produced vaccine from Sabin strains and also vaccine imported from the Soviet Union,[51] 93 per cent of Czechoslovakia's child population was vaccinated, roughly 3.5 million children between the ages of two months and fourteen years.[52] The mass vaccination was deemed to be an instant success: no confirmed poliomyelitis cases developed in the territory of Czechoslovakia in the first two epidemic seasons after the beginning of the campaign.[53]

Although less widely known than the field trials and early mass-immunisation programmes in the Soviet Union and Czechoslovakia,

Hungary was also among the Sabin vaccine pioneers. A growing disillusionment with the inactivated vaccine initiated a switch to Sabin's live poliovirus vaccine, making Hungary the first country in the world to begin mass immunisation with the new vaccine on a national level in early December 1959.[54] Hungarian virologists and public health authorities had been following oral vaccination trials closely throughout the year, and some had been in touch with Albert Sabin personally, meeting regularly at conferences and sharing results.[55] A turning point in developing serious interest came with the epidemic of the summer of 1959. Trials with vaccine imported from the Soviet Union began in Győr-Moson-Sopron County in 1959 on 3 and 4 November, during which the population between the ages of three months and fifteen years[56] was vaccinated. Virologists reported the average acceptance rate of the vaccine to be 96 per cent.[57]

The trial was short, and not much time was spent on evaluating the results. The National Public Health Institute analysed 127 stool samples before and after the trial to investigate the presence of the attenuated virus after vaccination; but the overall evaluation of the vaccine and the decision to introduce the vaccine was based on the large-scale field trials conducted by the Soviet Union, as well as the experiences of Czechoslovakia and Singapore with the Sabin, and Poland and the Belgian Congo with the Koprowski strains.[58] Hungarian virologists, in this sense, drew on an international experiences with live vaccines that not only crossed the dividing lines of the Cold War, but also spanned across continents. They were able to do so thanks to access to international journals and a continuous presence at international polio conferences and symposiums.

On 14 December 1959, nationwide vaccination in Hungary began with the Sabin drops. Immunisation was mandatory for children between three months and two years; for all other age groups, the immunisation was voluntary.[59] Vaccination was organised in Mother and Infant Protection Offices by the district paediatricians. Children were also vaccinated in day care settings, kindergartens and schools,[60] which renders the term *voluntary* dubious. By 1960, Hungary had vaccinated 2.5 million people, more than the total in the two years of Salk vaccination. The country thus joined the Soviet Union and Czechoslovakia in being the first countries in the world to organise mass vaccination with the new, live -poliovirus vaccine.

East Germany followed suit with a field trial of the Sabin vaccine in April 1960, citing the favourable results in the Soviet Union, Czechoslovakia, Hungary and Poland as the basis for their own trial. The vaccination was free and voluntary, and German virologists reported a very favourable public acceptance, immunising around 86 per cent of the people between the ages of two months and twenty years. Vaccination with the oral vaccine became compulsory in 1961, reaching 43 per cent of the total population by 1962.[61]

It is important to note another large-scale field trial conducted in Poland, using Hilary Koprowski's live poliovirus vaccine. The vaccination began with a small-scale vaccination in October 1958, involving a total population of 8,716 in a small town and three villages. In the next step, after approval from the special committee appointed by the Ministry of Health, all children between the ages of six months and fifteen years were immunised with the type 1 (Chat) strain in two provinces, Krakow and Opole, totalling 643,000 people.[62] Beginning in autumn 1959, in a mass immunisation campaign, over 7 million people, mostly children, received type 1 (Chat) and type 3 (Fox) strains. By the end of 1960, 26 per cent of the total population was immunised with oral vaccine, including 76 per cent of children between the ages of six months and fifteen years.[63] Based on the decrease of the incidence rate of epidemics, Polish virologists determined the vaccine's efficacy to be 82.9 per cent.[64]

Mass vaccination campaigns with the live poliovirus vaccine soon followed in the rest of Eastern Europe: in Bulgaria in 1960, targeting about two million children between two months and fourteen years of age;[65] in Romania in 1961, administered to the whole population under the age of 30: around ten million people.[66] Yugoslavia carried out a small field trial with the Sabin vaccine from January to May 1960, involving about eight thousand pre-school children in the city of Kragujevac, and, following a relatively severe epidemic in 1960, began mass vaccination in 1961.[67]

Eastern European governments and the West alike saw the field trials and mass vaccinations in the region as something particular to communist states. On the one hand, participant states in the field trials and early mass vaccination campaigns saw the success in dramatically curbing polio as ultimate proof of the superiority of their ideological and political system. On the other hand, for many researchers and

public health officials of the West, intensive, mass field trials and vaccination campaigns, such as the ones conducted in Eastern Europe and
the Soviet Union were inextricably connected with authoritarianism
inherent in communist states.

As polio cases began to plummet, communist states were quick to
claim credit. This was especially true for the two countries leading vaccination efforts with the Sabin vaccine. Hungary emphasised the
importance of the overall communist enterprise in the success of the
Sabin vaccine.

At first, official communication on the Sabin vaccination re-evaluated
the state's role in vaccine procurement. In the case of the Salk vaccine,
the government was portrayed as a hero, which, in spite of all hardships
and even running into debt, managed to go out there and get much
needed protection for children.[68] This time, the significance of outside
help was emphasised, having arrived from the right side of the Iron
Curtain: according to daily newspaper Népszava, the Hungarian government. 'asked for the help of the Soviet Union and not without result:
We were granted 2.5 million doses of vaccine.'[69] There was no talk of
cost or debt or the feat of the state required to import the vaccine. Later,
communist officials contrasted the polio-free world of Eastern Europe
with struggling western nations, who, for the sake of free trade and
economic hardships were reluctant to switch to the Sabin vaccine and
thus were still experiencing polio epidemics.[70]

Czechoslovak scientists and public health officials chose to emphasise their own contribution to vaccine development and the role of the
communist state in the project. Vilém Škovránek, chief hygienist,
clearly declared the achievement of the Czechoslovak polio prevention
strategy to be an evidence of good governing: 'The success of the mass
vaccination was a proof of the highly developed organizing abilities of
the Czechoslovak Ministry of Health and the profound understanding
of our people for health problems. The vaccination campaign was
accomplished without any particular troubles and the attendance of the
population was very high.'[71]

The Czechoslovak sentiments highlight two important aspects of
Eastern European polio vaccination campaigns in the Cold War: the
question of voluntarism and the advantages of the authoritarian organisation of state and public health. First, as Škovránek emphasised, the
fact that citizens happily volunteered for trials and readily complied

with mass vaccination campaigns was crucial in the representation of successful public health interventions, and not only in Czechoslovakia. This fitted very well with western stereotypes of Eastern European citizens being either oppressed by the communist state or being uniform, obedient subjects.

However, it is very difficult to discover how voluntary and compliant the Eastern European population actually was. Official communication on vaccination hardly ever touched on problems or significant challenges, only when unexpected epidemic crises unfolded, did criticism and reluctance surface. Such a case was the 1959 epidemic in Hungary, when the government accused parents of carelessness and scolded them for not vaccinating their children.[72] Reports reveal that some parents did not trust the new vaccine and their distrust was shared with some physicians as well.[73] Since the debacle of 1959 was almost certainly not exclusively caused by low immunisation rates,[74] it is not clear if large numbers of parents were involved, or if they only became visible as a possible explanation as the government was trying to make sense of an inexplicable situation.

Second, the military-like organisation of preventive public health measures, such as vaccination and the compulsory participation of the population in such enterprises rang alarm bells in the immediate postwar years. In the wake of a horrible war against the Nazi dictatorship that organised itself with utmost efficiency, and with the looming threat of Soviet totalitarianism, engaging with anything remotely authoritarian caused uneasiness in the West when contemplating public health measures. Already in 1948 such sentiments were articulated at the First International Poliomyelitis Conference, where one participant pointed out the tensions between the legacy of dictatorships and the most effective ways of preventing and controlling disease through autocratic measures.[75] The merit of a high level of state authority in successfully implementing public health policies, especially in times of epidemics, and the frustrations this perception caused in Cold War thinking became a recurring issue in the history of polio.

Reservations about autocratic regimes, disease prevention and scientific knowledge production came to the forefront during the evaluation of the Soviet field trials in 1959. The American virologist, Dorothy Horstmann, representing the WHO in the assessment of the validity of the trials highlighted the role of a centralised and state-operated public health system in successfully organising such an endeavour. In her report, Horstmann spoke of live virus vaccination programmes and the Eastern European, military-like organisation of public health as being 'peculiarly fitted'.[76] In the Soviet case, a state and health care system that was centrally controlled top-down seemed ideal in organising a project on a mass scale and at the same time guaranteed that such scientific trials would be meticulous.

Conclusion

For the relatively young communist governments, polio pitted specific challenges to ideas of state paternalism, which permeated health care policies, in a decade that was burdened by Cold War thaws and frosts and revolutions. The stakes did not only regard the health of the population and epidemic control, but also the strength and capability of the new communist system.

Both East and West shared the perception of what the communist state was and its ideal role in polio prevention. Following the appearance and successful application of live poliovirus vaccines, Eastern European states saw themselves as particularly suited to achieve effectiveness in curbing – and eradicating – polio through their part in vaccine development and its distribution. The West, while not endorsing such political regimes ideologically, agreed. Indeed, Czechoslovakia, Hungary and Poland became pioneers in introducing, testing and applying live poliovirus vaccines on a mass scale, while their Eastern European peers were quick to follow in mass vaccination.

From a broader geopolitical perspective, polio raised uncomfortable questions about the positive side of communist regimes (i.e. effective epidemic control) and in a short time came to symbolise 'neutral' science that broke the barriers between East and West. The top-down organisation of vaccine trial organisation and immunisation, which was, at the time, seen as particularly communist and Eastern European, also came to be seen as the most effective way to eradicate polio on a global scale.

Eastern European trials and the mass vaccination methods applied in communist countries became reference points in scientific discussions on the safety and efficacy of the Sabin vaccine. The mass vaccination strategies developed in Hungary, Cuba and later in Brazil became models for the global polio eradication programme of the WHO.[77] The long-term effects of Eastern European states' role in live virus vaccine development and disease elimination carried the legacies of how communist states worked and the way in which they were imagined, over the boundaries of Europe and beyond the Cold War to global epidemic management strategies of the present.

Acknowledgements

I would like to express my gratitude to Jessica Reinisch, Ana Antic and David Bryan for inspiring conversations on Eastern Europe's place in the history of international public health. Furthermore, I would like to thank Paul Greenough for pointing out invaluable sources and references. This research was partially funded by the Wellcome Trust.

Notes

1 K. Žáček, E. Adam and V. Adamova, 'Mass Oral (Sabin) Poliomyelitis Vaccination. Virological and Serological Surveillance in Czechoslovakia, 1958–59 and 1960', British Medical Journal, 1:5285 (1962); D. Slonim, 'Global Eradication of Poliomyelitis. On the 80th Anniversary of the Founding of the National Institute of Health', Epidemiologie, Mikrobiologie, Imunologie; 54:3 (2005).

2 H. F. Hull et al., 'Progress toward Global Polio Eradication', Journal of Infectious Diseases, 175:1 (1997), S4.

3 See for instance N. Oreskes and J. Krige (eds), Nation and Knowledge: Science and Technology in the Global Cold War (Cambridge, MA: MIT Press, 2014): P. Erickson, The Politics of Game Theory: Mathematics and Cold War Culture (University of Wisconsin, 2006).

4 A. Pető, 'Women's Rights in Stalinist Hungary: The Abortion Trials of 1952–1953', Hungarian Studies Review, XXIX:1–2 (2002).

5 G. Kligman, The Politics of Duplicity: Controlling Reproduction in Ceausescu's Romania (Berkeley: University of California Press, 1998), p. 19.

6 D. Stenvoll, 'Contraception, Abortion and State Socialism: Categories in Birth Control Discourses and Policies', Kansai Univ. Rev. L. & Pol., 28 (2007); R. Dudova, 'Regulation of Abortion as State-Socialist Governmentality: The Case of Czechoslovakia', Politics & Gender, 8 (2012).

7 A. Klinger, 'Magyarország Népesedése Az Elmúlt Negyven Évben', in Magyarország Társadalomtörténete III (1945–1989) [Hungary's Population

in the Past Fourty Years, in *The Social History of Hungary III*], ed. Nikosz Fokasz and Antal Örkény (Budapest: Új Mandátum, 1999), p. 47.

8   C. Ionesco-Mihaiesti, 'Roumania', in M. Minculescu, *A Ragályos Betegségek Megelőzése És Leküzdése Gyermekeknél* [The Prevention and Treatment of Contagious Diseases in Children], ed. Eugen Rusu (Kolozsvár: Tudomány- és Kultúraterjesztő Társaság Könyvtára, 1957), pp. 53–5.

9   F. Prezmycki, 'Poland', in *ibid.*, pp. 52–3.

10 I. Dömök, 'A Hazai Járványügyi Helyzet az Élő Poliovírus Vakcina Bevezetése Előtt', in *A Gyermekbénulás Elleni Küzdelem. Beszámoló a Ma Már Múlttá Vált Betegség Ellen Folytatott Hősies Küzdelemről és Felszámolásának Lehetőségéről* [Epidemiological circumstances in Hungary Before the Introduction of the Live Poliovaccine, in Fight Against Poliomyelitis. Account of the Heroic Struggle against a Disease of the Past and the Possibilities of its Eradication], ed. Rezső Hargitai and Ákosné Kiss (Budapest: Literatura Medicina, 1994).

11 I. Vaptzarov, D. Bratovanov and T. Kristev, 'La Vaccination Contre La Poliomyélite en Bulgarie' [Vaccination against Poliomyelitis in Bulgaria], in *Anti-Poliomyelitis Vaccinations, Physio-Pathology of the Respiratory Disorder, Poliomyelitis of the 'Very Young Child'. VIth Symposium of the European Association Against Poliomyelitis*, ed. H. C.A. Lassen (Munich: European Association Against Poliomyelitis, 1960).

12 V. Skorvanek, 'Czechoslovakia. Zur Vakzination Gegen Polio' [Czechoslovakia. Of polio vaccination], in Minculescu, *A Ragályos Betegségek Megelőzése és Leküzdése Gyermekeknél*, pp. 28–9.

13 Žáček *et al.*, 'Mass Oral (Sabin) Poliomyelitis Vaccination'.

14 B. M. Moore, 'For the People's Health: Ideology, Medical Authority and Hygienic Science in Communist Czechoslovakia,' *Social History of Medicine*, 27:1 (2014).

15 *Ibid.*

16 S. L. Hoch, 'The Social Consequences of Soviet Immunization Policies, 1945–1980', ed. The National Council for Eurasian and East European Research (Washington DC, 1997).

17 Subcommittee on Health and Safety of the Committee on Interstate and Foreign Commerce, *Polio Vaccines*, First session on developments with respect to the manufacture of live virus polio vaccine and results of utilization of killed virus polio vaccine, 16 March 1961, pp. 3–4.

18 D. M. Oshinsky, *Polio: An American Story* (Oxford and New York: Oxford University Press, 2005), p. 203.

19 N. Nathanson and A. D. Langmuir, 'The Cutter Incident Poliomyelitis Following Formaldehyde-Inactivated Poliovirus Vaccination in the United

States During the Spring of 1955', *American Journal of Epidemiology*, 78:1 (1964).

20 Oshinsky, *Polio: An American Story*; Paul A. Offit, *The Cutter Incident: How America's First Polio Vaccine Led to the Growing Vaccine Crisis* (New Haven: Yale University Press, 2005); James Colgrove, *State of Immunity. The Politics of Vaccination in Twentieth-Century America* (Berkeley: University of California Press, 2006).

21 See for example, 'Safety and Antigenic Potency Testing of Poliomyelitis Vaccine: A Report from the Biologifal Standards Control Laboratory, Medical Research Council Laboratories, London, NW3', *The British Medical Journal*, 2:5037 (1957); 'Oral Poliomyelitis Vaccine', *The British Medical Journal*, 2:5247 (1961).

22 For the protocol of Salk vaccine production, see S. Koch, G. Veres and E. Farkas, 'Jelentés a Koppenhágai Tanulmányútunkról' [Report of our Study Trip to Copenhagen], in *The Papers of the Health Ministry* (Budapest: MOL, 1957).

23 'A Járványos Gyermekbénulás Elleni Védekezés Időszerű Feladatai. Előterjesztés a Magyar Forradalmi Munkás-Paraszt Kormányhoz' [The Timely Tasks of Polio Prevention. Proposal Presented to the Hungarian Revolutionary Workers-Peasant Party], ed. Minisztertanács (Budapest: Magyar Országos Levéltár, 1957).

24 V. Skovranek, 'Present State of Vaccination against Poliomyelitis in Czechoslovakia', in *Vaccination and Immunity. Neurophysical and Neuropathological Aspects of Poliomyelitis. Vth Symposium of the European Association Against Poliomyelitis*, ed. H. C.A. Lassen (Madrid: European Association Against Poliomyelitis, 1959).

25 *Ibid.*, p. 49.

26 *Ibid.*

27 A. Petrilla, *The Results of Intracutaneous Poliomyelitis Vaccination in Hungary, 1957*, Acta Microbiologica (Budapest: Akadémia Kiadó, 1958).

28 For more details on the history of polio vaccination in Hungary, see D. Vargha, 'Between East and West: Polio Vaccination across the Iron Curtain in Cold War Hungary', *Bulletin of the History of Medicine*, 88:2 (2014).

29 I. Szeri, P. Földes and S. Bognár, 'Adatok a Poliomyelitis Elleni Intrakután Védőoltás Kérdéséhez' [Data for the Problem of Intracutaneous Poliomyelitis Vaccination], *Orvosi Hetilap*, 100:38 (1959).

30 A. Kátay, 'Vaccination Against Poliomyelitis in Hungary'. Paper presented at the Eigthth European Symposium on Poliomyelitis, Prague, 23–6 September 1962.

31 Moldován, ' "Aki Még Nem Kapott" Áprilisban Jelentkezzék Gyermekbénulás Elleni Védőoltásra' ['If you have not yet received it', sign up in April

for the Polio Vaccination] *Népszava* (16 April 1958); Aladár Kátay, 'The Active Immunization against Poliomyelitis in Hungary and Its Three Years' Results', in *The Control of Poliomyelitis by Live Poliovirus Vaccine. Studies on Mass Vaccinations in Hungary, in the USSR, in Czechoslovakia and the German Democratic Republic. Papers Presented at the Hungarian-Soviet Medical Conference September 24–30, 1960*, ed. J. Weissfeiler (Budapest: Publishing House of the Hungarian Academy of Sciences, 1961).

32 F. Prezmycki, 'Poland', in Minculescu, *A Ragályos Betegségek Megelőzése És Leküzdése Gyermekeknél*, pp. 52–3.

33 F. Przesmycki, 'Vaccination against Poliomyelitis in Poland', in *Vaccination and Immunity. Neurophysical and Neuropathological Aspects of Poliomyelitis. Vth Symposium*, ed. Lassen.

34 Vaptzarov, Bratovanov and Kristev, 'La Vaccination Contre La Poliomyélite En Bulgarie' [Vaccination Against Poliomyelitis in Bulgaria].

35 Kukowa, 'Poliomyelitis-Schutzimpfung in Der Deutschen Demokratiscen Republik' [Poliomyelitis Vaccination in the German Democratic Republic].

36 A. Baicus, 'History of Polio Vaccination', *World Journal of Virology*, 1:4 (2012).

37 Koch, Veres and Farkas, 'Jelentés a Koppenhágai Tanulmányútunkról' [Report of our Study Trip to Copenhagen].

38 Oshinsky, *Polio: An American Story.*

39 See *ibid.*; S. Benison, 'International Medical Cooperation: Dr. Albert Sabin, Live Poliovirus Vaccine and the Soviets,' *Bulletin of the History of Medicine*, 56, Winter (1982); Albert B. Sabin, 'Role of My Cooperation with Soviet Scientists in the Elimination of Polio: Possible Lessons for Relations between the USA and the USSR', *Perspectives in Biology and Medicine*, 31:1 (1987).

40 M. P. Chumakov *et al.*, 'Some Results of the Work on Mass Immunization in the Soviet Union with Live Poliovirus Vaccine Prepared from Sabin Strains', *Bulletin of the World Health Organization*, 25:1 (1961).

41 A. A. Smorodintsev *et al.*, 'Results of a Study of the Reactogenic and Immunogenic Properties of Live Anti-Poliomyelitis Vaccine', *Bulletin of the World Health Organization*, 20 (1959).

42 Sabin, 'Role of My Cooperation with Soviet Scientists in the Elimination of Polio: Possible Lessons for Relations between the USA and the USSR', p. 61.

43 Chumakov *et al.*, 'Some Results of the Work on Mass Immunization in the Soviet Union with Live Poliovirus Vaccine Prepared from Sabin Strains'.

44 'Mass Immunization with the Live Poliovirus Vaccine in the Soviet Union,' *British Medical Journal*, 1:5187 (1960), p. 1729.

45 Žáček *et al.*, 'Mass Oral (Sabin) Poliomyelitis Vaccination'.
46 A. B. Sabin, 'Letter from Sabin, Albert B. to Rivers, Thomas M. Dated 1958'10'06,' in *Correspondence, NFIP* (Cincinnati: Hauck Center for the Albert B. Sabin Archives, 1958).
47 A. B. Sabin, 'Letter from Sabin, Albert B. To Raska, Karel Dated 1958–09–25', in *Correspondence, OPV International* (Cincinnati: Hauck Center for the Albert Sabin Archives, University of Cincinnati, 1958).
48 D. Slonim *et al.*, 'History of Poliomyelitis in the Czech Republic – Part III', *Central European Journal of Public Health*, 3:3 (1995); Vilem Skovranek, 'Letter from Skovranek, Vilem to Sabin, Albert B. Dated 1958–11–10', in *Correspondence, OPV International* (Cincinnati: Hauck Center for the Albert B. Sabin Archives, 1958).
49 V. Skovranek and K. Zacek, 'Oral Poliovirus Vaccine (Sabin) in Czechoslovakia. Effectiveness of Nation-Wide Use in 1960,' *JAMA*, 176:6 (1961).
50 *Ibid.*
51 V. Skovranek, 'Present State of Poliomyelitis after Nation Wide Vaccination with Live (Oral) Vaccine in Czechoslovakia', in *Programs of Vaccination, Encephalitis and Meningitis in Enteroviral Infections, Virological and Clinical Problems. VIIth Symposium of the European Association Against Poliomyelitis*, ed. H. C.A. Lassen (Oxford: Europ. Assoc. Poliomyelitis and Allied Diseases, 1962).
52 Škrovánek and Žážek, 'Oral Poliovirus Vaccine (Sabin) in Czechoslovakia'.
53 Skovranek, 'Present State of Poliomyelitis after Nation Wide Vaccination with Live (Oral) Vaccine in Czechoslovakia.'
54 'December 14 – Én Kezdődnek a Gyermekbénulás Elleni Sabin-féle Védőoltások' [Sabin Vaccinations Against Poliomyelitis begin on December 14] *Népszava*, November 22 1959.
55 A. B. Sabin, 'Letter to Sabin, Albert B. To Ivanovics, George Dated 1957'02'1,' in *Correspondence, Individual* (Cincinatti: Hauck Center for the Albert B. Sabin Archives, 1957).
56 'Az Egészségügyi Minisztérium Tájékoztatója Az Ország 1959. Évi November Havi Járványügyi Helyzetéről,' [The Report of the Health Ministry of the Country's Monthly Epidemiological Situation in November 1959] in the Papers of the Public Health and Epidemiological Division of the Health Ministry (Budapest: Magyar Országos Levéltár, 1959).
57 I. Dömök, E. Molnár and Á. Jancsó, 'Virus Excretion after Mass Vaccination with Attenuated Polioviruses in Hungary,' *British Medical Journal*, 1:5237 (1961), p. 1410.
58 Dr T. Bakács, 'Az Eddigi Poliomyelitis Vaccinatio Eredményeinek Értékelése,' [The Evaluation of the Current Poliomyelitis Vaccination] *Orvosi Hetilap* 101:20 (1960), p. 690.

59 'Budapesten December 14–15–16–án Kapják a Gyerekek a Gyermek-bénulás Ellen Védő Sabin-Oltóanyagot,' [in Budapest Children Receive the Sabin Vaccine Against Poliomyelitis on December 14–15–16] *Népszava* (26 November 1959).

60 *Ibid.*

61 T. Kima and W. A. Belian, 'National Report of Immunisation Program of German Democratic Republic,' in *Programs of Vaccination, Encephalitis and Meningitis in Enteroviral Infections, Virological and Clinical Problems. VIIth Symposium.*

62 F. Przesmycki and J. Kostrzewski, 'Evaluation of Oral Poliomyelitis Vaccine Prepared from Koprowski's Type 1 (Chat) and Type 3 (Fox) Strains', in *Programs of Vaccination, Encephalitis and Meningitis In Enteroviral Infections, Virological and Clinical Problems. VIIth Symposium.*

63 H. Wior, 'Vaccination against Poliomyelitis in Poland', in *Programs of Vaccination, Encephalitis and Meningitis In Enteroviral Infections, Virological and Clinical Problems. VIIth Symposium.*

64 Przesmycki and Kostrzewski, 'Evaluation of Oral Poliomyelitis'.

65 S. Rangelova *et al.*, 'Epidemiological and Serological Evaluation of Results of Mass Vaccination with Live Vacine in Bulgaria', in *Vaccination and Epidemiology of Poliomyelitis and Allied Diseases, New Developments in the Programs of Vaccination, Virological and Serological Studies, Clinical Problems. VIIIth Symposium of the European Association Against Poliomyelitis and Allied Diseases*, ed. H. C. A. Lassen (Prague: European Association on Poliomyelitis and Allied Diseases, 1963).

66 I. Spinu, S. B. Moroianu and S. Popa, 'Considérations Épidémiologiques Et La Vaccination Contre La Poliomyélite En Roumanie' [Epidemiological Considerations and the Vaccination against Poliomyelitis in Romania] *Vaccination and Epidemiology of Poliomyelitis and Allied Diseases, New Developments in the Programs of Vaccination, Virological and Serological Studies, Clinical Problems. VIIIth Symposium.*

67 M. V. Milovanovic, 'Poliomyelitis in Yugoslavia', *Vaccination and Epidemiology of Poliomyelitis and Allied Diseases, New Developments in the Programs of Vaccination, Virological and Serological Studies, Clinical Problems. VIIIth Symposium.*

68 J. Faragó, 'Mindannyiunk Felelőssége' [All of our Responsibility] *Népszabadság* (24 July 1959).

69 *Ibid.*

70 V. Kapos, 'Jelentés a Főváros Közegészségügyi Járványügyi Helyzetéről,' in *MSZMP Budapesti pártértekezletei 1957–1989* [Report of Budapest's Public Health and Epidemiological Situation, in the Budapest Party Meetings of the HSWP 1957–1989] (Budapest: Budapest Főváros Levéltára, 1966).

71 V. Škovránek, 'The Organization and Results of Mass Vaccination Against Poliomyelitis in CSSR', in J. Weissfeiler (ed.), *The Control of Poliomyelitis by Live Poliovirus Vaccine. Studies on Mass Vaccinations in Hungary, in the USSR, in Czechoslovakia and the German Democratic Republic. Papers Presented at the Hungarian-Soviet Medical Conference September 24–30, 1960.* (Budapest: Akadémiai Kiadó, 1961), p. 43.

72 J. Faragó, 'Mindannyiunk Felelőssége'.

73 S. Tóth, 'Gyermekbénulás Elleni Védőoltásokkal Kapcsolatos Felmerült Problémák', in *Egészségügyi Minisztérium Állami Közegészségügyi Felügyeleti és Járványvédeli Főosztály* [Problems in Vaccination Against Polio, in the Papers of the Health Ministry's Public Health and Epidemiological Division] (Debrecen: Magyar Országos Levéltár, 1957).

74 Contemporary sources point to several factors, including inefficient organisation and unrealistic expectations from the Salk vaccine's efficacy.

75 H. J. Seddon, 'Economic Aspects of the Management of Poliomyelitis', in *First International Poliomyelitis Conference* (New York: Lippincott, 1948), p. 35.

76 D. Horstmann, *Report on Live Poliovirus Vaccination in the Union of Soviet Socialist Republics, Poland and Czechoslovakia* (World Health Organization, 1959), p. 99.

77 G. J. Ebrahim, 'Polio Eradication, and After ...' *Revista Brasileira de Saúde Materno Infantil*, 2:2 (2002).

4

'A vaccine for the nation': South Korea's development of a hepatitis B vaccine and national prevention strategy focused on newborns

Eun Kyung Choi and Young-Gyung Paik

Introduction

When the scale of hepatitis B infection in South Korea came to light in the 1970s, the emerging public debate on the disease centred on the method of transmission. South Korean medical doctors focused on blocking the transmission routes and on campaigning for a hygienic lifestyle. In the end, public fear and arguments about hepatitis B meant the authorities had to produce a national prevention strategy. This national strategy proceeded in three phases that were closely related to the political developments and changes Korea was facing as a nation. First, a campaign against hepatitis B virus (HBV) transmission was initiated as a way to save the nation from the dishonour of being an underdeveloped country. Second, a domestic HBV vaccine was developed to forge a more independent path for modernisation, although with international assistance. Third, the first national prevention strategy using the vaccine was implemented. Later, in 1985, the vaccination programme was modified to focus on the vaccination of newborn babies, the future of the nation.

This chapter follows the construction of the national hepatitis B vaccination plan in the 1980s. For the implementation of this vaccination plan, the Korean government had to try not only to develop a less costly vaccine but also to justify its plan to the public and to overcome disagreements in the medical community. The first of these challenges was closely connected to international vaccine strategy, while the second one also drew on resources from outside Korea. This chapter shows how the idea of 'building the future health of the nation', even if it was actually an idea originated outside Korea, has exercised a major influence on the country's vaccination strategy. Moreover, throughout the implementation of the vaccination plan, as we will see, it was hardly a univocal one: there was deep confusion and disagreement among doctors, vaccine manufacturers, the mass media and the authorities. Yet, it should be noted that the final outcome was not entirely random; not so surprisingly, the national strategy pretty much coincided with a reflection of the nation's future-oriented, developmentalist imaginaries.

The 1950s: Korea becomes a favoured place to conduct hepatitis research

The symptoms of hepatitis, and its effects on the liver, have been known since ancient times. However, in the late nineteenth century, the possibility that this may not be a single disease began to be raised. In fact, most of the earlier descriptions were of what is now known as hepatitis A, or 'infectious hepatitis'.[1] By the 1940s, 'serum hepatitis' or hepatitis B began to be identified as a distinctive disease. It was later discovered that these two different types of hepatitis are actually caused by separate viruses. Infection by the hepatitis B virus might rapidly lead a person towards death, but it is also possible that the infected person would first develop cirrhosis or cancer of the liver. In the aftermath of the Second World War viral hepatitis attracted increasing research attention. An extensive hepatitis epidemic, which was noticed by US Army health officers, occurred among American troops stationed in Germany, but the transmission route of viral hepatitis was highly uncertain. It was not only in Germany that viral hepatitis was then found to be prevalent, however. It was found also to occur in China, the South Pacific region and around the Mediterranean. The high prevalence rate of hepatitis among American soldiers stationed abroad was understood as being mostly related to frequent contact with local civilians and the hepatitis epidemic among soldiers was regarded as reflecting local civilian hepatitis rates.[2]

The Korean War (1950–53) provided an opportunity for a large-scale survey of viral hepatitis. The US Army built a 'Hepatitis Center' at its military hospital in Kyoto (Japan), where it intensively treated and researched hepatitis among the US troops in East Asia. Nearly 1,000 US soldiers suffering from acute hepatitis received medical care in the centre. In addition, by the spring of 1951, a 'hepatitis team' had been organised by the army, established to study cases of viral hepatitis among military personnel. The accelerated epidemic, which reached 34,000 cases during the Korean War, led to this extensive hepatitis research by the US Army.[3]

This quote from Dr M. E. Conrad, Director of the Walter Reed Army Research Institute in Washington, DC, illustrates how Korea was seen as a vantage point for the US research on hepatitis.

> Korea was selected for the performance of this study because it is an Asian country where 50,000 US soldiers are assigned yearly for a 13-month tour of military duty, all soldiers arrive in Korea through a single airport, all patients with hepatitis are hospitalized at one of two military hospitals, peacetime operations provide a greater chance of success and the incidence of hepatitis was sufficient to permit perform-ance of the study within two or three years.[4]

The Korean medical elites were extremely cooperative towards US health officers, and, due to the Korean conscription system, large numbers of Korean males were available as research subjects. The US Army, in particular the 406th Medical General Laboratory, together with Korean doctors, carried out a large-scale Serum glutamic pyruvic transaminase test, a test which in the clinic is used to diagnose hepa-tocellular injury. Here 1,906 recruits at a training centre in Korea were tested. The thirty-two cases with abnormal results were taken to an army hospital and liver biopsies were performed on them. The hepatitis researches in the 1950s mostly focused on *anicteric hepatitis*, a relatively chronic form of hepatitis, seldom visibly showing the signs of jaundice.

In 1964, a US military programme was established to protect all military personnel stationed in Asia against hepatitis for the first time.[56] Under this programme all American military personnel in Asia were administered gamma globulin made from human plasma, which had been found to confer a degree of protection. The programme was based upon the results of hepatitis research in Korea. It confirmed ongoing research in Korea that gamma globulin could lower the hepatitis rate in an area where viral hepatitis was endemic.[7]

In 1964 Dr Baruch Blumberg, an American geneticist, found a strange protein in the blood of an Australian aborigine while analysing blood samples from around the world. This substance, which became known as the Australia antigen, proved to be a protein from the hepatitis B virus. This discovery made research into viral hepatitis much easier, since a simple blood test could now be used in place of an invasive liver biopsy. By using the blood of an asymptomatic layperson, serological diagnosis and epidemiological studies of hepatitis also became possible. With aid of the serological advance, prominent hepatitis researcher Dr Chung Young Kim could study epidemiology in Korea, where viral hepatitis was endemic. Although the validity of Dr Kim and other physicians' research could not be fully established at this point, the medical doctors started gaining the status of experts leading the nation's way into 'modernity'.

Although viral hepatitis was endemic in Korea, the term hepatitis was not widely known to the public and, in this sense, it was not a well-recognised disease among the general population. Therefore, Korean medical elite carried out various studies with an intention of raising awareness about hepatitis. Dr Chung Young Kim was a key figure in Korean hepatitis research at this time.

After finishing a residential course in internal medicine in 1964, he had trained as a research fellow at Harvard University Medical School and Boston City Hospital. He had researched the connection between the Australia antigen and viral hepatitis with the aid of grants from the National Institutes of Health, the Office of the Surgeon General, and the US Department of the Army.[8] After returning to Korea, he continued this work, in 1971 reaching the conclusion that 9 per cent of the blood in Korean blood banks was contaminated by the hepatitis virus.[9]

However, at the time this assertion did not attract much attention. The mass media in Korea paid more attention to his later work on the serum-hepatitis virus and on antibodies. In 1977, he developed a hepatitis B vaccine, which became known as 'Kim's vaccine', using serum from the blood of HBV-infected patients. Although he made use of clinical data, his research contained no data from experiments on primates.

Two years later, the hepatitis rate in Korea became a prominent issue. In 1979, Dr Kim and Dr Hong, his pupil, researched sero-epidemiological patterns of hepatitis B in Korea.[10] There had been some previous sero-epidemiological research into hepatitis B in Korea, but it had been limited to very specific populations, such as primary liver cancer patients (1972),[11] health care workers (1975),[12] and prostitutes (1979).[13] In addition, one researcher other than Kim had already demonstrated the prevalence rate of the hepatitis B antigen among the patients in a hospital in 1977. But unlike these earlier studies, the media expressed intensive interests in Kim's findings of '66% of Koreans being hepatitis B patients' and framed it as 'a dishonor of being an underdeveloped country with high rates of an epidemic disease'. In this way, hepatitis B turned into a test bed judging the extent of the nation's development.

Dr Kim's epidemiological results also came later than those from other Asian countries, including Singapore (1972)[14] and Thailand (1973).[15] Nor did he present data on the actual occurrence rate of hepatitis B revealed by follow-up research, limiting himself only to the prevalence of the hepatitis B antigen in blood samples. Nonetheless, his results showed that 66.3 per cent of patients had anti-HBc, which indicated previous infection. Dr Kim and Dr Hong publicly announced that '66% of Koreans have hepatitis B virus'. The mass media in Korea were shocked by this announcement.[16]

The 1970s: controversy over the transmission route emerges

In 1975 studies of 1,000 birth mothers in Taiwan showed that hepatitis B virus could be transmitted by the maternal-fetal route.[17] This work suggested that the maternal transmission of the hepatitis virus could be more prevalent in a hepatitis-endemic area than the transmission through sexual contacts or through the use of a contaminated needle. However, maternal transmission had not been proven in Korea and doctors were unwilling to assume that results from Taiwan could be extrapolated to South Korea. The first study of vertical transmission in Korea concluded that, 'Vertical transmission of HBsAg seems to be unimportant to the high prevalence of hepatitis in Korea.'[18] HBsAg, or the surface antigen of HBV, which can indicate current hepatitis B infection, was more prevalent in children than in infants in South Korea, which indicated that transmission of the hepatitis virus mostly occurred through daily social interactions within the family rather than at birth.

Dr Kim's study indicated not only the high prevalence of HBV but also the role of intrafamilial transmission. The sero-epidemiological study by Kim and Hong showed that the HBV prevalence rate was highest in the first year of life (which could be due either to intrafamilial transmission or to maternal-fetus transmission) but that there was also an increase in the prevalence rate after eight years. This might be due to the children's admission to elementary school. Scientists thought that the results pointed to the likelihood of transmission through everyday social life in the family or at school.[19]

Not all Korean doctors were convinced, though. Some did not even believe that maternal-fetus transmission and intrafamilial transmission were the main transmission routes, and there was substantial support for this view. For example, Dr I. M. Kim showed that there were many opportunities for infection outside the family.[20] Dr J. M. Lee found that only 30 per cent of newborns from HBsAg-positive mothers became HBV-positive, which did not correspond with the maternal-fetal transmission theory.[21] Dr J. H. Park also reported negative evidence for the maternal-fetal transmission theory and suggested the possibility of transmission in other ways, such as acupuncture.[22] For most scientists in Korea, the main cause of the hepatitis B epidemic needed further investigation, and daily life of cherishing 'pre-modern' collectivity more than 'modern' individuality in Korea seemed more suspect than the family. Although the theory of maternal-fetal transmission as the main cause of HBV transmission in endemic areas was widely accepted outside Korea, Korean doctors did not all agree with it. For example, Dr J. J. Koo said, 'There is a huge difference in the hepatitis carrier rate between ethnic groups and countries.'[23] With these research outcomes, the opinion of South Korean doctors was skewed toward the position that the South Korean situation could be different from the Taiwanese one.

While Korean people feared that the hepatitis virus could be transmitted at high rates through everyday activities, public panic focused particularly on transmission through indirect oral contact, especially through saliva. Most commentary in the media drew attention to the habit of sharing glasses in Korean drinking culture. Most social drinking in the workplaces or family gatherings tended to involve shared glasses, leaving individuals almost no choice. Then, after the emergence of the hepatitis B epidemic, public panic arose about the possibility of viral transmission through the sharing of glasses. Some scientists also demonstrated the risk of transmission in this way, through a simple clinical experiment featuring twenty subjects.[24] Since this ritual of sharing glasses was seen as symbolic of hierarchy in every organisation, some could find an excuse to resist abandoning this 'pre-modern' custom. Although some epidemiological studies later revealed that sharing glasses was not a major transmission route in Korea, the panic and suspicion did not diminish and the popular belief of sharing glasses as a major source of transmission has not completely disappeared even today. In some way, as the ordinary people had become more conscious about the individual hygiene, they tended to find the hierarchical and collectivist culture of sharing glasses even more uncomfortable and held it responsible for the persistence of hepatitis B.

The 1980s: the campaign for a hygienic lifestyle

A year after public awareness of the hepatitis B epidemic had arisen, the Korean Medical Association (KMA) initiated its own campaign against HBV transmission, alongside that of the public health authority. The KMA decided to prioritise the anti-hepatitis campaign among its major campaigns against major diseases in South Korea and established an anti-hepatitis task force team to take charge of it.[25] Professor J. M. Yang, at the school of public health, stated that 'physicians have only protected their own interests with treatment and have neglected the prevention of disease through lifestyle changes'.

When he emphasised that 'today we should adopt a more hygienic lifestyle and pursue public health education and enlightenment', it was to underscore the importance of lifestyle changes rather than the necessity of introducing vaccines and treatment. The KMA was the first to adopt and espouse the idea of the campaign and pursue it, which embarrassed the public health authority.[26] Japan also conducted a similar campaign during 1980s.[27]

The main goal of the KMA campaign was to promote a hygienic lifestyle and public awareness. The campaign mainly targeted behaviour such as hand washing and the use of disposable syringes. Dr Kim emphasised that hand washing was of the upmost importance in blocking transmission. The KMA also tried to ensure that physicians' material interests were protected in the campaign. For example, it sought to guarantee that doctors would be reimbursed for the costs of using disposable syringes. Moreover, it tried to shift blame from the medical practices at their own clinics to the 'unhygienic' ones at barbershops, acupuncture clinics or dental clinics.[28]

While the campaign underlined the high rates of hepatitis B among adults, it paid less attention to vertical transmission. However, some public health officials, such as Mr S. W. Shin, doubted the value of the campaign, arguing that 'the campaign is focusing upon washing hands, and not sharing glasses ... There was no campaign about vertical transmission.'[29] On the other hand, Dr J. D. Lew, who headed the anti-hepatitis task force of the KMA, responded by stating, 'I did not know that vertical transmission was that much important.'[30] The physicians in the KMA neglected maternal-fetal transmission at first.

Initially, the government limited its intervention only to supporting the KMA campaign. However, soon after, in preparation for the 1988 Olympic Games, which would bring thousands of visitors to Seoul, the government decided to establish a comprehensive anti-hepatitis policy focusing on hygiene issues. Major actions taken by the government included the mandatory use of disposable syringes, sterilisation of medical instruments and public campaign to raise awareness about the importance of maintaining the hygiene of razors and dishes. The introduction of a hepatitis vaccine and the proclamation of hepatitis as a legally designated infectious disease were also discussed, though inconclusively.[31] The campaign by the government and the KMA was criticised for the lack of supporting evidence, such as epidemiological data. Later, some epidemiological results even contradicted the premises of the campaign.[32] Some epidemiologists openly denounced the assumption that an HBV-antigen-positive rate was indicative of the prevalence of the disease, which underlay the government and the KMA's measures. Instead, these epidemiologists insisted on the necessity of researching infection history; otherwise, the size of the epidemic would be overestimated. Nonetheless, the lifestyle-focused campaign prevailed until the full-scale vaccination campaign was introduced. From this point, the focus shifted from overcoming backwardness to becoming an advanced country.

Developing inexpensive vaccine: influences from international agencies

The hepatitis-prevention policy in Korea had originally emphasised behavioural change; however, the policy began to change, albeit slowly, with the possibility of developing a vaccine and in response to pressure from the World Health Organization (WHO) and overseas specialists. It is notable that, for various reasons, the health professionals in international agencies identified South Korea as a suitable country to produce inexpensive vaccine products.

At this point, most vaccine products including hepatitis B vaccine in South Korea had been imported. As of 1983, two Korean pharmaceutical companies, Joong Wae Pharmaceutical and Dong-A Pharmaceutical, were in charge of importing foreign vaccines. Yet, the cost of vaccination was around $140 per person, which made it virtually unavailable for the large proportion of the public.[33] The sheer estimated cost of imported vaccines deterred the Korean government from purchasing the products at their current price as well as from implementing the vaccination programme for the public.

Under these circumstances, some medical professionals in Korea began to turn their attention to developing vaccines using the 'Korean' technology, which would also provide an opportunity to demonstrate their expertise. The Korean Green Cross, whose specialty was a blood fractionation technology, started developing a vaccine (later named Hepabox) with the aid of Dr Jong Young Kim. A primate experiment was said to be the chief obstacle to developing a vaccine by Green Cross, because it was not possible in Korea.[34] For this reason, Green Cross contracted an American company and the Kitasato Institute of Japan to conduct tests. Finally, in 1983, after studies in the USA were completed, Hepabox received approval for sale.[35]

Meanwhile, foreign hepatitis experts started developing interests in finding a company that could produce a vaccine on a large scale on their behalf. A company based in South Korea would be a suitable candidate for their purposes because the country had a high rate of hepatitis and a large number of subjects as well as several vaccine companies, such as Green cross, Cheil Sugar and LG Industry, competing for sales. In the early 1980s Dr Alfred Prince of the New York Blood Center, who was famous for having discovered the importance of HBsAg, worked with Cheil Sugar to develop vaccines using his own technology, a heat-process method.[36] Having a humanitarian interest in supplying a low-priced vaccine to the Third World, he developed the Cheil vaccine, which was evaluated in 1985 by the Catholic University in Korea, a WHO-authorised research centre.[37] It could be made in a highly pure form and in high volume in compliance with WHO standards.[38]

At the early stage of development, the Korean government guaranteed the profitability of the domestic hepatitis vaccine technology to the companies. When Green Cross developed Hepabox, the government ordered the protection of its copyright for five years under the New Medicine Protection Rule. In addition, the government approved the Cheil vaccine for export.[39] An official of the Ministry of Health said, 'It is helpful to public health for a big company such as Cheil Sugar (with Samsung) to produce vaccines at low cost.' The Cheil vaccine was principally intended for foreign markets, such as those of Southeast Asia, rather than the domestic market. The mass export of the Cheil vaccine met the WHO's need for a cheap hepatitis vaccine across Asia. After Cheil Sugar began to market HepaxinB in Southeast Asia, Green Cross began to sell Hepabox in Indonesia.[40] Following Cheil's success in developing a second-generation vaccine, the price of the vaccine fell sharply.

Despite intense competition among Korean vaccine companies, they shared a common interest in mass sales and vaccination. They sought ways to sell their vaccines on the global markets as well as on the domestic one. At first they thought that, rather than vaccinating several high-risk groups of adults, vaccinating all newborns could be a much more efficient approach. They constantly held lectures and symposia, and invited foreign scholars to promote a newborn-vaccination policy.[41]

Their interest coincided with the WHO's strategy of a newborn-vaccination policy in order to control more effectively; the Organization had emphasised the need to vaccinate newborns from the early stages of the campaign. Since 1983 WHO had focused on hepatitis prevention, with later studies showing the relationship between hepatitis B and primary liver cancer.

The WHO's hepatitis-prevention strategy recommended vaccination of all newborns in high endemic areas and vaccination of high-risk groups in low endemic areas.[42] The WHO regarded the HBV as a 'carcinogen next to smoking'.[43] In the view of the WHO, the Asia-Pacific region, including Korea, was a strategically important one among WHO regions for its goal to develop a vaccine and a prevention strategy. The programme in the Asia-Pacific region proposed to dramatically control the disease both by lowering the cost of vaccine by mass production and by vaccinating all newborns.[44] Korea had been a key country in the WHO's strategy, and could hardly be left out.

Modifying the path and targeting the 'Future Generation'

After the development of a domestic vaccine, the Korean government quickly implemented a national hepatitis B prevention strategy in late 1983.[45] The plan was accelerated by the forthcoming Olympic Games, which made the Korean government eager to decrease the hepatitis rate. It was a five-year plan with its main goal of vaccinating 40 per cent of the entire Korean population. Groups frequently interacting with the public, such as officials and teachers, were to be targeted first, with a low-cost vaccine. Prostitutes, industrial employees and infants below the age of 6 were to be the next target group. The free vaccination of newborns from HBV-positive parents was to be achieved after 1985. In addition, every official institution was to conduct a hepatitis test on new staff prior to employment. The programme was clearly intended to decrease the prevalence rate quickly, mainly targeting adults who worked with the public.

As soon as this policy was implemented, it attracted harsh criticism, both from Korean scientists abroad and from the WHO. WHO specialist Dr J. E. Maynard, who visited Korea in 1985, pointed out that the WHO's hepatitis policy was about public promotion, mass vaccination, hepatitis tests upon birth mothers, and mandatory newborn vaccination. He reminded his audience that Korea was among those countries with a large number of carriers, which the WHO recommended should vaccinate all newborns. He dismissed concerns that had arisen in Korea about the dangers of the vaccine, saying that, 'The hepatitis vaccine is generally perfectly safe.'[46] He also urged the Korean government to withdraw its protection of the Green Cross vaccine patent in favour of the Cheil vaccine.[47]

The pressure from the WHO not only induced the mass production of the vaccine in Korea but also led to a change in hepatitis policy. Reversing the approach adopted by Korean doctors until that point, the decision was taken to vaccinate all newborns. Most Korean doctors had preferred behavioural control and adult-inclusive vaccination at individual clinics after a serological test, and they distrusted mass vaccination without prior testing. Some physicians were annoyed when nurses inoculated students with the hepatitis vaccine in schools, following the introduction of mass vaccination in schools by Seoul's education council. The doctors insisted that 'Mass vaccination should be avoided because hepatitis vaccination needs an immunisation test and medical examination.[48] They objected to mass vaccination because it meant unskilled personnel would administer the vaccine. Korean doctors continued to distrust mass vaccination thereafter; on one occasion, they reported a nursing school hospital to the KMA ethics committee for vaccinating at a reduced price.[49]

Korean doctors overseas also criticised the South Korean government's hepatitis-prevention policy. They insisted that universal newborn vaccination was the most effective approach for future generations and condemned the adult vaccination policy as a waste of money. Dr Jae-Ha Kim, the head of the committee of Korean scientists resident in Japan, was a key opponent of the national policy. In his article 'Modifying the Path', published in 1985, he asserted that: 'The program neglects infants below the age of three and promotes unnecessary mass vaccination upon adults.' He also said, 'Prevention of transmission from the carrier population should be altered by the non-creation of a carrier population.'[50] He submitted his opinion letter to the government in late 1984.

In a 1985 paper, Dr J. H. Kim showed the importance of changing the target of the policy (see figure 4.1). If hepatitis B patients are assigned to group A, hepatitis carriers to group B, and non-infected people to group C, the government's five-year plan would only benefit the people in group C and would have no effect on group A. He argued that the non-creation of antibody among new members in groups A and B was critical, and that this could best be done by targeting the vertical transmission responsible for 30 per cent of the transmission route. In his theory, horizontal transmission, which accounted for 70 per cent of transmission, could be reduced by an increased level of education and hygiene habits. For the future health of Korea, rather than focusing on the health of group C (the non-infected), it was important that in the next generation there should be no new members of groups A and B. In his account, only the problem of vertical (maternal-fetal) transmission would remain, and targeting vertical transmission would be the only efficient way of reducing the HBV-positive population.

Dr J. H. Kim's argument gained attention before the causes of hepatitis B transmission in Korea had been clearly ascertained. He believed that even if vertical transmission was not the chief cause in Korea, newborn vaccination was the most effective way of improving the

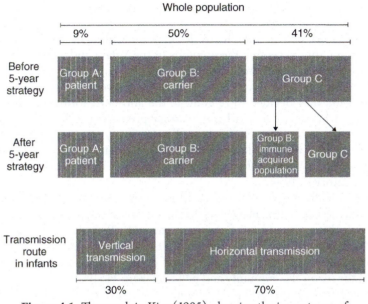

Figure 4.1 The graph in Kim (1985), showing the importance of changing the target population.

health of the country, saying, 'In adulthood, viral infection will just be transient, whereas in childhood it produces permanent carriers.'[51]

Dr J. H. Kim offered a similar view to the KMA's newspaper in 1985. According to him, current policy would require additional purchase of foreign vaccines, which would cost an extra trillion won ($100 million). Consequently, the vaccination of infants below the age of 3 was more practical and efficient.[52] Dr Whan Gook Chung disputed his opinion, pointing out that adults are infected with hepatitis, too, and that testing all birth mothers for HBeAg, the extracellular form of HBcAg, would be too expensive. He also criticised the vaccine industry for its greed.

Dr W. G. Chung's objections exemplified the attitude of Korean physicians to vaccination. They were wary of vaccinating all newborns without prior testing. In their view, it was better to vaccinate high-risk adult groups first and only then to extend the vaccination programme. Physicians accused the government and mothers mainly for ignoring hepatitis testing during pregnancy.[53] They expressed distrust of the vaccination-centred hepatitis-prevention programme, disagreeing with the vaccine industry.[54]

In December 1985 the KMA decided to recommend newborn vaccination, thus accepting the opinions of the WHO and foreign scientists. They formally agreed that total newborn vaccination was a more safe and effective approach for the future. However, along with this decision, they decided to re-evaluate the anti-body formation rate of the newborn vaccination before further promoting it.[55] In fact, total newborn vaccination was achieved only slowly: the recommended infant vaccination guidelines from the Korean paediatrics society first included HBV vaccination in 1991, and the government only made it mandatory in 1994.

Gradually, hepatitis B ceased to be regarded as an 'adult disease'. Public opinion also changed in that infant care came to be regarded as having been a significant factor in the hepatitis B epidemic, and hepatitis B infection as mainly due to mothers. Placing the responsibility for transmitting hepatitis B on the back of mothers had many advantages for the medical community and policy makers. Firstly, it seemed easier to isolate the target group. Also, mothers were a very compliant group, ready to do anything for the sake of their babies. Most of all, the prevention campaign gained a momentum as now it was framed as a scheme to save the nation's future. From this point, Korean society became silent about the risk of transmission among adults. Newborn vaccinations in paediatric clinics and health centres proceeded quietly. Meanwhile, public concerns have surfaced that the HBV vaccine is not effective enough to provide protection over a sufficiently long period, and that revaccination would be required. Some Korean epidemiologists are also concerned about the decline of immunity with time, the absence of a prevention programme, and the lack of a re-vaccination programme in schools.[56]

Conclusion

After the Korean War, Korea was classified as a hepatitis-endemic area. Because of the war, it became a favourable location to research hepatitis B, which was an important research subject at that time. The US Army and Korean medical elite jointly researched viral hepatitis in Korea, producing the latest information about hepatitis for the army and providing Korean doctors with appropriate hepatitis-related research skills. However, for a long time, this active hepatitis research environment paid attention to the occurrence of hepatitis in clinical settings but not so much to hepatitis epidemiology in Korea. For example, Dr C. Y. Kim, who pioneered hepatitis research in Korea, made a hepatitis B vaccine prior to understanding the epidemiology of the disease in Korea. Public attention also tended to concentrate only on the technology, and not on the epidemiological model.

However, after the public announcement of an epidemic, in the 1980s public concerns arose about the transmission of hepatitis B. In particular, the habit of sharing drinking glasses was regarded as a problem, a symbol of backwardness, and Korea's culture of collectivist eating and hierarchical social drinking was heavily criticised. Although it is hard to prove these concerns scientifically, they did not subside for a long time. Meanwhile, researchers disagreed about the principal transmission route – whether maternal, intrafamilial, or socio-cultural. Maternal-fetal transmission had been proven to be the main transmission route in other high endemic areas like Taiwan, but had not been demonstrated in Korea. Korean doctors initiated a public anti-hepatitis campaign focusing on the promotion of a hygienic lifestyle. At least at first, it was a good opportunity to establish medical practitioners' hegemony in the public health field.

Korean doctors were eager to develop a domestic anti-hepatitis vaccine using their own technology, but the development of a vaccine in Korea was subordinated to the international vaccine strategy of promoting a cheap and safe vaccine. The Green Cross, and Cheil, vaccines were developed under these conditions, ensuring competition in the market. Prominent foreign scholars connected with the WHO were deeply involved in their development.

In 1985, the Korean government initiated five-year strategy against hepatitis B, targeting the adult population in preparation for the 1988 Olympics. The goal of this approach was clearly to reduce the prevalence of hepatitis among the working population. However, harsh criticism occurred just after the implementation of the national plan, not from inside the country, but from abroad. The WHO and foreign scholars persistently emphasised newborn vaccination. In WHO's view, Korea was an outpost of a worldwide vaccination plan. Therefore, a massive newborn hepatitis vaccination plan had to be introduced and established in Korea. On the other hand, Dr J. H. Kim, a Korean doctor residing in Japan, urged a change in strategy, arguing that total newborn vaccination would be the most efficient option for the '조국의 미래' (future of Korea). His argument rested on the prioritising the future of the nation and, thus, the future generation, rather than the working population in the present. The role of the current generation was to develop economy and vaccines for the bright future of the nation.

To begin with, Korean doctors had focused on changes to what were seen as unhygienic social practices rather than vaccination. As the vaccination strategy became increasingly significant, their position conflicted with that of the vaccine industry. Whatever physicians may have thought, newborn vaccination was justified in terms of promoting the nation's health and in the interest of future generations. In this sense, when an anti-hepatitis plan was finally introduced in South Korea, it was not just a reaction to the prevalent hepatitis B but also a reflection of the nation's future-oriented, developmentalist imaginaries.

Notes

1 W. Muraskin, 'The Silent Epidemic. The Social, Ethical, and Medical Problems Surrounding the Fight Against Hepatitis B', *Journal of Social History*, 22 (1988), pp. 277–98.

2 J. R. Paul, 'Endemic Hepatitis Among US Troops in Post-War Germany', *Proceedings of the Royal Society of Medicine*, 43:6 (June 1950), pp. 438–40.

3 T. C. Chalmers, R. D. Eckhardt, W. E. Reynolds *et al.*, 'The Treatment of Acute Infectious Hepatitis: Controlled Studies of the Effects of Diet, Rest, and Physical Reconditioning on the Acute Course of the Disease and on the Incidence of Relapses and Residual Abnormalities', *Journal of Clinical Investigation*, 34:7, Pt 2 (1955), p. 1163.

4 M. E. Conrad, 'Endemic Viral Hepatitis in US Soldiers: Causative Factors and the Effect of Prophylactic Gamma Globulin', *Canadian Medical Association Journal*, 106:Special Issue (1972), p. 456.

5 W. K. Chung, S. K. Moon, R. K. Gershon, A. M. Prince, Y. C. Park and Y. S. Cho, 'Anicteric Hepatitis in Korea: I. Clinical and Laboratory Studies', *Archives of Internal Medicine*, 113:4 (1964), pp. 526–34.

6 A. M. Prince, F. Hiroshi and R. K. Gershon, 'Immunohistochemical Studies on the Etiology of Anicteric Hepatitis in Korea', *American Journal of Epidemiology*, 79:3 (1964), pp. 365–81.

7 M. E. Conrad, A. L. Ginsberg, M. E. Conrad *et al.*, 'Prevention of Endemic HAA-Positive Hepatitis with Gamma Globulin: Use of a Simple Radioimmune Assay to Detect HAA', *New England Journal of Medicine*, 286:11 (1972), pp. 562–6; S. Krugman, 'Viral Hepatitis: Overview and Historical Perspectives', *The Yale Journal of Biology and Medicine*, 49:3 (1976), pp. 199–203.

8 R. Kater, C. Y. Kim and C. S. Davidson, 'Australia Antigen and Viral Hepatitis', *Journal of Infectious Diseases*, 120:3 (1969), pp. 391–92; C. Y. Kim and D. M. Bissell, 'Stability of the Lipid and Protein of Hepatitis-Associated (Australia) Antigen', *Journal of Infectious Diseases*, 123:5 (1971), pp. 470–6.

9 C. Y. Kim *et al.*, 'HAA Expression Rate in Korean – Especially in Whole Blood Donor, Village and Medical Practitioners. The 23rd Korean Association of Internal Medicine Symposium (15 October 1971); "9% of Blood Donors Have Hepatitis Virus"', *Maeil Business Newspaper*, 5:8 (1972).

10 W. S. Hong and C. Y. Kim, 'Seroepidemiology of Type A and Type B Hepatitis in Seoul Area', *Korean Journal of Medicine*, 25:1 (1982), pp. 19–26.

11 C. Y. Kim, 'Occurrence of HBsAg in Korean populations and medical personnels', *Korean Journal of Medicine*, 18:9 (1975), pp. 705–10.

12 K. Y. Yoon, *et al.*, 'The Observation about Occurrence Rate of HBs Antigen to Waitress Entertaining at Restaurant Business', *Korean Journal of Environmental Health Sciences*, 6:1 (1979), pp. 47–52.

13 H. H. Kwon and D. J. Suh, 'The Changing Pattern of Occurrence of HBsAg in Korean Patients During a Period of 5 Years', *Korean Journal of Medicine*, 5:20 (1977), pp. 423–38.

14 E. H. Yap, Y. W. Ong, M. J. Simons, K. Okochi and M. Mayumi, 'Australia Antigen in Singapore. II. Differential Frequency in Chinese, Malays and Indians', *Vox Sanguinis*, 22:4 (1972), pp. 371–5.

15 S. Punyagupta, L. C. Olson, U. Harinasuta *et al.*, The Epidemiology of Hepatitis B Antigen in a High Prevalence Area', *American Journal of Epidemiology*, 97:5 (1973), pp. 349–54.

16 '66% of Korean People are Hepatitis B Patients', *Dong-A Ilbo* (15 October 1979).

17 C. E. Stevens, R. P. Beasley, J. Tsui and W. C. Lee, 'Vertical Transmission of Hepatitis B Antigen in Taiwan', *New England Journal of Medicine*, 292:15 (1975), pp. 771–4.

18 D. K. Chung, H. S. Sun and H. K. Chung, 'General Presentation: Vertical Transmission of Hepatitis B', *The Korean Journal of Gastroenterology*, 6:1 (1974), pp. 93–4.

19 'The research by Dr Kim and his colleagues in SNU hospital: Hepatitis B is transmitted by mother', *Kyunghyang Shinmoon* (9 October 1980).
20 I. M. Kim and J. J. Lee, 'Intrafamiliar Spread of Hepatitis B Virus Infection', *Korean Journal of Medicine*, 25:11 (1982), pp. 1191–8.
21 J. M. Lee, H. S. Kim, Y. Oh *et al.*, 'General Presentation: Hepatitis in Pregnant Women and Newborn Infection', *The Korean Society of Obstetrics and Gynecology Symposium*, 51 (1983), pp. 55–6.
22 J. H. Park, S. D. Yoon, C. Y. Kim and S. K. Lee, 'The Effect of Maternal HBs Antigenemia on Neonatal Health', *Korean Journal of Preventive Medicine*, 17:1 (1984), pp. 47–55.
23 J. J. Koo, D. H. Hwang, W. J. Kim and Y. M. Kim, 'Status of Vertical Transmission of HBs Antigen and HBs Antibody in Korean Term Pregnant Women', *Korean Journal of Obstetrics & Gynecology*, 27:2 (1984), pp. 168–74.
24 'Don't Share Glasses in Drinking: Research Team in Kyungpook Medical School Identified Infection Through Saliva and Mouth with Experiment', *Dong-A Ilbo* (2 February 1982).
25 'Anti-Hepatitis Public Campaign will Start', *Ui-Hyub Shinbo* (5 October 1981).
26 'How to do Public Health Campaign', *Ui-Hyub Shinbo* (16 November 1981).
27 'Anti-Hepatitis Public Campaign will Start'.
28 'Medical Society Supports Anti-Hepatitis Public Campaign', *Ui-Hyub Shinbo* (19 October 1981).
29 'Discussion After the 2nd Anti-Hepatitis Campaign', *Maeil Business Newspaper* (30 July 1983).
30 *Ibid.*
31 'KMA's Anti-Hepatitis Campaign will be Expanded to the Campaign by Authorities', *Ui-Hyub Shinbo* (19 August 1982).
32 'Sharing Acupuncture and Toothbrush is the Chief Cause of Hepatitis Transmission', *Ui-Hyub Shinbo* (23 June 1983).
33 'Ministry of Health and Society Approves Anti-Hepatitis Vaccine', *Maeil Business Newspaper* (13 July 1982).
34 'Green Cross Succeeded in Developing Anti-Hepatitis Vaccine: Approval is Uncertain', *Ui-Hyub Shinbo* (16 November 1981).
35 'Domestic Anti-Hepatitis Vaccine will be in Market from September', *Dong-A Ilbo* (26 August 1983).
36 W. A. Muraskin, *The War Against Hepatitis B: A History of the International Task Force on Hepatitis B Immunization* (Philadelphia: University of Pennsylvania Press, 1995), pp. 22–4.
37 *Ui-Hyub Shinbo* (*The KMA News*, 19 August 1985).

38 'Live at International Symposium of Cancer and Hepatitis B', *Maeil Business Newspaper* (23 October 1984).

39 'Large Amounts of Domestic Hepatitis Vaccines will be Exported to South East Asia', *Dong-A Ilbo* (9 May 1986).

40 *Ibid.*

41 'Dong-A Pharmaceutical Held a Lecture About Viral Hepatitis', *Ui-Hyub Shinbo* (5 November 1982).

42 A WHO Meeting, 'Prevention of Hepatocellular Carcinoma by Immunization', *Bulletin World Health Organization*, 61:5 (1983), pp. 731–44.

43 J. E. Maynard, 'World-Wide Control of Hepatitis B', *International Journal of Epidemiology*, 13:4 (1984), p. 406; WHO, *WHO Technical Report Series, No. 691* (Geneva: WHO, 1983).

44 WHO, *WHO Second Technical Advisory Group Final Report* (Geneva: WHO, 1985); WHO, *WHO Expert Committee on Biological Standardization: Thirty-first report. Annex 4. Requirements for Hepatitis B* (Geneva: WHO, 1983).

45 '40% of all People will take Vaccine', *Maeil Business Newspaper* (2 December 1983).

46 *Ui-Hyub Shinbo* (2 September 1985).

47 Muraskin, *The War Against Hepatitis B*, p. 30.

48 'Urging Mass Inoculation of Anti-Hepatitis Vaccine', *Kyunghyang Shinmoon* (20 May 1986).

49 'Quarrel on a Low Cost of Anti-Hepatitis Vaccination', *The Hankyoreh* (27 July 1988).

50 J. H. Kim, 'Modifying the Path of Anti-Hepatitis Policy', *Science & Technology*, 18:12 (1985), pp. 61–6.

51 'Nonselective Mass Vaccination is Ineffective and Unsafe', *Dong-A Ilbo* (17 April 1985).

52 'Reader Contribution', *Ui-Hyub Shinbo* (20 June 1985).

53 H. K. Suh, 'Hepatitis B Carrier and Prevention Methods', *Secondary U-ri Education*, 11 (1990), pp. 511–12.

54 'Responding to Dr Kim's Opinion', *Ui-Hyub Shinbo* (4 July 1985).

55 *Ui-Hyub Shinbo* (16 December 1985).

56 M. R. Ki, M. H. Kim, H. K. In and J. K. Oh, *Seroepidemiology on Hepatitis B Virus in Elementary School Students Cohort in Kyonggi Province* (Seoul: National Science Foundation, 2003).

II

Nationality, vaccine production and the end of sovereign manufacture

5

Vaccine production, national security anxieties and the unstable state in nineteenth- and twentieth-century Mexico

Ana María Carrillo

Introduction

Since pre-Columbian times, Mexico has experienced notable periods of progress in science and technology. Political, economic and social problems have, however, often interrupted these developments, thus the country has been forced to rebuild its science and technology capacity time and time again. Since 1821, when the country began its independent life, Mexican government investment in education and research has been essential for modern science to flourish. In its search for self-determination, the Mexican state has employed science both to legitimise itself and to serve society.

This chapter deals with the development and production of vaccines in Mexico from the last third of the nineteenth century to 1989, when the erosion of this sector began. Along with discussing Mexican physicians' reception of discoveries in microbiology and immunology, it highlights the existence of a network of relationships between Mexican institutions and others around the world. The chapter shows that vaccine development and production did not follow a constant ascendant path, but that it also suffered declines and regressions. It describes the field's achievements and limitations and reveals its relationships with the political, economic and social conditions of the country in different historical moments. Finally, the chapter evaluates the importance of attaining national self-sufficiency in vaccine development and production for the building of the state in pre- and post-revolutionary Mexico, and seeks to provide some answers to the questions of how and why the erosion of this strategic field occurred.

For three centuries (1521–1821) Mexico – then, New Spain – was part of the Spanish Empire. In New Spain, the arrival of modern science late in the colonial period was mediated both by the existence of a self-taught community of enlightened individuals interested in progressing towards applied science, and the imperialist economic reform of the Spanish state in the eighteenth century, which created institutions in order to offer scientific instruction, improve economic exploitation and better local conditions.[1]

It was in this context that vaccination against smallpox was officially introduced to New Spain in 1804 by the Spanish Royal Philanthropic Expedition – supported by King Charles IV of Spain and led by Francisco Javier de Balmis – though the vaccine had in fact arrived earlier.[2] That year, officials established the first vaccination centre in Mexico City; according to Miguel E. Bustamante – epidemiologist and historian – this signalled the beginning of governmental action in the area of preventive medicine.[3]

The War of Independence (1810–21) affected all national institutions, and medical practice was no exception. After 1821, the formation of the modern state began, which included attempts to control economic processes and create a strong political system. Mexican independent governments considered science a matter of public interest, and utilised it to build a national culture in a context of the increasing secularisation of society.[4]

In the case of smallpox, for example, for more than a hundred years only five people managed the vaccine in Mexico, so that its purity was guaranteed.[5] Public health officials administered the vaccine in areas as remote as Texas[6] – which was part of Mexican territory until 1836 – but service was not always continuous because between 1810 and 1876 the country suffered constant political instability.

In addition to the War of Independence, Mexico underwent two French interventions (1838–39 and 1862–67), the Mexican–America War – which began in 1846 and ended two years later, culminating in Mexico's loss of more than half of its territory to the United States – as well as indigenous groups' insurrections and struggles between liberals and conservatives. For all these reasons, in this period at least fifty smallpox epidemics occurred in the country.[7]

The beginning of vaccine production

A relative pacification of the country arrived with the authoritarian regime of Porfirio Díaz (1876–1910), one marked by the modernisation of society and the economy and by a growing concentration of federal political power. Strong central government brought improvements in mining, industry and also public health. Vaccination laws were part of this health policy, and by the end of the Díaz regime smallpox vaccination was mandatory in most states in the Mexican republic.[8] But, as Stern and Markel have stated, 'vaccines are powerful medical interventions that induce powerful biological, social and cultural reactions', including insurrections.[9] While Mexico does not appear to have experienced any medical movements opposed to smallpox vaccination, a century after its introduction there was still public opposition. Perhaps the most significant case was in the state of Oaxaca, where compulsory vaccination was established in 1903, but five years later a popular rebellion achieved its cancellation.[10]

Vaccination in this period was not limited to the prevention of smallpox. Several nineteenth-century Mexican physicians were in direct contact with international scientists, and through them the introduction of bacteriological thinking and practices took place in Mexico in the late nineteenth and early twentieth centuries. Eduardo Liceaga – president of the Superior Board of Health – visited the Pasteur Institute in France in 1888, was given personal instruction, and learned to prepare the rabies vaccine. Early that year, he inoculated a Mexican boy[11] and established the Anti-Rabies Preventive Inoculation Service, as a branch of the Superior Board of Health.[12] From 1888 to 1910, the board administered 11,177 inoculations – with only thirteen deaths recorded among the recipients.[13] By 1909, five states of the Mexican republic had created anti-rabies centres.

In 1895, the Pathological Anatomy Museum was founded. Upon applying for its creation, Rafael Lavista, its first director, assured President Díaz that as well as demonstrating to visitors to the Second Pan-American Medical Congress (to be held in Mexico two years later) that science was being cultivated in the country, it was also required for the study of the symptoms manifested by diseases modified by climate, elevation and other characteristics peculiar to Mexico. Almost from the beginning, the museum had a bacteriology section, which continued working after 1899 when the Pathological Anatomy Museum was transformed into the National Pathology Institute.[14]

At the end of 1902, a plague epidemic affected some ports and cities in northwest Mexico. The sanitary campaign organised by the Superior Board of Health to combat the outbreak was a watershed moment, signalling the beginning of modern public health in Mexico.

This was the first sanitary campaign in the country in which a state government ceded public health authority to the federal government, and also the first to be based on the emerging scientific fields of microbiology, immunology, tropical medicine and epidemiology. The sanitary bureaucracy sought to control the outbreak through persuasive methods, but relied mostly on coercion, including a mandatory vaccine policy that generated various forms of popular resistance.[15] M. J. Rosenau, Head of the Hygiene Laboratory of the Marine Hospital Service of the United States, sent two cultures of *Bacillus pestis* to Mexico free of charge,[16] and the Bacteriology Section of the National Pathology Institute produced and certified doses of the Haffkine and Besredka vaccines, the latter of which underwent its first extensive testing in Mexico (the Haffkine vaccine was first tested in India).[17] The institute also prepared sera for curative purposes, and exported some doses of the Besredka vaccine to Chile and El Salvador.

The Bacteriology Section played such an important role in the sanitary campaign against plague that, along with the Medical Chemistry Section, it was separated from the Pathology Institute in 1905 to create the National Bacteriology Institute. The new institute was made up of sections for bacteriology, serum preparation, biological chemistry and veterinary medicine.[18] As similar institutes around the world, it combined research with biological production. In addition to plague vaccines, the institute produced tetanus, diphtheria, dysentery, gangrene and pneumococcus sera, and supplied these to public health authorities.[19] Early in the twentieth century, the Superior Board of Health, with the support of the National Bacteriology Institute, established bacteriology stations in some ports, in order to diagnose cases of plague and cholera and vaccinate against both illnesses; in the case of cholera, with Jaume Ferran's vaccine.[20] Smallpox and rabies vaccines were excluded from the Bacteriology Institute's responsibilities, as the Superior Board of Health produced them itself.

In 1900, life expectancy in Mexico was only 25 years, and infant mortality was 288 per 1,000 live births. Smallpox, measles, pertussis (whooping cough) and diphtheria were common among children, and the two leading causes of death were diarrhoeal and respiratory diseases, preceded almost always by malnutrition.[21] At the time, some countries, particularly the United States, threatened Mexico with exclusionary quarantines due to its infectious disease burden, and pushed it – along with other countries – to adopt hygienic measures in its ports and in other areas strategic for international trade. In order to protect commercial activities, the Mexican Superior Board of Health actively fought plague outbreaks when they arrived at the country's ports, and prioritised the campaign against yellow fever.[22] However, they also organised campaigns against malaria, tuberculosis and syphilis, which were endemic in Mexico.

At the time, specialisation in bacteriology was, generally speaking, only available in some foreign laboratories, though some individuals were trained in Mexico under the direction of a bacteriologist, Mexican or otherwise. Much depended on the individual training of young Mexican scientists or on the interest of foreign bacteriologists on conditions in Mexico; as a result no country dominated and French, German and American influences flowed into Mexico by singular routes. French influence was strong, both because of the fact that several French scientists were working in Mexico, but also more commonly because Mexican physicians had received training there.

The first head of the National Bacteriology Institute and the pioneer of microbiology in Mexico, Ángel Gaviño, had been trained by Roux and Duclaux at the Pasteur Institute,[23] while Joseph Girard, a French bacteriologist who interned at the Pasteur Institute, worked from 1906 to 1913 as the assistant director of the Laboratory of the National Bacteriology Institute in Mexico.[24] But that period also saw a great diversification of influences. Manuel Toussaint – who was for a time in charge of both histological and bacteriological work at the Pathological Anatomy Museum, and would later serve as the head of the National Pathology Institute – studied for several years in Germany.[25] Most of Gaviño's scientific training had also taken place in Germany, and he went to the United States and Canada several times to attend American Public Health Association meetings. Octaviano González Fabela – bacteriologist of the Superior Board of Health – took courses at the universities of Harvard and Pennsylvania, and during the revolutionary years he studied in Bern, Switzerland.[26] A US scientist, Howard Taylor Ricketts – professor at the universities of Pennsylvania and Chicago – died in Mexico while conducting research on typhus at the National Bacteriology Institute with his colleague Russell M. Wilder.[27] Despite all these international influences, the National Bacteriology Institute and all Mexican scientific institutions were financially and therefore also scientifically, independent of any foreign country.

The revolution and the beginnings of national reconstruction

The research and public health programme active at the beginning of the twentieth century was abruptly interrupted by the revolution that broke out in Mexico in 1910, as peasants throughout the country rose up against poor living conditions and the lack of local democracy. The civil war lasted a decade, during which most sanitary campaigns were abandoned and many scientific institutions, among them the National Pathology Institute, were forced to close. The revolutionary governments that ruled during this time not only ceased to support basic medical sciences, but actively opposed to them and favoured applied science.[28]

The National Bacteriology Institute survived for a few more years, but in 1913 it too suspended all original research and one year later interrupted its production of sera and vaccines. In 1913 and 1914, Gaviño reported on several occasions that budget constraints and the lack of test animals had made further research on typhus and diphtheria impossible. In 1914, he was fired from his position as director of the Institute. This matter involved both jealousy between colleagues and political conflict, because Gaviño had collaborated with the government of Victoriano Huerta, who had risen to power after a coup d'état against the revolutionary government of Madero. After Huerta was defeated, Gaviño was sacked by the new revolutionary government when González-Fabela stated – after a one-hour visit to the Institute – that he distrusted domestic sera. At the time, Gaviño warned the minister of Government of the danger of eliminating the stock of national sera, including the significant holdings stored at the National Bacteriology Institute, and argued that the country needed them – especially during a period when Europe was at war and sera prices were exorbitant. He further asserted that the sera of the National Bacteriological Institute enjoyed great prestige, both inside the country and beyond its borders.[29]

When the revolutionary state finally established a degree of stability, it sought to centralise sanitary activities, professionalise the public health sector and reorganise vaccine production. In 1918, Gaviño was called once again to direct the National Bacteriological Institute, which by that time was producing only smallpox vaccine. Yet another plague epidemic affected various states of the republic in 1920, and despite the terrible conditions that reined at the institute, Gaviño managed to extinguish the epidemic by providing thousands of doses of both sera and vaccines.[30] In 1921, the Rockefeller Foundation began to play an important role in public health in Mexico. It taught health workers at two training stations established in the country, and sent sixty-eight Mexican fellows to North American universities, most of whom later occupied high-ranking posts in the Mexican federal public health bureaucracy or headed research institutes.[31]

Following the prolonged period of civil armed struggle, the process of state reconstruction included the creation of institutions, among them some related to the health sector. Though the civil war profoundly affected the National Bacteriology Institute, in 1920 it was reorganised as the Institute of Hygiene, an offshoot of the Public Health Department – which at the end of the revolution had replaced the Superior Board of Health – and was engaged in both research and the production of sera and vaccines. In 1925, only four years after Albert Calmette and Camille Guéran had prepared a vaccine for tuberculosis (the BCG) in France, and the first clinical trial with *Bacillus Calmette-Guérin* took place, Fernando Ocaranza – then head of the Institute of Hygiene – received strains of attenuated *Bacillus* from Calmette, and in 1931 began production of the BCG in Mexico.[32] This was despite the fact that in 1929, over a hundred vaccinated children died in a German town due to accidental contamination of the vaccine with a virulent strain.[33]

Both Hans Zinsser (Harvard University) and Herman Mooser (University of Zurich, who also worked at Harvard) supported the participation of North American universities in Mexican medicine. Their Mexican disciples, Maximiliano Ruiz Castañeda and Gerardo Varela, were awarded fellowships by the Rockefeller Foundation and opened the door to post-Pasteurian bacteriology in Mexico.[34] Ruiz Castañeda had studied microbiology at the University of Paris and the Pasteur Institute between 1924 and 1925. He then travelled to the United States, where he discovered, together with Mooser and Zinsser, that rats serve as a reservoir for murine typhus, and that the vehicle of transmission is the flea. In the early 1930s, Zinsser and Ruiz Castañeda developed a serum that was tested on hospitalised patients and the general population in times of epidemics, as well as a vaccine against typhus.[35]

Vaccines: a means to an end

The true pacification of Mexico took place under the government of Lázaro Cárdenas (1934–40), which included a social project designed to fulfil the promises that the Revolution had made to the peasants and workers who had participated in it. Cárdenas granted 49,605,673 acres of fertile land to one million peasants, and accompanied this measure with credits, as well as water, and educational and medical services.[36]

Cárdenas' regime brought about the creation of the Institute of Public Health and Tropical Diseases, which was at the forefront in integrating research teams in protozoology, helminthology, entomology, anatomo-pathology, bacteriology, pharmacology, chemistry, epidemiology and statistics. For almost two decades, the Institute of Hygiene had carried out basic research, but this research ceased when the Institute of Public Health and Tropical Diseases was established. However, the Institute of Hygiene continued producing vaccines and sera, and extended its laboratories to satisfy the demand for biological products.[37] The Anti-Rabies Institute of Mexico survived until 1938, the year in which Pasteur's classical method was replaced by that of Sample, and rabies vaccine production was entrusted to the Institute of Hygiene.[38]

Other centres were also conducting vaccine research and development. Ruiz Castañeda returned to Mexico at the end of the 1930s, founded the Experimental Laboratory of Immunology at the General Hospital of Mexico City, and with his team developed another vaccine against typhus, this one based on *Ricketsia prowasekii* attenuated in rats's lungs. To investigate the value of the vaccine, medical experimentation was carried out on prisoners and general paralytics, while the Germans repeated the experiments on Jews in the Warsaw ghetto during the Second World War.[39] The ethical aspects of conducting medical experiments at concentration camps have been analysed elsewhere,[40] but these episodes of clinical experimentation in Mexico should be examined as well. This particular typhus vaccine was, however, destined to be forgotten, because scientists began to utilise DDT to destroy lice and fleas, and antibiotics to treat clinical forms of the disease.[41]

In 1943, the American Academy of Paediatrics approved for routine use the pertussis vaccine – developed by Pearl Kendrick and her partner Grace Eldering at the Michigan Department of Health Laboratory – and a year later the American Medical Academy recommended its use. According to Shapiro-Shapin, Kendrick and Eldering shared their vaccines, plates, cultures and research with scientists around the world, and helped them to establish vaccine programmes.[42] This was also the case in Mexico, where pertussis vaccine production began as early as 1940 under the supervision of Dr Kendrick.[43] In general, vaccine production remained at low levels, in accordance with the demands of health services; but in the case of the pertussis vaccine, demand grew rapidly, so production had to as well: in 1940, the laboratory produced 19,365,000 ml, and in 1944, 215,545,000 ml, to be used in large-scale vaccination campaigns.[44]

In 1943, the Public Health Department (which was responsible for public health activities) amalgamated with the Ministry of Welfare (which had been in charge of public hospitals), to form the Ministry of Health and Welfare. The Laboratory of the Pharmaceutical Industry, previously part of the Ministry of Welfare, was incorporated into the Institute of Hygiene, but closed when the National Chemical Pharmaceutical Industry was born.[45]

Cárdenas had proposed to combat the causes of infant mortality, as well as the roots of epidemic and endemic diseases that plagued the population, by improving diet and housing and emphasising the importance of preventive medicine, but the governments that followed gradually abandoned these projects and changed the focus to curative medicine.[46] This was most likely one of the reasons why the number of smallpox cases increased between 1943 and 1945, presenting a challenge for Mexican health workers.

Mexican sanitary authorities reorganised the Anti-Smallpox Campaign in 1950, and brigades spread out across the country. Scientists had obtained the technique for producing glycerinated pulp through the Research Institute in Lagos, Nigeria, and had managed to increase and conserve its potency. Nevertheless, at the request of the Pan-American Health Organization (PAHO), they agreed to conduct experiments in Mexico with dried smallpox lymph. The last case of the illness in the country was reported in February 1951. On 16 June 1952, the World Health Organization (WHO) declared that smallpox had been officially eradicated from Mexico, twenty-six years before it was totally eradicated worldwide. Vaccine production and smallpox vaccination nevertheless continued until the end of the 1970s.[47] In 1982, at the suggestion of Dr Arita – chief of the WHO Smallpox Eradication Unit – Mexican sanitary authorities destroyed their remaining stocks of the virus.[48]

Other vaccines experienced interrupted development in Mexico. The Campaign against Tuberculosis had included BCG vaccination since the 1930s, but in 1950 several newborn babies, vaccinated with oral BCG during the first ten days of life, died of generalised tuberculosis. Though physicians knew that the intravenous vaccination was safer, they opted for the oral vaccine because parents accepted it more easily. The BCG Laboratory's director, specialists, and even the mission chief in Mexico for the International Campaign against Tuberculosis deliberated the subject. After thorough research, the Consultant and Technical Body of the BCG of the Ministry of Health and Welfare reported that all of the deceased babies had been breastfed and none had a family history of tuberculosis, and thus concluded that the deaths were due to the vaccine, adding that: 'The magnitude of the disaster caused by the oral administered BCG in Mexico still needs to be clarified.'[49] They pointed out that infant mortality had significantly risen in Mexico City just after the introduction of oral BCG vaccination, and a newspaper campaign against the vaccine drew on evidence from independent physicians and sanitary personnel who were opposed to the oral BCG. Oral vaccination was suspended, as it was in most countries at the time, but the controversy also affected intravenous vaccination. Those opposed to oral BCG suggested returning to sanitary methods of control sanctioned by experience, and it took ten years for tuberculosis vaccination advocates to be able to bring vaccination back to Mexico.[50]

In 1951, the Institute of Hygiene informed the Ministry of Health and Welfare that it was possible to produce the yellow fever vaccine in Mexico, though a laboratory and equipment would be required. Dr

Rake of Squib Laboratories in the United States had provided them with plans for the installation of such a laboratory,[51] which was finally developed,[52] though there were periods in which the country did not produce the vaccine.

As mentioned previously, scientists had produced the simple pertussis vaccine since 1940. Eight years later, they achieved a successful combination with diphtheria toxoid, and in 1954 it finally became possible to include the tetanus toxoid.[53] Armed with this combination vaccine, DPT, in 1960 Mexican health authorities began massive vaccination campaigns.

The population had received news of the first poliomyelitis epidemics in Mexico with enormous anxiety. In 1953 – the year of one of the most severe epidemics – the National Campaign against Poliomyelitis was declared in the national interest and on the same day the National Committee for the Fight against Poliomyelitis was established.[54] The problem of poliomyelitis could only be solved by preventive vaccination, since treatment capacity was severely limited. In 1960, for example, the Children's Hospital of Mexico had only a dozen beds and a dozen iron lungs for sick children, as well as a department of rehabilitation and physical therapy, at a time when hundreds of children and adults were already suffering the paralytic effects of the disease, and hundreds more would be added every year.[55]

In April 1955, when the Francis Report declared Jonas E. Salk's 'killed or inactivated' polio vaccine (IPV) safe and efficacious, it was considered timely to begin production in Mexico.[56] The general director of the Chemical Pharmaceutical Industry and the Centre for the Study of Poliomyelitis – a private group formed to support research and fight the illness – promoted the commencement of vaccine production in Mexico, funded by the Ministry of Health and Welfare and the National Institute for Child Welfare. In 1956, the National Chemical Pharmaceutical Industry produced the first poliomyelitis vaccine, following the methods proposed by Salk and his collaborators.[57] After two years of vaccination and the application of 1,055,229 doses, Mexican sanitary authorities stated that the vaccine prepared in Mexico was effective in 80 per cent of cases.[58]

Studies with the Sabin 'weakened or attenuated' oral polio vaccine (OPV) began in Mexico in 1957. The vaccine was tested first on orphan children housed in an orphanage, then with children in public day care centres and poor communities, and finally in children from the upper social classes. For a time, both vaccines were applied simultaneously due to the need to finish the series initiated with the Salk vaccine,[59] but health authorities eventually decided to replace the Salk vaccine with the Sabin vaccine. After that, doctors only used the oral vaccine, on the recommendation of the WHO and – as Stuart Blume has shown – due to considerations that were more practical and economic than scientific.[60] In 1960, the National Institute of Virology was established to make epidemiological diagnoses of illnesses caused by viruses. By 1962, the Sabin vaccine was being produced in Mexico under the supervision of Sabin himself. This is when mass vaccination really began in Mexico.[61]

Though there were difficulties with the production of various vaccines, the most challenging for Mexican scientists was the polio vaccine, and on several occasions Mexico lost and recovered its licence to produce it. It was revoked, for example, in 1970 because virulence tests were not satisfactory, according to the WHO adviser Milan V. Milošević. But production commenced again in 1977 under the aegis of the WHO. After visiting the Mexican National Institute of Virology in 1979, Albert Sabin wrote to Frank T. Perkins – chief of biologics at the WHO – and to Charles Cockburn – also from the WHO – stating: 'If I were still the official assessor, I would certainly approve this lot of [polio] vaccine.'[62]

The potential risks of the OPV were soon discovered, and in the end scientists had to recognise that some cases of polio were related to vaccination,[63] which is why, after analysing cases in the UK, the Netherlands and West Germany, Lindner and Blume asked themselves whether scientific and epidemiological data determine vaccine policy or, on the contrary, scientific, epidemiological and economic data are subject to construction and reconstruction by political actors.[64] In Mexico, sanitary authorities only began to switch to IPV at the beginning of 2007.

Crisis, reorganisation and erosion of national capacity in vaccine development

Advances in therapeutics in the mid-twentieth century and especially the discovery of penicillin gave rise to the generalised opinion that chemotherapy and the antibiotic treatment of infectious diseases were so effective that they had made the utilisation of immune-prophylactic measures unnecessary. This notion resulted in decreased support from the private sector and even government entities for institutes or laboratories producing vaccines. These institutions suffered a progressive deterioration as a result. This abandonment came to be felt at the Pasteur Institute in France, and at the Latin American institutes that followed its leadership.[65]

In Mexico, the Institute of Hygiene reflected this abandonment most dramatically, as in 1970 an accident with fatal consequences forced it to temporarily interrupt activities: early that year many children died after being immunised with DPT. Colima, on the Pacific coast, was one of the states most severely affected. At first, sanitary authorities thought it was sabotage, but later it turned out that the problem lay in the institute's procedures. Investigators from the Institute of Hygiene discovered active *clostridium tetani* (the causative agent of tetanus) in the beakers and test tubes used for the production of the DPT vaccine; a batch of non-detoxified toxin had been mixed in with the vaccine. This contaminated vaccine batch had also been used in the offices of the Civil Registry in Mexico City, where it caused seventy-five deaths. The head of production at the Institute of Hygiene would later declare that it was not a case of negligence, but was due to the lack of material, equipment and adequate installations that she had previously reported to her superiors, in a place where no expense or resource should be spared.[66]

The investigation of the incident was entrusted to the veteran bacteriologist Gerardo Varela, as well as to the head of the Department of Microbiology of the Faculty of Medicine of the National Autonomous University of Mexico, and the dean of the National School of Biological Sciences, at the National Polytechnic Institute. They concluded that there were profound problems at the Institute of Hygiene, such as the reutilisation of animals that had survived other tests, a lack of discipline with respect to international norms of control, dependence on the control laboratory of the institute's production department, which constrained its independence, and lack of capacity on the part of administrative personnel.

The Institute of Hygiene was temporarily closed for reorganisation.[67] This reorganisation coincided with a worldwide reconsideration of the utility of immune-prophylaxis, and with regional projects by the PAHO and others by the WHO. In Mexico, the reorganisation included aid in obtaining strains through agreements with producing laboratories. In addition, staff underwent training, either travelling to international centres or receiving leading scientists at Mexican institutions (frequently with WHO or PAHO support). Help also came in the form of the standardisation of biological products, as well as the implementation of external control of domestically produced vaccines and sera.

Many foreign scientists and institutions collaborated with Mexicans and advised them, such as Tatsuichiro Hashimoto in a new BCG laboratory, and Frank T. Perkins in the production of viral vaccines, particularly against poliomyelitis. The Institute of Immunology of Zagreb provided the Edmonston-Zagrev strain for the production of measles vaccine, and Dr Drago Ikić – the institute's head – advised on the components of DPT. In addition, Jacques Laiuthud of the Institut Mérieux (Lyon, France) helped create a new section of blood derivatives, and Eduardo Fuenzalida aided in the production of a rabies vaccine through an accord with the Bacteriological Laboratory of Chile. Other international institutions that collaborated with Mexico at the time were the Serum Institute of Copenhagen, the Sclavo Laboratories of Siena, the National Institute for Biological Standardisation and Control of London, and the Wellcome Laboratories of the UK.[68] Between 1983 and 1989, thirty experts from the Pasteur Institute in France, the WHO, the PAHO, the Centers for Disease Control and Prevention, the Food and Drug Administration, and the National Institutes of Health of the United States, visited Mexican institutions to advise on technical activities. There were also reciprocal visits with Colombia, Peru, Chile, Argentina and Brazil.[69]

The Institute of Hygiene had three main functions: production of vaccines and sera, for both national consumption and export; certification of all biological products in accordance with WHO norms; and experimentation with new techniques and methods for the production and administration of biological products. The Institute of Virology, meanwhile, became a laboratory for viral vaccine production against poliomyelitis, measles and rabies. The Reagents Central Laboratory was created.[70] A decade later, the Institute of Hygiene, the Institute of Virology, and the Central Laboratory were all grouped together as the General Management of Biologics and Reagents, which became virtually the sole producer of biological products in the country.

In the late 1980s, Mexico was the only Latin American country to produce all of the vaccines included in the United Nations Children's Fund (UNICEF) Extended Vaccination Programme (tuberculosis, diphtheria, pertussis, tetanus, poliomyelitis and measles), as well as human and canine rabies and typhoid fever vaccines, and others in the field of veterinary medicine (a total of twenty-five products).[71] The Mexican Ministry of Health confirmed that Mexico was also the only developing country that had the equipment, technology and human resources required to produce vaccines against poliomyelitis that were approved by the WHO. The vaccine against measles was produced at the National Institute of Virology, with a methodology first partly, and then wholly, developed there. While the internationally recognised technique required the use of chicken embryos, the methodology developed in Mexico utilised human diploid cells as the substrate, inoculated with a previously adapted vaccine strain of the Edmonton-Zagrev virus.[72] In 1979, the General Management of Biologics and Reagents was designated by the PAHO as a Regional Centre of Reference for Latin America. As such, it evaluated vaccine lots from twelve countries: Argentina, Brazil, Costa Rica, Chile, El Salvador, Guatemala, Honduras, Nicaragua, Panama, Peru, Dominican Republic and Uruguay, and provided technological support to them all.[73]

Mexico had therefore achieved self-sufficiency in vaccine production, control, storage and distribution, except in the case of the poliomyelitis vaccine, whose production did not always fulfil national demand, and by the end of the 1980s was exporting biological products (including vaccines, mainly for rabies) to fifteen countries in the Caribbean and Central and South America. Domestic vaccine production was a political priority, because politicians saw that imports were expensive and also because national security dictated protecting public health. 'Artisanal' procedures for making vaccines were replaced by industrial methods of production, for which Mexican as well as Dutch manufacturers supplied the needed equipment. In 1983, the Mexican government launched National Vaccination Days, and shortly afterwards it introduced National Vaccination Weeks; these eventually evolved into the nationwide Universal Vaccination Programme.[74]

In 1989, health officials began to compare public and private vaccine production. For some, like Garza Ramos, the former responded to the needs of public health programmes, while the latter obeyed commercial interests. Public production focused on the vaccines that were required, even if their production was not cost-effective (e.g. BCG, DPT and viral vaccines), while private production focused on those that generated economic benefits. Public production entailed national technology, private production utilised imported technology. In the former, the research carried out created scientific and technological holdings that served the country, while in the latter most research took place outside Mexico and the benefits were accrued by parent industries. In public production, prices were set in relation to costs, unburdened by extra charges for attractive presentations and propaganda, while private production depended on supply and demand and their prices definitely included such charges. Public production assured that currency remained in Mexico, while private manufacturing increased capital flight. Public production concentrated on products that resolved local problems, which was of little or no concern to private production. In public production, all products were generated within the country, while private production required importing finished products or products shipped in bulk. In the public sector, the technical and administrative personnel were Mexican, in the private sector they were foreigners (with the exception of Myn y Zapata Laboratories).[75]

For all these reasons, Garza Ramos wrote that, 'National production of these goods constitutes a priority, since their acquisition in foreign markets is tremendously onerous, and doing without said products would bring as a consequence the deterioration of the population's health.'[76] Producing biologics in Mexico meant taking advantage of human and technological resources and of the installed capacity at both the National Institute of Hygiene and the National Institute of Virology of the General Management of Biologics and Reagents.

Mexican scientists also controlled the quality of imported vaccines that were not yet produced in the country: those for rubella, mumps, cholera, yellow fever (for people travelling abroad), a serum against coral snake venom (for high-risk zones), and the rabies vaccine elaborated with diploid cells.[77] The government placed emphasis on national self-sufficiency in vaccine production, as well as on efforts to diagnose and control disease, especially those of greatest epidemiological importance.

In 1990, human and technological resources existed in the country, and both the National Institute of Hygiene and the National Institute of Virology had the capacity to produce, certify, store and distribute quality biological products in the required quantities in a timely fashion. In other words, self-sufficiency had been achieved. Since 1990, there have been no reported cases of unvaccinated poliomyelitis and since 1991 no cases of diphtheria.[78]

But things were already beginning to change. On the one hand, there was a high demand for biological products owing to the existence of ambitious vaccination programmes; vaccines were becoming more complex, and new ones were being developed. On the other hand, as in several other countries, there was also growing pressure from international industry (organised into ever more powerful consortiums), which had succeeded in lowering costs and improving quality. These were advances that the public sector could not achieve, in particular, because reduced budgets for health care came with the application of neo-liberal policies in the area of health services (this process is thoroughly analysed by Blume in Chapter 6 in this book).[79] Private enterprises had begun to invest in vaccines and sera production: their 5.5 million peso investments in 1983 rose to 51 million in 1990.[80] In 1989, a period of 'expansion and confusion' – in Garza Ramos words – began, and it ended up diminishing the production of some fundamental biologics, and in its eventual disappearance. This signalled the beginning of the erosion of Mexican vaccine production.[81]

The General Direction of Biologics and Reagents and the Ministry of Health (renamed in 1985) decided to transform the institutes into a privatised industry. They began with Biomex – though this measure never surpassed the project phase – at great cost to the health administration. In 1991, Birmex, an entity mostly based on state-level participation, was created. Thereafter, Mexico suspended fabrication of most vaccines: BCG, measles, pertussis, diphtheria and tetanus for children, and rabies. BCG, for example, ceased to be produced domestically, because from one day to the next the Ministry of Health requested bottles with fewer dosages, which was impossible to achieve immediately. Today Mexico imports all these vaccines. Consequently, it had lost self-sufficiency in vaccine supply by the beginning of the new millennium.[82] Some raised their voices against the new government policy – such as former head of the Institute of Hygiene, Manuel Servín Massieu – and many Mexican epidemiologists and scientists disagree with this loss, but they were unable to organise against it.

Birmex only produces poliomyelitis and tetanus and diphtheria for adult vaccines, though it does market products from private enterprises. When the switch from OPV to IPV is complete, they will also stop producing the polio vaccine. Birmex's functionaries have participated in PAHO and WHO Good Manufacturing Programmes, which offer training and specialisation aimed at health authorities and the academic and industrial sectors.[83]

This later period has also seen changes in Mexico's routine vaccination schedule. In 1998, the number of vaccines on the schedule rose from six (*Bacillus* Calmette-Guérin [BCG], oral polio vaccine [OPV], diphtheria, pertussis and tetanus [DPT] and measles) to eight, as mumps and rubella were added. Then, in 1999 it increased to ten, with the addition of the *H. influenzae* b (Hib) and hepatitis B vaccines. In 2006 and 2007, respectively, pneumococcus and retrovirus vaccines were added. Since 2009, the human papilloma virus vaccine has been applied to 9-year-old girls. In 2000, authorities initiated programmes to vaccinate the adolescent and young adult population (measles, rubella, hepatitis B and influenza), those over 60 years of age (influenza, pneumococcus, diphtheria, tetanus and hepatitis B) and pregnant women (diphtheria, pertussis and tetanus).[84]

Final reflections

Since the early nineteenth century, vaccination in Mexico was a matter of state concern regarding public welfare (as in Brazil, discussed by Benchimol: Chapter 7 in this book), but it also reflected an elite concern with national security. In a country frequently beset with political violence, it is no coincidence that disease immunity was often considered an element of political strategy. Mexico had foreign enemies with a habit of invasion, and Mexican sanitary authorities always pointed out that vaccine production was as old as the production of ammunitions, meaning that both were needed to protect the Mexican people against their enemies.

In its dependence on foreign institutes and manufacturing laboratories for training and models of manufacture, and in its repeated stopping and starting of vaccine production under conditions of revolutionary instability, Mexico's experience anticipated, by at least fifty years, the similar difficulties that institutions of science and technology experienced in new countries in Asia and Africa following decolonisation.

The end of the nineteenth century saw the birth of modern public health and the production of public sector vaccine, which would be the start of a long tradition. Although separated by a decade of civil war, the government of Porfirio Díaz and the post-revolutionary governments formed part of the same process of capitalist development, and they all considered science to be congruent with their goals. The Díaz regime laid the foundations of modern public health, while post-revolutionary governments sought to make public health an integral part of nation-state formation. As a result, it became possible for the country to develop in its own individual path, with the support of advances in Europe and the United States.

Many of the researchers who worked in the production of vaccines studied in institutions abroad. Mexican scientists established many ties, regardless of the nationality of those who could train them. In the last third of the nineteenth century, several of them studied at French, German, and US institutions, and then introduced the bacteriological thinking and practices they learned there back at home; the main influence was the Pasteur Institute in France. By contrast, in the twentieth century the Rockefeller Foundation and the WHO exerted dominant influence.

This building of relationships with scientists from many countries brought the early introduction of the BCG, pertussis and polio vaccines. This was not a simple transfer of science to the periphery. The reception of new ideas and theories was active as Mexicans maintained direct contact with vanguard scientists through several means, including participation in congresses, personal correspondence and research exchange programmes; they also created institutes where they carried out original, basic and applied research.[85]

Between 1895 and 1905, Mexico founded the Anti-Rabies Preventive Inoculation Service, the National Pathology Institute and the National Bacteriology Institute, and they combined research with the production of vaccines and sera. The Civil War interrupted these works almost completely, but in 1920 they were reorganised and for the following five decades played a fundamental role in building and strengthening the nation. The years between 1921 and 1934 brought the first efforts at national reconstruction in Mexico, in which government policies regarding public education and health played an important role. The Mexican government was concerned with achieving levels of production that were sufficient to satisfy its immunisation programmes in the hope of assuring future healthy generations.

Over the course of the twentieth century, state builders created several institutions devoted to the production of vaccines: the Institute of Hygiene, the Laboratory of the Pharmaceutical Industry, the National Institute of Virology and the Central Laboratory of Reagents, all attached to the Ministry of Health. They considered that national production of vaccines and sera were not only a matter of national pride, but also a priority, because of the high costs of importing them, because they were needed to protect the population and to help lower morbidity and mortality due to infectious diseases, and last but not least, for reasons of national security, namely to assure the availability of biological products in order to avoid the economic and technical dependence that came with imported products and the transfer of foreign methodologies.[86]

Today, this development has practically disappeared; though this was no linear history, as this chapter has sought to demonstrate, and in the past there were cases of what Marcos Cueto has called scientific excellence in the periphery.[87] Indeed, it was not intellectual or technical incapacity that influenced the disappearance of national vaccine production but rather economic, political and cultural factors, including strong governments, revolution and civil war, controversies among physicians, rebellions against vaccines, accidents, and the creation, reorganisation and dissolution of institutions. As Saldaña would say, these were particular experiences of science, which turned out as they did due to their local history; one manifestation, among many others, of Mexican science thinking on its own.

Acknowledgements

I am grateful to Stuart Blume for his perseverance in conducting collective research on the history of vaccines and vaccination around the world, and to Blume, Christine Holmberg and Paul Greenough for their invitation to write this chapter, as well as for their critiques and extremely helpful suggestions. I also benefited from the advice of Elizabeth O'Brien.

Notes

1 J. J. Saldaña, *Las revoluciones políticas y la ciencia en México* [*Political revolutions and science in Mexico*], 2 vols (Mexico, Conacyt, 2010), 1, pp. 32–7.

2 The vaccine had been brought to Puerto Rico from the Danish island of Saint Thomas. The arrival in Cuba of a woman who had recently been vaccinated in Puerto Rico led the professor of medicine Tomás Romay to begin vaccination on the island. The fluid had also arrived in New Spain, carried by two ships coming from La Habana. Díaz de Iraola, G ... *La vuelta al mundo de la Expedición de la Vacuna (1803–1818)* [*The Round the World Voyage of the Smallpox Vaccine (1803–1818)*] (Spain: Consejo Superior de Investigaciones Científicas/Escuela de Estudios Hispano-Americanos de Sevilla, 1948).

3 M. E. Bustamante, 'Consecuencias médico-sociales de la viruela y de su erradicación' [Socio-medical Consequences of Smallpox and its Eradication], *Gaceta Médica de México*, 113 (1977), pp. 564–73.

4 D. Tank-de-Estrada, 'Justas florales de los botánicos ilustrados. Ciencia y tecnología en la historia de México' [Public Contests of the Enlightened Botanists. Science and Technology in Mexican history], *Diálogos*, 106 (1989), pp. 19–31; J. J. Saldaña, 'Acerca de la historia en la ciencia nacional' [Regarding History in National Science], in J. J. Saldaña (ed.), *Los orígenes de la ciencia nacional* [*The Origins of National Science*] (México: Universidad Nacional Autónoma de México/Sociedad Latinoamericana de Historia de las Ciencias y la Tecnología, 1992), pp. 9–54.

5 J. M. Oropeza, 'Apuntes para la historia de la vacuna en México' [Notes for the History of the Vaccine in Mexico], Archivo Histórico de la Secretaría de Salud, México [Historical Archive of the Ministry of Health, Mexico] (hereafter, AHSSA), salubridad pública [Public Health], Inspección de la Vacuna [Vaccine Inspection], 3/ 20, f. 49–182, 1921–2.

6 *Ibid.*

7 J. Álvarez-Amézquita, M. E. Bustamante, A. López-Picazos and F. Fernández-del Castillo, *Historia de la salubridad y de la asistencia en México* [*History of Health and Welfare in Mexico*], 4 vols (México: Secretaría de Salubridad y Asistencia, 1960), 2.

8 A. M. Carrillo, 'Por voluntad o por fuerza. La lucha contra la viruela en el porfirismo' [Voluntary or by Force. The Fight Against Smallpox During Porfirian Times], in C. Cramaussel and M. A. Magaña-Mancillas (eds), *El impacto demográfico de la viruela en México de la época colonial al siglo XX. La viruela después de la introducción de la vacuna* [*The demographic impact of smallpox from colonial times to the 20th century. Smallpox after vaccine introduction*], 3 vols (Zamora: El Colegio de Michoacán, 2010), pp. 91–111.

9 A. M. Stern and H. Markel, 'The History of Vaccines and Immunization: Familiar Patterns, New Challenge', *Health Affairs*, 24:1 (2003), pp. 611–21.

10 Gobierno del Estado de Oaxaca, *Historia de la salud en Oaxaca* [*History of Health in Oaxaca*] (Oaxaca: Gobierno del Estado de Oaxaca, 1993).

11 A. C. Rodríguez de Romo, 'La ciencia pasteuriana a través de la vacuna antirrábica: el caso mexicano' [Pasteurian Science Through the Rabies Vaccine: The Mexican Case], *Dynamis*, 16 (1996), pp. 291–316.

12 A. Reyes, 'Inoculaciones preventivas de la rabia' [Preventive Rabies Vaccine], *Gaceta Médica de México*, 24:18 (1889), pp. 344–7.

13 E. Liceaga, *Algunas consideraciones acerca de la higiene social en México* [*Some reflections about social hygiene in Mexico*] (México: Vda. de F. Díaz de León, 1911).

14 Archivo Histórico de la Universidad Nacional Autónoma de México [Historical Archive of the National Autonomous University of Mexico], Escuela Nacional de Medicina [National School of Medicine], institutos y sociedades médicos [Medical Institutes and Societies], Museo Anatomo-Patológico–Instituto Patológico Nacional [Pathological Anatomy Museum–National Pathology Institute], 40/1, f. 1v, 1895.

15 A. M. Carrillo, '¿Estado de peste o estado de sitio? Mazatlán y Baja California 1902–1903' [State of Plague or State of Siege? Mazatlan and Baja California, 1902–1903], *Historia Mexicana*, 54:4 (2005), pp. 1049–103.

16 Archivo Histórico de la Secretaría de Relaciones Exteriores, México [Historical Archive of the Secretary of Foreign Affairs, Mexico], Embajada de México en los Estados Unidos de América [Mexican Embassy in the United States of America], 164/4, 115 f.: 46–7, 1900–4 and 1907–8.

17 I. J. Catanach, 'Plague and the Tensions of the Empire 1988: India 1896–1918', in D. Arnold (ed.), *Imperial Medicine and Indigenous Societies* (Manchester: Manchester University Press, 1988), pp. 149–71.

18 'Ley constitutiva del Instituto Patológico Nacional y del Instituto Bacteriológico Nacional' [Constitutive Law of the National Pathology Institute and the National Bacteriology Institute], *Diario Oficial* [*Official Gazette*] (ciudad de México, 17 October 1905), pp. 629–31; M. Servín-Massieu, *Microbiología, vacunas y el rezago científico de México a partir del siglo XIX* [*Microbiology, vaccines and scientific lag in Mexico from the 19th century on*] (Mexico: Instituto Politécnico Nacional/Plaza y Valdés, 2000).

19 A. M. Carrillo, 'La patología del siglo XIX y los institutos nacionales de investigación médica en México' [19th Century Pathology and the National Medical Research Institutes in Mexico], *Laborat-ACTA*, 13:1 (2001), pp. 23–31.

20 A. Garza-Brito, 'El Instituto Nacional de Higiene' [The National Institute of Hygiene], AHSSA, Instituto de Higiene [Institute of Hygiene], trabajos de concurso [professional concourse], 2/22 [88 f.], 1989.
21 Álvarez-Amézquita et al., Historia de la salubridad.
22 A. M. Carrillo and A. E. Birn, 'Neighbors on Notice: National and Imperialist Interests in the American Public Health Association', Canadian Bulletin of Medical History/Bulletin Canadien d'histoire de la Medicine, 25:1 (2008), pp. 225–54.
23 Servín-Massieu, Microbiología, vacunas..
24 Archivo Histórico de la Facultad de Medicina de la Universidad Nacional Autónoma de México [Historical Archive of the Faculty of Medicine of the National Autonomous University of Mexico], Escuela de Medicina y Alumnos [School of Medicine and Students], 204/19, 38 f.
25 R. Silva, 'Muerte del socio honorario D. Manuel Toussaint' [Death of the Honorary Member D. Manuel Toussaint], Gaceta Médica de México, 58:12 (1927), pp. 787–90.
26 AHSSA, salubridad pública, expedientes de personal [staff records], 35/1, 2 and 3; 113, 220 and 167 f.; 1896–1900, 1900–7 and 1907–29.
27 Gaceta Médica de México, 5:5 (1910), p. 187.
28 I. Costero, 'Desarrollo de la anatomía patológica en México' [Development of Pathological Anatomy in Mexico], in E. Beltrán (ed.), Memorias del I Coloquio de Historia de la Ciencia [Proceedings of the History of Science Symposium] (México: Sociedad Mexicana de Historia de la Ciencia y la Tecnología, 1964), pp. 349–69.
29 A. M. Carrillo, 'La influencia de la bacteriología francesa en la mexicana en el periodo de su institucionalización' [The Influence of French Bacteriology on Mexican Bacteriology in the Period of its Institutionalisation], Quipu. Revista Latinoamericana de Historia de las Ciencias y la Tecnología, 14:2 (2012), pp. 93–119.
30 A. De-Garay, 'En memoria del Dr. Ángel Gaviño' [In memory of Ángel Gaviño], Salud Pública de México, 2:4 (1960), pp. 899–903.
31 A. E. Birn, Marriage of Convenience. Rockefeller International Health and Revolutionary Mexico (Rochester: University of Rochester Press, 2006).
32 J. Garza-Ramos, C. Viesca and G. Franco-de-Guzmán, 'Les vaccins au Mexique' [Vaccines in Mexico], in J. Garza-Ramos (ed.), Symposium. Progres a l'usage de vaccins, 1885–1985 [Symposium. Progress in the Use of Vaccines, 1885–1985] (México: Gerencia General de Biológicos y Reactivos/Secretaría de Salud, 1986), pp. 260–9.
33 A. M. Moulin, 'The International Network of the Pasteur Institute: Scientific Innovations and French Tropisms', in C. Charle, J. Schriewer and P. Wagner (eds), The Emergence of Transnational Intellectual Networks and the

Cultural Logic of Nations (New York: Campus Verlag, 2004), pp. 135–62.

34 A. Pérez-Miravete, 'La producción mexicana de reactivos y vacunas' [Mexican Production of Reagents and Vaccines], in M. Urbina-Fuentes, A. Moguel-Ancheita, M. Muñiz-Martelón and J. A. Solís-Urdaibay (eds), *La experiencia mexicana en salud pública. Oportunidad y rumbo para el tercer milenio* [*The Mexican Experience in Public Health. Opportunity and Direction for the Third Millennium*] (Mexico: Secretaría de Salud/Organización Panamericana de la Salud/Sociedad Mexicana de Salud Pública/Fundación Mexicana para la Salud/Instituto Nacional de Salud Pública/Fondo de Cultura Económica, 2006), pp. 177–89.

35 H. Zinsser and M. R. Castaneda, 'Mexican Typhus Fever', *Journal of Experimental Medicine*, 57:3 (1933), pp. 381–90.

36 Birn, *Marriage of Convenience*.

37 *Seis años de gobierno al servicio de México 1934–1940* [*Six Years of Government Service to Mexico 1934–1940*] (Ciudad de México: Talleres Gráficos de la Nación, 1940). R. Vargas-Olvera, 'Introducción', in Y. Trejo, R. Vargas-Olvera, D. Molina-Alamilla *et al.*, *Guía del Fondo del Instituto de Salubridad y Enfermedades Tropicales* [Guide of the Institute of Public Health and Tropical Diseases Collection] (México: Secretaría de Salubridad y Asistencia, 1993), pp. i–xii.

38 AHSSA, Instituto de Higiene, trabajos de concurso, 2/22 [88 f.], 1989.

39 E. Landa, 'Las primeras aplicaciones del suero antitifoso de Ruiz Castañeda y Zinsser' [The First Applications of the Ruiz Castañeda and Zinsser Anti-Typhus Serum], *Gaceta Médica de México*, 66:3 (1933), pp. 123–32.

40 T. Taylor, 'The Doctor's Trial and the Nuremberg Code. Opening Statement of the Prosecution, December 9, 1946', in G. J. Annas and M. A. Grodin (eds), *The Nazi Doctors and the Nuremberg Code: Human Rights in Human Experimentation* (New York: Oxford University Press, 1992), pp. 67–93.

41 Garza-Ramos, Viesca and Franco-de-Guzmán, 'Les vaccins au Mexique'.

42 C. G. Shapiro-Shapin, 'Pearl Kendrik, Grace Eldering, and the Pertussis Vaccine', *Emerging Infectious Diseases*, 18:8 (2010), pp. 1273–8.

43 A. De-la-Garza Brito, 'El Instituto Nacional de Higiene', AHSSA, Instituto de Higiene, trabajos de concurso, 2/22 [88 f.], 1989.

44 Silvermann, quoted in Pérez-Miravete, 'La producción mexicana de reactivos y vacunas'.

45 AHSSA, Instituto de Higiene, trabajos de concurso, 2/22 [88 f.], 1989.

46 A. M. Carrillo, 'Salud pública y poder en México durante el Cardenismo, 1934–1940' [Public Health and Power in Mexico During Cárdenas' Times,

1934–1940], *Dynamis*, 25 (2005), pp. 145–78: Birn, *Marriage of Convenience*.

47 Garza-Ramos, Viesc and Franco-de-Guzmán, 'Les vaccins au Mexique'.

48 AHSSA, Secretaría de Salubridad y Asistencia [Ministry of Public Health and Welfare], Gerencia General de Biológicos y Reactivos [General Management of Biological Products], 20/8, 270 f., 1982.

49 AHSSA, Secretaría de Salubridad y Asistencia, Subsecretaría de Asistencia [Underministry of Welfare], 53/1, 248 f. [n.fol.n], 1950–79.

50 *Ibid.*

51 AHSSA, Secretaría de Salubridad y Asistencia, 13/ 5, 232 f., 1946–80.

52 Garza-Ramos, Viesca and Franco-de-Guzmán, 'Les vaccins au Mexique'.

53 *Ibid.*

54 *Diario Oficial*, Mexico, 27 April 1953, p. 1.

55 F. Gómez, 'Symposium sobre examen de los conocimientos actuales sobre vacunación en la poliomielitis. Introducción' [Symposium on Current Knowledge About Poliomyelitis Vaccination], *Gaceta Médica de México*, 91:12 (1961), pp. 1051–3.

56 L. Gutiérrez-Villegas, 'Resultados de la vacuna contra la poliomielitis tipo Salk elaborada en México' [Results of the Poliomyelitis Salk Vaccine Produced in Mexico], *Gaceta Médica de México*, 88:5 (1958), pp. 82–93.

57 J. Muñoz-Turnbull, 'Observaciones sobre la vacuna antipoliomielítica preparada en México. Conocimientos recientes sobre su aplicación' [Observations Regarding the Poliomyelitis Vaccine Produced in Mexico. Recent Knowledge About its Application], *Gaceta Médica de México*, 87:5 (1957), pp. 337–44.

58 Gutiérrez-Villegas, 'Resultados de la vacuna contra la poliomielitis tipo Salk elaborada en México'.

59 'Carta del Comité Nacional de Lucha contra la Poliomielitis al ministro de la Secretaría de Salubridad y Asistencia' [Letter from the National Committee for the Fight against Poliomyelitis to the Minister of Health and Welfare], Mexico, 30 April 1954, AHSSA, Secretaría de Salubridad y Asistencia, Secretario Particular [Particular Secretary], 95/ 1, 186 f.

60 S. Blume, 'Lock in, the State and Vaccine Development: Lessons from the History of Polio Vaccines', *Research Policy*, 34 (2005), pp. 159–73.

61 C. Calderón and C. Campillo, 'Epidemiología de la poliomielitis en México. Mecanismos de inmunización' [Epidemiology of poliomyelitis in Mexico. Immunisation mechanisms], *Boletín Epidemiológico* [*Epidemiological Bulletin*], 24:4 (1960), pp. 117–25.

62 AHSSA, Secretaría de Salubridad y Asistencia, Subsecretaría de Salubridad [Underministry of Health], caja 38, exp. 1, 313 f., 1979.

63 J. I. Santos, 'Cambios en los esquemas de vacunación y la vacunación en adultos' [Changes in Vaccination Schedule and in Adult Vaccination], in M. Urbina-Fuentes, A. Moguel-Ancheita, M. Muñiz-Martelón and J. A. Solís-Urdaibay (eds), *La experiencia mexicana en salud pública. Oportunidad y rumbo para el tercer milenio* (México: Secretaría de Salud/Organización Panamericana de la Salud/Sociedad Mexicana de Salud Pública/Fundación Mexicana para la Salud/Instituto Nacional de Salud Pública/Fondo de Cultura Económica, 2006), pp. 191–223.

64 U. Lindner and D. Blume, 'Vaccine Innovation and Adoption: Polio Vaccines in the UK, the Netherlands and West Germany, 1955–1965', *Medical History*, 50 (2006), pp. 425–46.

65 A. Escobar, J. L. Valdespino and J. Sepúlveda, quoted in Pérez-Miravete, 'La producción mexicana de reactivos y vacunas'.

66 O. L. Galicia Aguilar, 'Un accidente doloroso' [A painful accident]: Pérez-Miravete, 'La producción mexicana de reactivos y vacunas'.

67 AHSSA, Secretaría de Salubridad y Asistencia, Gerencia General de Biológicos y Reactivos, 2/4, 280 f., 1965–70.

68 AHSSA, Secretaría de Salubridad y Asistencia, Gerencia General de Biológicos y Reactivos, 10/6, 148 f, 1970; 12/3, 158 f., 1970–71; 19/1, 239 f., 1980–81, 20/8, 380 f., 1982: Pérez-Miravete, 'La producción mexicana de reactivos y vacunas'. AHSSA, Instituto de Higiene, trabajos de concurso, 2/22, 88 f., 1989.

69 Interview with Juan Garza Ramos, Director of the General Management of Biologics and Reagents between 1983 and 1988, and now Director of the National Producer of Veterinarian Biologics (conducted by the author, Mexico City, March 2014).

70 A. Garza-Brito,'El Instituto Nacional de Higiene', AHSSA, Instituto de Higiene, trabajos de concurso, 2/22 [88 f.], 1989.

71 A. Homma, J. L. di Fabio and C. de Quadros, 'Los laboratorios públicos productores de vacunas: el nuevo paradigma' [Public Laboratories for Vaccine Production: A New Paradigm], *Revista Panamericana de Salud Pública* [Pan American Journal of Public Health], 4:4 (1998), pp. 223–32, www.scielosp.org/scielo.php?script=sci_arttext&pid=S1020-49891998001000001 (accessed 31 August 2016).

72 J. Garza-Ramos, 'La producción de biológicos y reactivos en México', AHSSA, Instituto de Higiene, trabajos de concurso, 2/22 [88 f.], 1989.

73 Interview with Juan Garza Ramos (conducted by the author, Mexico City, March 2014).

74 Pérez-Miravete, 'La producción mexicana de reactivos y vacunas'. AHSSA, Instituto de Higiene, trabajos de concurso, 2/22 [88 f.], 1989.

75 AHSSA, Secretaría de Salubridad y Asistencia, Gerencia General de Biológicos y Reactivos, 17/6, 219 f., 1977–1978.

76 Garza-Ramos, 'La producción de biológicos y reactivos en México', AHSSA, Instituto de Higiene, trabajos de concurso, 2/22 [88 f.], 1989.

77 *Ibid.*

78 AHSSA, Secretaría de Salubridad y Asistencia, Gerencia General de Biológicos y Reactivos, 17/ 6, 219 f., 1977–78.

79 S. Blume, J. Jagrati and S. Roalkvam, 'Saving Children's Lives: Perspectives on Immunisation', in S. Roalkvam, D. McNeill and S. Blume (eds), *Protecting the World's Children. Immunisation Policies and Practices* (Oxford: Oxford University Press, 2013), pp. 1–30.

80 Garza-Ramos, 'La producción de biológicos y reactivos en México'.

81 Interview with Juan Garza-Ramos (conducted by the author, Mexico City, March 2014).

82 Pérez-Miravete, 'La producción mexicana de reactivos y vacunas'.

83 www.paho.org/HQ/index.php?option=com_content&view=article& id=1589%3Agrupo-de-trabajo-en-buenas-pruecticas-de-manufactura& catid=1157%3Ahss-pandrh-technical-working-grou&Itemid= 1686&lang=en (accessed 15 September 2013).

84 http://web.ssaver.gob.mx/saludpublica/files/2014/02/mensajero-SNSalud.pdf (accessed 20 October 2014).

85 F. T. Glick, 'La transferencia de las revoluciones científicas a través de las fronteras culturales' [The Transfer of Scientific Revolutions Through Cultural Boundaries], *Ciencia y Tecnología*, 12:72 (1987), 77–89.

86 AHSSA, Secretaria de Salubridad y Asistencia, Subsecretaria de Asistencia, 13/5, 232 f., 1946–80.

87 M. Cueto, *Excelencia científica en la periferia* [*Scientific Excellence in the Periphery*] (Perú: GRADE CONCYTEC, 1989).

6

The erosion of public sector vaccine production: the case of the Netherlands

Stuart Blume

Introduction

Despite earlier resistance to compulsory smallpox vaccination, by 1900 the possibility of protection against diphtheria was greeted with hopeful anticipation. Diphtheria, a bacterial infection of the respiratory tract, caused the deaths of many children. At the end of the nineteenth century it was discovered that the disease could be treated with an antitoxin. Subsequently, Emil von Behring found that combining a small amount of the diphtheria toxin with the antitoxin produced a serum that offered long-term immunity to the disease. As states increasingly concerned themselves with public health (though in ways and to extents that varied greatly from one country to another)[1] a variety of institutions set about meeting demand for the new public health technologies. Some were commercial manufacturers. In Germany, in 1904, von Behring established Behringwerke to produce them. In Italy Achille Sclavo founded the *Istituto Sieroterapico e Vaccinogeno Toscano 'Sclavo'* in Siena in the same year. In Britain, the Burroughs-Wellcome pharmaceutical company, established in 1880, began producing diphtheria anti-toxin in 1894. Some were state institutions. Thus, the Danish Statens Serum Institut (State Serum Institute or SSI) was established to produce diphtheria antitoxin in 1902, and a Swedish institute (SBL) in 1909. In the Netherlands, production of the anti-toxin began in a private institution, the Bacterio-therapeutisch Instituut. However, problems in meeting national needs during the First World War, coupled with political anxieties regarding security of supply and a sense of political responsibility, led the Dutch government to take over the Institute in 1919.[2]

Driven in part by the economic and political interests of the colonial powers, new public health technologies and practices also diffused far beyond Europe and North America.[3] Inter-governmental organisations, and private foundations such as the Rockefeller Foundation and the Pasteur Institute all played important roles in this process.[4] A consequence was that institutes combining bacteriological research with the production of vaccines and sera were established in much of Asia, in parts of Africa and in Latin America (as discussed by Carillo and Benchimol in Chapters 5 and 7). Many of these institutes were established by (colonial) governments, and many of their directors had been trained at one of the leading European institutes.

A hundred years ago, in other words, states' demands for the new bacteriology-based tools of public health were met by a mix of public and private institutions. In some countries primary responsibility lay with state institutes of bacteriology or of public health. Indeed, in the Netherlands and the Scandinavian countries this remained the case until well after the Second World War. Since the 1980s, however, various governments (including those of Sweden and the Netherlands), have abandoned vaccine and serum production. Because vaccines have become ever more central to public health programmes, this seems odd. How should we understand this withdrawal of states from vaccine production? I argue here that in trying to answer this question we must attend to the complex interplay of a number of factors, operating over a period of two or more decades.

Changing technology and a changing industry

With the exception of those against smallpox and yellow fever, the vaccines in widespread use before the Second World War offered protection against bacterial diseases: diphtheria, tuberculosis, whooping cough (pertussis) and tetanus. Experimental vaccines against other viral diseases, notably polio, had been disastrous failures.

However, in the late 1940s research by John Enders and his Harvard colleagues showed how polio virus could be safely cultured. This vital breakthrough opened the way to development of vaccines against a variety of viral diseases. A vaccine against polio, that 'dread disease', was the first priority, and – encouraged in the USA by President Roosevelt – it attracted the attention of numerous research groups, in universities as well as in pharmaceutical companies. Jonas Salk, at the University of Pittsburgh, developed the first polio vaccine to be successfully tested and licensed (in 1955).[5] By the 1960s, with vaccines against both polio and measles in production and others under development, the vaccine business looked promising. Pharmaceutical companies increased their commitment. However, by the 1970s this was changing. Vaccines were proving more difficult to develop and produce than drugs. Because their production involved handling live pathogens they carried particular risks, and required particularly stringent testing. Some pharmaceutical companies abandoned vaccine production. In the USA, in particular, this was becoming a matter of political concern. The Office of Technology Assessment of the US Congress (OTA), investigating the matter, felt that: 'The apparently diminishing commitment – and possibly capacity – of the American pharmaceutical industry to research, develop, and produce vaccines ... may be reaching levels of real concern.'[6] As far as nineteen vaccines, including the polio vaccine, were concerned, the USA was dependent on only a single American pharmaceutical company. What if that producer decided to exit the vaccine field?

In the 1980s more American pharmaceutical companies left the vaccine business, influenced not only by the resources and risks involved, but now also by fear of punitive liability claims if anything went wrong. In 1986, driven largely by widespread popular concern at side effects of the pertussis vaccine, and the resulting surge in damage actions against manufacturers, the US Congress passed legislation establishing the National Childhood Vaccine Injury Compensation Program. This limited the liability of manufacturers and established a public fund from which possible compensation claims could be paid. Reassured by the protection this Act afforded, pharmaceutical firms began to reconsider their commitment to vaccines. However, another change was also taking place, and one which affected vaccine development worldwide. In the 1980s new, biotechnology-based ways of making vaccines emerged. Expertise in this area tended to lie not with the old, established manufacturers, but with small biotechnology firms. Because these new methods promised to reduce the safety concerns in vaccine production, and allow more 'targeted' development, accessing them became important to large pharmaceutical companies.[7] Frequently, the easiest way of doing so was by purchasing the small companies that possessed it. And finally, patents, which had previously played no role in the vaccines field, were becoming increasingly important. Looking at the structure of the US vaccine industry, in the mid-1990s Mowery and Mitchell noted that 'the extent of acquisitions and alliance formations among vaccine manufacturers during the past decade, especially from 1990 to 1993, is staggering'.[8] A brief look at the European industry shows a similar process of alliances and increasing concentration. The pioneers, their names and their companies, have vanished.[9] Nor have public sector institutes been immune to this process of agglomeration. For example Sweden's State Biological Laboratories (SBL) had been producing vaccines and sera since 1909. In 1993 its production department was separated from the Institute's other functions and turned into a private company, SBL-Vaccin.[10] In 2006 SBL-Vaccin was acquired by the Dutch biotechnology company Crucell.[11]

Something similar happened in the Netherlands, though more recently. In 2009 the Dutch government decided to terminate public sector vaccine production and sell the production facilities. But negotiations with potential purchasers took time, and it was only in July 2012 that the government announced that a buyer had been found.

Bare facts like these show the outcome of the process, but they reveal very little about underlying rationales. The reason given by the Dutch Minister of Health was a financial one.[12] The costs of producing vaccines for the small Dutch population (around 180,000 births per year) were too great. Meeting the ever more stringent international standards of 'good manufacturing practice' for so small a market resulted in prices far above those on the commercial market. However, this official explanation is by no means the whole story. The processes of which these privatisations and acquisitions are the outcomes can better be viewed as the outcome of a cascade of events that began years before. In order to understand how and why welfare states like the Netherlands and Sweden, justly proud of their long and successful records in public health, decided to divest themselves of the capacity to develop and produce vaccines, we have to dig deeper. This question is addressed in the remainder of this chapter, with specific reference to the Dutch situation.

Public sector vaccine development and production in
the Netherlands

RIV from the Second World War to the 1970s

The Bacterio-therapeutisch Instituut, which the Dutch government had
taken over in 1919, was soon renamed the Rijks-Serologisch Instituut.
It was later merged with the central public health laboratory, and in
1934 became the Rijks Instituut voor Volksgezondheid (State Institute
for Public Health), or RIV. Then followed the Second World War and
the country's occupation. As in much of Europe, the years after 1945
were a time of reconstruction. RIV was to produce vaccines against
pertussis and diphtheria, but lack of facilities, space and manpower
hindered its attempts to do so. In 1950 the Institute was reorganised, its
tasks more clearly set out, and new staff appointed.[13] By 1952 the Institute had succeeded in producing a combined diphtheria pertussis and
tetanus (DPT) vaccine. A new facility for smallpox vaccine was constructed, and the Institute was later to be given an important role in the
WHO smallpox eradication campaign. A 1956 polio epidemic, to which
more than 2,000 people succumbed, had two important consequences.
It led to the establishment of a centralised national vaccination programme. It also led the RIV to begin work on the production of viral
vaccines.

The Netherlands started its national vaccination programme in 1957
using the DPT vaccine produced by the RIV. However, production on
a sufficiently large scale demanded personnel with new skills: people
who would be able to develop the production technology required.
When the Dutch government decided to vaccinate against polio, problems became still more acute. Polio vaccine was first purchased from
the RIT in Belgium. In 1959 the RIV received government permission
to produce polio vaccine itself. This would be the killed virus vaccine,
or IPV, developed by Jonas Salk. (Alternative live vaccines were still
undergoing field trials. Albert Sabin's live oral vaccine – OPV – would
only be licensed in the USA in 1960.)

With the aid of new technology developed in the Institute, within a
relatively short time RIV had an innovative system in which polio virus
was grown continuously on layers of monkey kidney cells, themselves
growing on minute beads or 'microcarriers'.[14] Hans Cohen, head of the
Institute's vaccine department[15] saw that by combining the polio vaccine

with the DPT already in use, it should be possible to avoid additional vaccinations and so maintain coverage levels. Thus, a start was made, in parallel, with development of a combination DPT-P vaccine, and by 1962 RIV had succeeded in producing it. Success in controlling polio with IPV was such that the Netherlands felt no need to switch to the Sabin OPV as almost all other manufacturers, and countries (except Sweden and the other Scandinavian countries) were doing in the 1960s. On the contrary, the Institute invested considerable resources in further improving the production process and in enhancing the potency of the vaccine.[16]

The crucial point is that RIV production, and also the research and development (R&D) carried out, were wholly shaped by the interests of the national immunisation programme (NIP). The decision not to switch to OPV, whatever the rest of the world was doing, reflected the country's high coverage rate and near-success in controlling the disease.[17] Polio vaccine was combined with the existing DPT vaccine in order to avoid the need for an additional visit to the doctor or child health centre, which could have brought down the coverage level. A stronger ('enhanced') IPV was developed in order to reduce the number of vaccinations required. Sustaining the national vaccination programme and avoiding any changes were at the heart of the Institute's strategy. There was little or no interest in developing markets outside the Netherlands – a non-commercial culture which some members of staff would later find uncongenial.[18]

In the mid-1960s, and in parallel with many institutions elsewhere, RIV turned its attention to two other viral diseases: measles and rubella (German measles). As with polio vaccine development, these vaccines could be produced either by *inactivating* the virus, so producing a 'killed' virus vaccine, or by *attenuating* it by passing it through an appropriate cell culture. Salk's polio vaccine had been produced in the former manner, Sabin's in the latter. While many virologists had always been sceptical about the efficacy of killed virus vaccines, they did seem to be safer. There was no chance of their reverting to virulence, as occasionally happened with the live polio virus vaccine. Still, whichever route was chosen difficult decisions were unavoidable. How best to inactivate the virus? Or, if it were to be attenuated, in what medium, and how much attenuation was required to produce a vaccine that was both safe and effective?

Influenced by their earlier successes with inactivated polio vaccine, both Dutch and Swedish scientists began work on inactivated measles vaccine.[19] The Dutch researchers hoped to combine an inactivated measles vaccine with the four component vaccine then being used in the national vaccination programme. This work was continued despite an emerging consensus in the USA that the protection provided by inactivated vaccine was unacceptably short, and that the vaccine could even induce an unusual form of measles.[20] Erling Norrby in Sweden, who had been working on an inactivated measles vaccine since 1959, believed that a different inactivation process from that used in the USA could yield an effective vaccine. The RIV adopted Norrby's method of inactivation, and by 1967 had established a production process.

In December 1967 the Dutch Health Council (the government's principal advisory body on medical research and innovation) issued a report on measles vaccines.[21] The Council argued that the country should wait before beginning measles vaccination on a national scale. It was still unclear which vaccine should best be used, and how disruption of the NIP could best be avoided. The Council recommended that further studies, particularly of the inactivated vaccine, should first be carried out. Meanwhile, import of both live and inactivated vaccines should be permitted. Individual medical practitioners could decide whether or not to recommend measles vaccination to their patients, and with which vaccine.[22]

In 1971 the RIV was ready to begin a clinical trial of its pentavalent DPTP-M vaccine. The results of the trial were, however, so disappointing that this line of work was aborted in 1973.[23] In 1974 live *Attenuvax* was purchased from Merck, and in 1976 mass measles immunisation began in the Netherlands. The country's very high immunisation rate was not compromised, and measles incidence declined rapidly.

By 1976, a vaccine against another potentially serious viral disease was added to the NIP. This was rubella, or German measles. RIV had begun studying the possibilities of producing a rubella vaccine in the early 1960s, more or less at the same time as work on a measles vaccine began. It had been established long before that rubella contracted during pregnancy could lead to spontaneous abortion, to central nervous system defects, or to one of a range of other serious and debilitating conditions in a new-born child (congenital rubella syndrome, or CRS). The epidemic that struck the USA in 1963–65 was said to be responsible for some 20,000 fetal deaths and a similar number of brain-damaged children. There was growing public and political pressure to produce a vaccine.[24]

Attempts to develop an inactivated virus rubella vaccine were soon abandoned. However, because investigators in different places used different virus strains, and attenuated them in different ways, competing vaccines emerged. These included the 'HPV77' developed at the NIH Division of Biologics Standards; the 'Cendehill' developed at RIT in Belgium (soon to be taken over by SmithKline & French); and 'RA27/3' developed by Stanley Plotkin in Philadelphia, using a culture made from aborted fetuses.[25]

By 1970 a number of rubella vaccines were commercially available. In the UK SmithKline's 'Cendevax' (using the Cendehill strain) and Burroughs Wellcome's 'Almevax' (an RA27/3 vaccine) were licensed. Discussion of the relative merits of these vaccines was more protracted and more complex than was the case with measles vaccines. Control of rubella presented a unique problem, because its 'ultimate goal … is a remote one, namely the protection of some future fetus against damage from intrauterine infection.'[26] This meant that the possibility of immunity declining with time was particularly important, since it could result in a more susceptible population of women of childbearing age.[27]

By 1971 the RIV had obtained an HPV77 strain from the USA and had attenuated it further. Trials suggested that this further attenuated vaccine was comparable with commercial vaccines in terms of effectiveness and safety, and by 1973 the RIV was convinced that it should be added to the NIP. Starting in 1974, 11-year-old girls (only) were vaccinated. Reported cases fell from 2,000–3,000 per year in the early 1970s to roughly 700–800 in the years thereafter. However, it was still unclear whether the protection would last until the time of an eventual pregnancy. Unlike most European countries, strategy in the USA was to vaccinate both boys and girls. The objective was then not protection of the individual woman, as in Europe, but to halt circulation of the virus. The relative benefits of the two approaches would become a matter for discussion in the Netherlands and in Europe more widely.[28]

RIVM in the 1980s and 1990s

In 1984 two other institutes, working in the field of environmental health, were merged with RIV, and the expanded institute was renamed the Rijksinstituut voor Volksgezondheid en Milieuhygiene (RIVM). Hans Cohen, Director General of RIV, became head of the RIVM. Internal reorganisations followed. What had previously been separate departments, one for vaccine production and the other for microbiology (diagnostics, epidemiology), were integrated. This would enable the Institute's vaccine work to more effectively reflect the changing disease patterns shown by epidemiological surveillance. As the ex-head of the vaccine sector later explained;

> That is both structurally and psychologically an important point because earlier vaccines had been something of a separate world within the RIV. The advantage now was that you could say: so, why are we making vaccines. Because we want to control the infectious disease problem in the Netherlands. So not as a kind of independent thing ... we're a vaccine producer, but also – and that is politically very important – you can say that infectious disease control in the Netherlands is possible partly because we have a RVP. And what do you need for that? Vaccines.[29]

Far-reaching changes were, however, taking place in the broader vaccine field. These included the new approaches to developing vaccines based on genetic engineering, and they included changes in the structure of the vaccine industry (the mergers that were starting to take place). Still more profound changes were taking place in the world of politics and business within which vaccine development and production took place. One such change was an increasingly aggressive attitude to the protection of intellectual property rights. Years before, knowledge and expertise had been freely exchanged, even between public and private sector vaccine institutions. By the 1980s this was no longer the case. Commercial vaccine producers were starting to patent everything they could, and to enforce secrecy on academic researchers whose work they funded.[30] The free play of market forces was coming to be seen as the only efficient way of allocating resources, and the role of the state (and public expenditure) was to be reduced as far as possible. All these developments, taking place in the 1980s, had inevitable implications for the Dutch Institute's functioning.

One consequence of the changing ideological climate was that in the early 1980s state production of vaccines came to be questioned for the first time. Given the ideologically inspired wave of free-market thinking that was then sweeping the world, it is hardly surprising that some

Dutch politicians began to question the Institute's role. For the first time, it was becoming necessary to defend the existence of RIVM as a state vaccine producer.

At about this time (the early 1980s) the Canadian Connaught Laboratories (not yet taken over by Pasteur Mérieux) talked with the agency that represented the Dutch Ministry of Economic Affairs in North America. It was suggested to Connaught that acquisition of RIVM's vaccine production could offer the firm a means of entering the European vaccine market. Whereas the Ministry of Economic Affairs appears to have encouraged the Connaught initiative, the RIVM, which fell under (and was funded by) the Ministry of Health, did not wish to be taken over. RIVM felt itself perfectly capable of meeting the country's vaccine needs. Resisting takeover, the RIVM was supported by its parent ministry. In the late 1980s Berna, a commercial producer based in Switzerland,[31] also attempted a takeover of RIV vaccine production. This too was successfully opposed. But it was clear that the Institute's future as a vaccine producer was far from secure.

This episode illustrates a change in how vaccines were perceived, politically. In the Netherlands they had been viewed almost exclusively as tools of public health: the tools with which the state could best protect its citizens against infectious disease. Paediatric vaccines were paid for by the state and provided freely. But vaccines could also be viewed as sophisticated technologies with economic/export potential. Friction between the ministries of health and of economic affairs (responsible for industrial policy) reflected the gap between these two perspectives, not easily bridged in the increasingly polarised ideological climate of the 1980s.

The changing political climate, and the threat of privatisation, led to a number of organisational initiatives being taken. Thus at the end of the 1980s vaccine production was separated from the RIVM's other responsibilities in vaccine R&D, regulatory control and epidemiological surveillance. Production was brought under a new entity, SVM. SVM was a foundation, wholly owned by RIVM, but no longer a government agency. The Director General of RIVM functioned also as chair of the board of the SVM. This restructuring was intended to protect public sector vaccine production against private sector challenges, but also to provide a buffer against fluctuations (reductions) in funding from the state budget. Moreover, it provided a clearer separation of vaccine production from the government's control function. A single institution that combined a quasi-commercial manufacturing role with both regulatory functions (ensuring that products were of proper quality) and advisory responsibilities (advising on which products were to be used) was coming to be seen as inappropriate.[32] The WHO insisted on the importance of independent quality control if safety were to be guaranteed. Others argued that state production represented an unacceptable interference with 'fair trade'.

RIVM began to explore the possibility of strategic partnerships with comparable institutions in Scandinavia. It might be possible to pool expertise, share production and benefit from some economies of scale. Discussion with sister institutes in Denmark, Finland, Norway and Sweden led to the idea of a Dutch-Nordic consortium, and this was formally established in 1990. One of its functions would be to facilitate technology transfer to developing countries. Thus, in 1991 an agreement was signed to jointly develop a conjugate pneumococcal vaccine for use in developing countries. Tasks were divided among the five countries according to their specific expertise.[33] However, problems soon arose. These included confusion over the ownership of the technology, a lack of funding and privatisation. The SBL, one of the participants in the consortium, was privatised in 1993. In Denmark there was talk of privatising the SSI's vaccine production (though this step was ultimately not taken). These accumulating difficulties led to collapse of the consortium. Nevertheless, under WHO auspices RIVM continued to emphasise and develop its role as a non-commercial centre of expertise for developing countries.[34]

However, to understand the challenges confronting the Institute from the 1980s onwards it is not enough to focus only on the macro politics. Resisting 'assaults' from the private sector, changing legal status and cooperation agreements were institutional responses to a profoundly changing world. But the fact is that the Institute's expertise and its functioning were being eroded by more subtle changes over which it could have no possible influence, and which it was powerless to resist. In order to see how this was so we need to look in more detail at the Institute's substantive work in the vaccine field.

Since 1974, Dutch girls had been vaccinated against rubella at the age of 11 with a vaccine produced by the Institute. By the early 1980s, there was a growing international consensus that the rubella vaccination strategy should aim not at protection of the individual woman before she became pregnant, but at stopping circulation of the virus. Further, research elsewhere suggested that this could only be done by vaccinating both boys and girls: the strategy followed by the USA.[35] Discussions in the Dutch government's Health Council were leading to a consensus regarding the need to change the rubella vaccination strategy. These discussions also challenged the Institute's choice of rubella virus strain.[36]

Whereas RIV made use of the HPV77 strain, commercial manufacturers were all switching to the RA27/3 strain, which was claimed to have a higher immunogenicity. Members of a Health Council committee urged the Institute to change its rubella vaccine. In response, in 1981, the RIV carried out a study in Rotterdam. Half of the girls in the study were given the existing RIV vaccine, and half were given a commercial RA27/3 vaccine. RIV researchers concluded from this study that both vaccines produced a more than adequate response and saw no reason to switch to an RA27/3 vaccine.[37] The Institute argued that both vaccines were perfectly good, a switch would be expensive and would yield virtually no benefit. Not everyone agreed. A Belgian member of the Health Council committee, a virologist, argued that the Netherlands *should* switch, as Belgium had done, mainly in the interests of public confidence. Whatever research showed, there was a risk of controversy and public loss of trust if people believed they were being given an inferior vaccine. Despite the results of its own studies in 1984 the Institute started working with the RA27/3 strain.

A further challenge followed. The Minister of Health had asked the Health Council to consider the desirability of beginning vaccination against mumps. Mumps mortality was minimal, and many general practitioners considered it an unpleasant but fairly routine phase in a child's development. Because of this RIV had not done any work on mumps vaccine. However, a number of manufacturers had, and commercial mumps vaccines had been available since the late 1960s.

By the early 1970s Merck had combined mumps vaccine with measles and rubella vaccines to produce MMR. In 1984 the Health Council advised the minister that vaccination against mumps was desirable, and that MMR vaccine be introduced in the Netherlands. Its arguments in support of this recommendation had nothing to do with mumps mortality (which remained minimal). They were in part economic (looking at the costs of school absences and treatment of children who contracted mumps), and in part they reflected the conviction on the part of some experts that the Netherlands should harmonise its immunisation practice with those of other European countries. This argument was to be made with increasing stridency in subsequent years.[38]

Foreseeing that it would ultimately be required to provide a vaccine against mumps, the RIVM had begun considering the options. They would try to provide an MMR vaccine which included their existing measles and rubella vaccines, and a mumps strain obtained from one of the commercial manufacturers. A number of different strains were being used in commercial vaccines. The preference was for the Jeryl Lynn strain, which was used by Merck. Negotiations with Merck's European subsidiary (MSD) regarding the production of mumps vaccine under licence began in 1982. They broke down, however, when it became clear that Merck would consider licensing its combined MMR vaccine, but not the single mumps component. When the Minister of Health, following Health Council advice, decided that the country would switch to a combined MMR vaccine, the Institute would have to provide it. How was this to be accomplished? Looking back, the then head of the RIVM's vaccine department recalls that

> The end of the story is that we had to forget about our own measles and rubella. We could only do it by producing the threefold vaccine under licence from one of the companies. That's what happened. I negotiated with the Belgians, and the French, and with Merck and we ultimately chose for Merck. It was impossible otherwise.[39]

This was not an isolated episode. Subsequent events show further erosion in the Institute's expertise. They also show that the Institute could no longer engage with commercial vaccine manufacturers in the way that it once had.[40] These developments, and the changing environment in which the Institute worked, are well illustrated by its involvement in the production of whooping cough vaccine.

Whooping cough (pertussis) vaccines had been in widespread use for decades. Nevertheless, they were known to have more side effects than most other vaccines. Though these were worrying for parents they were generally soon over and rarely serious. However, in the 1970s reports appeared suggesting that the vaccine could cause encephalitis.[41]

These reports were greeted with alarm, and in both Sweden and Japan vaccination against whooping cough was halted and numbers of cases rose rapidly.[42] In the USA hundreds of lawsuits were filed, claiming billions of dollars in damages from vaccine manufacturers. Fearful of crippling litigation, all but two US manufacturers of DTP withdrew from the market, provoking fears of a vaccine shortage. This was a major incentive to the establishment of the National Childhood Vaccine Injury Compensation Program in 1986. Vaccine manufacturers set about developing so-called 'acellular' pertussis vaccines which would not have these side effects, and by the early 1990s many were offering a new combination DTP vaccine in which the old 'whole cell' pertussis component had been replaced by the new acellular vaccine.

However, the results of the trials, in which different acellular vaccines were compared with each other but also with some of the older vaccines, were not easy to interpret. The problem of the side effects had been solved, but the efficacy of the new vaccines was less clear. Some of the old whole cell vaccines were more effective than the new vaccines, though not all were. What did this imply? What should public health authorities do? According to one authoritative review 'health authorities are thus faced with a difficult choice. Should the better efficacy of certain whole cell vaccines be traded for the better tolerance of acellular vaccines?'[43] Because this trade-off depends on the particular whole cell vaccine in use, there is no simple and unambiguous answer.

The fears that had led to suspension of pertussis vaccination in Japan and Sweden did not affect the Netherlands. In 1988 the Dutch Health Council advised that though a switch to an acellular vaccine might ultimately be desirable the time was not yet right. Too little was known of their efficacy. By the 1990s it was becoming clear that there was nevertheless a problem. Not only was the incidence of whooping cough rising, but there seemed to be a shift in the population groups principally at risk. What had been a disease largely of young children was coming to affect older children and adults.[44] From the late 1990s onwards, in a series of reports, the Health Council advised that, for whatever reason, the locally produced vaccine no longer worked. The Netherlands should switch to the acellular vaccine being used elsewhere, and the Institute was instructed to work towards introduction of an acellular vaccine.

The Institute's scientists were not all convinced that an acellular vaccine was the answer to the long-term control of pertussis.[45] Some believed that in the long term the answer lay with a good whole cell vaccine such as was still being used in the UK and France. However, manufacturers of these 'good whole cell vaccines' were unwilling to supply them under licence. Development of the new acellular vaccine had required a considerable investment, and it was being sold for approximately three times the price of the old vaccine. Manufacturers wished to phase out production of the old vaccine.

As the introduction of acellular vaccine became inevitable the Institute had two options: it could replace the whole combination DPTP, or else it could combine a commercial acellular vaccine with the other locally produced components. The Institute preferred the latter course, for reasons that had much to do with its perception of its status and functions.

> We could have just bought a vaccine of course but in the first place it's much more expensive. In the second place, if you buy it, you buy the whole combination then you lose all the knowledge and production here. Then you just become a sort of warehouse, no longer a knowledge institute. It could have been injected immediately, but that's less important.[46]

These views were not universally shared, even within the public sector itself:

> We found from the very beginning that a DTaP-P had to be imported and however important an RIVM/SVM/NVI is for all the knowledge and expertise that we have in the Netherlands, that the interest of children had to be the primary consideration, and that a more effective vaccine is always more important than maintenance of our own production capacity. We still believe that.[47]

The difficulties that the Institute confronted in the 1980s and (increasingly) in the 1990s, were of a different order from the technical difficulties they had previously faced in trying to develop an inactivated measles vaccine. By the mid-1980s the Institute was confronting a changed industry. Pharmaceutical companies, increasingly multinational, jealously guarded knowledge that had now become 'intellectual property'. They no longer offered the easy collaboration they had once done, and the relationships that RIV had enjoyed with Mérieux in the

1960s and early 1970s were unthinkable by the 1990s. Moreover, at the political level perspectives were also changing. Reflecting moves towards European integration, there was a growing sense that the Netherlands should do the same as neighbouring countries. The implications for policy making and for the evidence on which policy should be based were profound. Were national boundaries and national populations the best way to think about public health? Did national experience and local epidemiological data offer the appropriate evidential base for policy?

The Institute's experiences in the 1980s and 1990s highlight a number of developments which were increasingly influencing its functioning and reducing its room for manoeuvre. The first one derives from changes in technology, industry and economic ideology. New and improved vaccines were being produced by sophisticated biotechnological processes, and the technology involved had been appropriated – and patented – by large pharmaceutical manufacturers. In sharp contrast to earlier decades, these private corporations were no longer willing freely to collaborate or to share knowledge. Second, and largely based on surveys of public sector producers in developing countries, it was increasingly taken for granted that public sector producers lacked the resources, the freedom from political interference and the expertise to produce good quality vaccines.[48] The third development was an increasing emphasis on standardisation: on the harmonisation of immunisation policies between countries. The fourth development, clearly related to the third, concerns the declining weight attached to 'local' research evidence. RIVM's experience with the alternative rubella strains in the early 1980s fits in a pattern that has become clearer over time. Policy options based on national research are no longer a match for policies based on international research and promoted internationally.[49] Though the relations between these developments is still to be disentangled, the hypothesis that the third and fourth were a consequence of the first has a certain plausibility.

In 1991 Europe's commercial vaccine manufacturers joined together to form the European Vaccine Manufacturers,[50] as a special group within the European Federation of Pharmaceutical Industries Associations, an influential lobby in Brussels. Vaccine manufacturers began to criticise the idea of national immunisation programmes, in the light of moves to European integration.

EVM argued that given the free movement of persons within the EC (now EU) the concept of herd immunity had to be seen in a European context. Europe should move gradually towards a standardised immunisation schedule and a Europe-wide system for testing and evaluation of vaccines. This was not only desirable, in the view of manufacturers, but likely to occur anyway, since 'the availability of new vaccines, coupled to the development of more precise concepts in vaccinology ... drive separate national systems towards similarity in their respective approaches'.[51] The growing involvement of the EU in public health, and subsequent moves toward a European procurement system, are clearly in line with the views of European manufacturers.

By the mid-1990s it was starting to seem that further legal protection was required if the Institute's tasks were to remain a state responsibility. In 1996 legislation was passed, the Law on the RIVM ('Wet op de RIVM') giving a firmer legal basis to the Institute's functioning and independence.

RIVM-NVI: the new millennium

At the beginning of the new millennium the Dutch Cabinet was still committed to maintaining the close link between infectious disease control and vaccine development and supply that the RIVM/SVM structure represented. This commitment was made clear in early 2002. However, there was to be a reorganisation. The vaccine R&D, the responsibility of RIVM, and SVM's production facilities, would be integrated in a new entity to be called the Netherlands Vaccine Institute (NVI). There would be a clearer separation between entities with development/production and control/advice functions.

> The government would seek independent advice regarding the NIP and would arrange for a continuous evaluation of vaccination policy independent of the views of the NVI. The Health Council is the most important advisor in this area. The most important reason for ensuring such independent advice is that *because the government itself produces vaccines through the NVI, there is the danger of giving the impression that the interests of the producer weigh more heavily than those of the public health*. In fact it is impossible wholly to neglect the interests of the public sector producer. This is not only a matter of psychological factors, but also of material arguments such as the importance of continuity in production if the capacity to produce vaccines is to be sustained.[52]

The core tasks of the NVI would be: (1) provision of vaccines for the NIP, for influenza, for travellers, and in case of calamities such as an influenza epidemic; (2) vaccine R&D in the interests of the vaccination programme (including longer-term strategic research not coupled to a specific product); and (3) research to support policy development. The inter-departmental group that planned the restructuring acknowledged that changes in vaccine science and technology, and the costs of developing new vaccines (and vaccine combinations), had profound implications for how the new Institute would work. There would have to be more intensive collaboration, both with international research institutes and with private vaccine manufacturers:

> dependence on industry has increased in recent years, and the availability of (combination) vaccines is less easy to guarantee than was previously the case. In order to guarantee provision in the future, as effectively as possible, requires, among other things, strengthening of public sector collaboration (with the Scandinavian countries and England).[53]

Reorganisation took time, but by 2005 NVI was functioning as intended.

However, by this time the context within which the Institute had to function had become still more complex. The forces with which the Dutch institute had had to contend in the 1980s and 1990s derived from global changes in industrial organisation and economic ideology, and a pressure to standardisation. Now, however, domestic politics were increasingly impacting on vaccine policy. Many authors have written of the growing involvement of 'health care consumers' in policy making, and of an erosion of trust in official pronouncements regarding risks and benefits to public health. In the Netherlands too, it was starting to seem that popular trust in the vaccination programme could no longer be taken for granted. There was a growing reluctance to accept vaccine recommendations on trust and unquestioningly. While NVI's planners had foreseen conflict of interest issues, they had underestimated the extent to which the state's involvement in vaccine production came to be presented as biasing its public health policies.

Yet this is what happened in 2004, when a newly established Vaccination Damage Foundation (Stichting Vaccinatieschade) began a campaign against the whole cell pertussis vaccine then being used in the

Netherlands. In their view the government had for years ignored evidence for the dangers of the existing vaccine. 'The thing is that the old vaccine is being made by the government itself, in the Netherlands Vaccine Institute. If that cannot produce those 800,000 jabs per year, you can just as well close it down. So they are working on their own stuff. That will be available in 2008/2009 at best.'[54]

A few days later the controversy was aired on television and questions were asked in Parliament.[55] Growing numbers of parents were objecting to their children being obliged to accept what they had come to see as an old, inferior vaccine. More and more Dutch parents were demanding that their children be given the new (and therefore better) vaccine. However valid the reasons which led some Dutch scientists to question the long-term value of acellular vaccines, they had been unable to convince the general public. The Health Council, pointing out that the Institute had not been able to develop the vaccine it said was needed, once again advised the Minister that a commercial acellular vaccine be purchased.[56] The country should be brought into line with practice in other Western countries. The Minister of Health finally agreed that in 2005 commercial acellular pertussis vaccine would replace the old whole cell vaccine in the NIP. Explaining his decision in Parliament, he stated that he had been most concerned, and influenced, by the actions of parents. The crucial thing, and the ground for his decision, had been the need to reassure parents and to restore their faith in the vaccination programme as a whole.[57]

In 2009 the commitment that had been reiterated seven years previously – that the state should retain the capacity to produce vaccines – was given up. There was a different government of a different political complexion. In February 2009 the Minister of Health informed Parliament that public sector vaccine production would cease. The production activities were said to be losing money and 'for a small producer such as the NVI it is increasingly difficult to meet increasingly stringent quality standards at an acceptable cost':

> The Netherlands is one of the last European countries with vaccine production in the hands of the government. With this privatization the Netherlands is following the example of other European countries.[58]

Despite the initiatives taken by NVI 'profitable production within the framework of a public sector institution and above all without major investment, is not possible.' Therefore, and despite the opposition of left-wing parliamentary parties, the decision was taken to seek a purchaser for the NVI's production facilities, and in July 2012 their sale to the Serum Institute of India (a private corporation) was announced.

Conclusion

In the 1960s and 1970s the Dutch Institute of Public Health was a significant and respected participant in vaccine development and production. Though it enjoyed good relations with commercial manufacturers, Mérieux in particular, RIV was resolutely non-commercial. Its production and its vaccine development work were oriented to the needs of the country's national immunisation programme. It would provide the public health service with the tools with which the nation's children could best be protected against infectious diseases. Such tools would thus reflect the country's specific epidemiological patterns and threats, its resources, and the functioning of the NIP. As the example of the polio vaccines shows, these tools would not necessarily be the same as those most other countries were purchasing from commercial manufacturers.

In the course of the 1980s, a number of developments began to threaten the way in which vaccine production and development had been steered by the needs of national policy. They included changes in vaccine technology. There were new vaccines, produced by new biotechnological processes, and the technology involved had been patented by large pharmaceutical manufacturers. As a result of mergers and acquisitions, the industry was increasingly dominated by a few multinational corporations. In contrast to the more distinctively national companies that had come before, these multinational corporations were unwilling freely to collaborate or to share knowledge. An ideological shift – the growing influence of free-market economics – provided conceptual support for these giant corporations' attempts to capture global markets. So too did the increasingly aggressive defence – and enforcement – of rigorous intellectual property regimes. The old idea that knowledge essential to safeguarding people's health should be a public good (Salk's ironic 'Can you patent the sun?')[59] no longer held. Now it was 'intellectual property rights' which had to be safeguarded at all costs. It was becoming more and more difficult for the Dutch institute to access the knowledge with which it could provide the country with the new tools that the pharmaceutical industry was offering.

No less important, however, was a change on what, following economic convention, we can call the demand side. The officials and experts responsible for formulating Dutch vaccine policy not only insisted on the introduction of the new biotechnology-produced vaccines, but increasingly insisted that policy must be harmonised with the policies of neighbouring countries. Coincidentally or not, this was the view of the European pharmaceutical industry, with its interest in standardised markets. It was also justified by reference to European integration. The very idea of a nationally autonomous policy, reflecting the distinctive health needs and profile of the Netherlands, was losing credibility. It was because of this that local evidence – the results of local epidemiological studies – was of less and less relevance. Standardised decisions should best be based on 'international' studies from which 'place' had been stripped away and which claimed universal generalisability.

The Institute's history between the late 1980s and the first years of the new millennium is marked by a series of reorganisations, legal protections and struggles against commercial assaults, designed to preserve the Dutch state's ability to provide itself with the public health tools it required. These initiatives ultimately proved inadequate because the real challenge was conceptual and ideological. In a world in which talk of 'public health' is giving way to talk of 'global health' the responsibilities of nation-states are becoming subordinate to those of global institutions.[60] It follows that nation-states no longer require, or have any legitimate reason to seek to preserve, the tools or the competences with which national policies can be developed and pursued. It is, of course, conceivable that the relative weight of the arguments in political discourse will change again. As the 'securitisation', of public health proceeds, European states might feel a need to secure the competences with which to protect their populations against biological assault.[61] Moreover, mistrust provoked by recent insights into commercial influences on global policy making, as manifest in relation to the H1N1 'pandemic', may have more enduring consequences.[62] Time will tell.

Acknowledgements

The author would like to thank Jan Hendriks for his comments on an earlier version of this chapter and the Wellcome Trust for supporting much of the research on which it is based.

Notes

1 See for example P. Baldwin, *Contagion and the State in Europe, 1830–1930* (Cambridge: Cambridge University Press, 1999); J. Colgrove, *State of Immunity. The Politics of Vaccination in Twentieth-Century America* (Berkeley and London: California University Press, 2006).

2 H. van Zon, *Tachtig Jaar RIVM* (Bilthoven: Rijksinstituut voor Volksgezondheid en Milieuhygiëne, 1990), pp. 85–96.

3 See for example D. Arnold, *Colonizing the Body. State Medicine and Epidemic Disease in Nineteenth Century India* (Berkeley and Los Angeles: California University Press, 1993); A. Bashford, 'Foreign Bodies. Vaccination, Contagion and Colonialism in the 19th Century', in A. Bashford and C. Hooker (eds), *Contagion. Historical and Cultural Studies* (New York and London: Routledge, 2001), pp. 39–60.

4 See for example M. Cueto (ed.), *Missionaries of Science. The Rockefeller Foundation & Latin America* (Bloomington, IN: Indiana University Press, 1994); A.-M. Moulin, 'The International Network of the Pasteur Institute, Scientific Innovation and French Tropisms', in C. Charle, J. Schriewer and P. Wagner (eds), *The Emergence of Transnational Intellectual Networks and the Cultural Logic of Nations* (New York: Campus Verlag, 2004), pp. 135–62.

5 See J. S. Smith, *Patenting the Sun. Polio and the Salk Vaccine* (New York: William Morrow and Co., 1990).

6 Office of Technology Assessment (OTA), *Review of Federal Vaccine and Immunization Policies* (Washington, DC: US Government Printing Office, 1979), p. 27.

7 S. S. Blume and I. Geesink, 'Vaccinology: an Industrial Science?' *Science as Culture*, 9:1 (2000), pp. 41–72; L. Galambos L. with E. Sewell, *Networks of Innovation: Vaccine Development at Merck Sharp and Dohme and Mulford, 1895–1995* (Cambridge: Cambridge University Press, 1995).

8 D. C. Mowery and V. Mitchell, 'Improving the Reliability of the US Vaccine Supply: an Evaluation of Alternatives', *Journal of Health Politics, Policy and Law*, 20:4 (1995), p. 978.

9 For example, Burroughs Wellcome (now GlaxoSmithKline), Sclavo (Novartis), Behringwerke (CSL).

10 Interview with P. Olin, Swedish Institute for Infectious Disease Control, Stockholm, conducted by D. Rose, 22 April 1998.

11 In 2011 Crucell was itself acquired by Johnson & Johnson.

12 Tweede Kamer der Staten-Generaal, *Toekomst van het Nederlands Vaccin Instituut*, vergaderjaar 2011–2012, 32 589 nr 4. The Hague.

13 Van Zon, *Tachtig Jaar RIVM*, pp. 169–89.

14 S. S. Blume, 'Lock In, the State and Vaccine Development. Lessons from the History of the Polio Vaccines', *Research Policy*, 34:1 (2005), p. 167.

15 Cohen became Director General in 1979.

16 These developments are discussed at length in Blume, 'Lock In, the State and Vaccine Development'.

17 'Near success' because in deference to the beliefs of the country's highly orthodox Protestant community, immunisation was and is voluntary. Orthodox communities in the country's so-called Bible Belt generally do not vaccinate their children and are subject to epidemics that the rest of the country escapes.

18 It is worth noting that Jonas Salk and the Institut Mérieux, RIV's collaborators in improving the IPV, *did* have an interest in markets outside the Netherlands. In order to restore IPV as a credible alternative to the then dominant OPV, clinical trials in tropical countries would have to show that there was some formulation of the enhanced IPV which was as effective as OPV, and less sensitive to temperature. See F. C. Robbins, 'Polio – Historical', in S. A. Plotkin and E. A. Mortimer (eds), *Vaccines* (Philadelphia: W. B. Saunders, 1988), pp. 98–114.

19 This section is based on J. Hendriks and S. S. Blume, 'Measles Vaccination Before the Measles-Mumps-Rubella Vaccine', *American Journal of Public Health*, 103:8 (2013), pp. 1393–401.

20 See W. H. Foege, O. S. Leland *et al.*, 'Inactivated Measles – Virus Vaccine. A Field Evaluation', *Public Health Reports*, 80:1 (1965), pp. 60–4; V. A. Fulginiti and C. H. Kempe, 'Killed Measles Virus Vaccine', *Lancet*, 290:7513 (1967), p. 468.

21 Gezondheidsraad (Health Council of the Netherlands) *Rapport Inzake de Vaccinatie tegen Mazelen*. Report 68–430–6 (The Hague, 1968).

22 M. F. Polak, 'Mazzelenvaccinatie', *Nederlands Tijdschrift voor Geneeskunde*, 112:42 (1968), pp. 1905–6.

23 R. Brouwer, 'Vaccination of Infants in Their First Year of Life with Split Inactivated Measles Vaccine Incorporated in a Diphtheria-Pertussis-Tetanus-Polio (Inactivated) Vaccine (DPYP-M) Compared with Live Measles Vaccination', *Journal of Biological Standardization*, 4:1 (1976), pp. 13–23.

24 Galambos, with Sewell, *Networks of Innovation*, p. 105.

25 S. A. Plotkin, 'History of Rubella Vaccines and the Recent History of Cell Culture', in S. Plotkin and B. Fantini (eds), *Vaccinia, Vaccination, Vaccinology. Jenner, Pasteur and their Successors* (Paris: Elsevier, 1996), p. 276.

26 D. M. Horstmann, 'Controlling Rubella. Problems and Perspectives', *Annals of Internal Medicine*, 83:3 (1975), pp. 412–17.

27 P. D. Parkman, 'Making Vaccination Policy: the Experience with Rubella', *Clinical Infectious Diseases*, 28:2, Supplement (1999), pp. S140–S146.

28 E. G. Knox, 'Strategy for Rubella Vaccination', *International Journal of Epidemiology*, 9:1 (1980), pp. 13–23.

29 Interview with J. Ruitenberg conducted by the author and Ingrid Geesink, Amsterdam, 21 December 1998.

30 W. W. Powell, K. W. Koput and L. Smith-Doerr, 'Inter-Organizational Collaboration and the Locus of Innovation: Networks of Learning in Biotechnology', *Administrative Science Quarterly*, 41:1 (1996), pp. 116–45; Blume and Geesink, 'Vaccinology: an Industrial Science?'.

31 In 2006 Berna merged with the Dutch biotechnology company Crucell, the same year in which Crucell acquired SBL-Vaccin.

32 In the interview with Olin it was suggested that this was a major issue in the separation and/or privatisation of SBL-Vaccin.

33 J. Hendriks, in *Report of a Meeting of International Public Sector Vaccinology Institutions* (Geneva: World Health Organization, 16–17 March 2000), p. 24.

34 J. Hendriks, 'Technology Transfer in Human Vaccinology. A Retrospective Review on Public Sector Contributions in a Privatizing Science Field', *Vaccine*, 30:44 (2012), pp. 6230–40.

35 Interview with E. Miller, Centre for Infectious Diseases, London, 15 October 2007.

36 This decision is discussed at greater length in S. S. Blume and J. Tump, 'Evidence and Policymaking: the Introduction of MMR Vaccine in the Netherlands', *Social Science & Medicine*, 71:6 (2010), pp. 1049–55.

37 RIV(M) *Berichten uit het RIV(M)*, 1981.

38 See Blume and Tump, 'Evidence and Policymaking', p. 1054.

39 Interview with J. Ruitenberg, 21 December 1998.

40 Notes on an interview with a senior scientist who had resigned from RIVM to join (what was then) SmithKlineBeecham. 'We talked about the relations between commercial and state institutes. At one point he used the word "versus" … about which I asked him "why one *versus* the other?" He corrected himself: "Of course it's not like that but that is how it was seen in RIVM"' (interview by the author, Amsterdam, 10 November 1997).

41 G. T. Stewart, 'Vaccination Against Whooping Cough. Efficacy Versus Risk', *Lancet*, 1:8005 (1977), pp. 234–7.
42 E. J. Gangarosa, A. M. Galazka, C. R. Wolfe *et al.*, 'Impact of Antivaccine Movements on Pertussis Control: The Untold Story', *Lancet*, 351:9099 (1988), pp. 356–61.
43 S. A. Plotkin and M. Cadoz, 'The Acellular Pertussis Vaccine Trials: an Interpretation', *Pediatric Infectious Disease Journal*, 16:5 (1997), pp. 508–17.
44 Dutch work on pertussis vaccines is discussed in more detail in S. S. Blume and M. Zanders, 'Vaccine Independence, Local Competences and Globalization. Lessons from the History of Pertussis Vaccine', *Social Science & Medicine*, 63:7 (2006), pp. 1825–35.
45 Their doubts were partly based on the theory that the pertussis bacterium was mutating (as the influenza virus is known to do) so that the more precisely a vaccine was tailored to strains in circulation at any one time, the lower its efficacy in the long term. This theory was, and remains, controversial. See NRC, 'Stammenstrijd om kinkhoest', *NRC Weekend* (23–4 March 2013), pp. 4–5.
46 Interview with laboratory scientist responsible for quality control of biological products, quoted in Blume and Zanders, 'Vaccine Independence, Local Competences and Globalization', p. 1831.
47 Interview with public health physician, government adviser, quoted in Blume and Zanders 'Vaccine Independence, Local Competences and Globalization', p. 1831.
48 For example, an inquiry by the Children's Vaccine Initiative (CVI) found: 'The private sector, particularly commercial pharmaceutical and vaccine manufacturers in industrialized countries, research institutions which were characterized by outdated technology and facilities, cheap labour and uncertain and unreliable products'. The indicators with which Milstien and colleagues evaluated local producers – including the right to hire and fire and to set salary levels, and a multi-year business plan – could be seen as unfavourable to public sector producers. See J. Milstien, A. Batson and W. Meaney, 'A Systematic Method for Evaluating the Potential Viability of Local Vaccine Producers', *Vaccine*, 15:12–13 (1997), pp. 1358–63.
49 D. Behague, C. Tawiah, M. Rosato *et al.*, 'Evidence-Based Policy-Making: the Implications of Globally-Applicable Research for Context-Specific Problem-Solving in Developing Countries', *Social Science & Medicine*, 69:10 (2009), pp. 1539–46.
50 Now renamed Vaccines Europe.
51 European Vaccine Manufacturers (EVM), *Study on Vaccines for Human Use and their Rational Use in Europe and Worldwide* (Brussels: European Federation of Pharmaceutical Industries' Associations, 1994) p. 48.

52 Nederlands Vaccin Instituut (NVI), *Kaderstelling Externe Sturing. Project Vorming NVI.*(Bilthoven: NVI, 2002) p. 12. Author's translation, italics added.

53 *Ibid.*, p. 17.

54 *Het Parool*, *Stichting vindt vaccine kinkhoest gevaarlijk* (5 January 2004), p. 4.

55 Tweede Kamer der Staten Generaal, *Aanhangsel van de Handelingen*, vergaderjaar 2003–4. Vragen 683–86.

56 Gezondheidsraad, *Vaccinatie tegen kinkhoest*. The Hague, document 04, 2004.

57 Blume and Zanders, 'Vaccine Independence, Local Competences and Globalization', p. 1833.

58 Tweede Kamer der Staten-Generaal, Brief van de Minister van Volksgezondheid, Welzijn en Sport 22 894, 'Preventiebeleid voor de volksgezondheid'. Vergaderjaar 2008–2009, Nr. 213 Den Haag 2009.

59 'Jonas Salk', in Wikipedia. See also Smith, *Patenting the Sun*.

60 T. M. Brown, M. Cueto and E. Fee, 'The World Health Organization and the Transition from International to Global Public Health', *American Journal of Public Health*, 96:1 (2006), pp. 62–72; D. P. Fidler, *SARS, Governance and the Globalization of Disease* (London and New York: Palgrave Macmillan, 2004); S. Roalkvam, D. McNeill and S. Blume (eds), *Protecting the World's Children: Immunisation Policies and Practices*. Oxford, Oxford University Press, 2013).

61 On securitisation see for example S. E. Davies, 'Securitizing Infectious Disease', *International Affairs*, 84:2 (2008), pp. 295–313; S. Rushton, 'Global Health Security: Security for Whom? Security from What?', *Political Studies*, 59:4 (2011), pp. 779–96.

62 Among many critical responses to decision-making around the 2009–10 H1N1 outbreak see for example D. De Wit, *Dossier Mexicaanse Griep. Een Kleine Griep met Grote Gevolgen* (Rotterdam: Lemniscaat, 2010); H. Engelenburg, 'Beleid grieppandemie ruikt verdacht', *Financieel Dagblad* (31 March 2010), p. 7 (on the Netherlands) and R. Ramesh, 'Report Condemns Swine Flu Experts' Ties to Big Pharma', *Guardian* (4 June 2010) (on the UK).

7

Yellow fever vaccine in Brazil: fighting a tropical scourge, modernising the nation

Jaime Benchimol

Introduction

In the wake of the Pasteurian revolution, vaccines and serums were developed for yellow fever in many countries. Yellow fever was one of the key public health challenges in Brazil for at least a century, from the 1850s to the 1950s. During this period, the most notable developments were the Domingos Freire vaccine in the last quarter of the nineteenth century, the vaccine and serum created by Hideyo Noguchi in the 1920s and – beginning in 1928 – a succession of experiments that culminated in large-scale production of the vaccine from 1937 onwards in a Rockefeller Foundation laboratory at the Oswaldo Cruz Institute in Rio de Janeiro (a laboratory which was later taken over by the Institute). In the last quarter of the twentieth century it became a cornerstone for major transformations in vaccine production capacity and regarding the use of vaccines to fight other diseases in Brazil.

I see these vaccines as complex sociotechnical constructs involving many different phenomena: the interactions of microorganisms, culture media and other physico-chemical and biological components that produce substances with alleged or proven immunisation effectiveness; unique dynamics in the understanding of the aetiology, pathogenesis and transmission of yellow fever; established traditions for fighting the disease in which vaccines play different roles; and different levels of institutionalisation in scientific research, public health, and the production and use of immunological products. Freire and Noguchi's vaccines and the vaccine produced by the Rockefeller Foundation/Oswaldo

Cruz Institute were fraught with controversies that galvanised not only specialists but also various other social actors whose interests were helped or hindered by the route these products took from the laboratory to the public domain. The first two vaccines dwindled from a position of considerable social standing to mere inventions that died out with their respective creators. The 1937 vaccine, after much dispute, became a relatively stable part of the public health machinery, though it is now being overtaken by new developments.

Focusing on the successive yellow fever vaccines, while also alluding to other immunological products, I seek to show how they have influenced the construction of the Brazilian nation state in three distinct periods: the patriarchal oligarchic state (1822–1930), the national developmentalist state (1930–80), and the state which has since then oscillated between liberal dependency and national interventionism.[1]

Yellow fever: from miasma to microbes

Although the New World had seen yellow fever outbreaks ever since its colonisation by Europeans, it was only in the nineteenth century that it became the scourge of the continent, turning two cities, Havana and Rio de Janeiro, into 'infectious volcanoes'.[2] Public hygienists blamed the environment, citing both the nature of the 'torrid latitudes', considered unhealthy for European settlers, and the artificial environment created by urban society. Epidemics developed as regularly as seasonal fruit, always during the hot, rainy periods. Yellow fever seemed perfectly adapted to coastal lowlands, especially the port cities, which were filled with rotting matter. Various interventions were proposed, focusing on the different environmental components seen as the culprits of the disease, depending on the local topography.

In the second half of the nineteenth century, the second Industrial Revolution – of steam trains and ships – made England a world power and led to other consequences in the Americas: the abolition of the slave trade, the consolidation of nation states, the advance of agro-export economies, the growth of port cities and increased migration to these ports. This in turn aggravated the sanitation problems in these cities, where yellow fever was a serious threat precisely because it struck immigrants the hardest. At a time when virulent epidemics were the norm, a new social actor emerged: the microbe.

In December 1879, Domingos José Freire of the Rio de Janeiro School of Medicine announced his discovery of *Cryptococcus xanthogenicus*, and it was not long before he had developed a vaccine for yellow fever. João Batista de Lacerda, the long-serving director of the National Museum of Rio de Janeiro, claimed that *Fungus febris flavae* was the true agent of the disease. Meanwhile, in Mexico, Manoel Carmona y Valle developed another vaccine with *Peronospora luteum*. Juan Carlos Finlay identified *Micrococcus tetragenus* while he was using mosquitoes infected by yellow fever sufferers as live immunising agents. In the 1890s, bacilli were also considered possible causative agents of the disease, and curative serums were developed.[3]

The impact of Freire's vaccine was partly due to the proliferation of microbe hunters, medical and scientific associations and periodicals, colonial and commercial interests, in addition to Freire's zeal in fostering social alliances at a time when science was helping to transform Brazil's political and social structures.

Freire's vaccine

In 1883, the Central Board for Public Health authorised Freire to inoculate people with an attenuated form of *Criptococcus xantogenicus*. At first, the yellow fever vaccine was administered at the Instituto Vacínico, which was responsible for smallpox vaccination, but soon it was taken out to the *cortiços* (slums) and other working-class areas. In the late nineteenth century, Rio de Janeiro was the capital of an imperial slavocracy governed by Emperor Pedro II, and its economy depended on exports of agricultural commodities. Soon, a committee set up by the Imperial Academy of Medicine endorsed the opinion of Jules Rochard of the Academy of Science in Paris: vaccinations should be suspended since the immunity they conferred was still dubious. Nevertheless, vaccination continued, surrounded by controversies that involved an intricate web of personalities and institutions in Brazil and abroad. Britons J. H. Sutton and J. B. Harrison, Frenchmen Félix Le Dantec, Hyacinthe Vincent, Paul Gibier and Victor Cornil, Romanian Victor Babès, and American George Sternberg are a few of the experts involved in verifying the work conducted by Freire and other bacteriologists. All of them favoured their own microbes and ruled out those of the others.

In 1886, Freire presented his ideas at leading French scientific institutions in Paris with the assistance of Claude Rebourgeon, a veterinary surgeon hired by the Brazilian government to introduce the animal smallpox vaccine to Brazil, and Paul Gibier from the Museum of Natural History in Paris.[4] When Freire returned to Brazil in June 1887, he was acclaimed by delegations from different educational and health institutions and by republican and slavery abolitionist groups. Weeks later, he travelled to Washington to take part in the Ninth International Medical Congress, which drew attention to his vaccine among countries affected by yellow fever.[5]

In 1890, George Sternberg, President of the American Public Health Association, published damning conclusions about Freire's vaccine and other discoveries made in Central and South America.[6] His conclusions were endorsed by the Pasteur Institute.[7] This did not prevent the expansion of Freire's vaccine in Brazil, however, which was undergoing a transition from monarchic rule to republicanism, a period marked by political power struggles, rapid economic and demographic changes, and unprecedented devastation caused by yellow fever and other epidemics in Brazilian cities.

Initially, only the poor were given the vaccine, but soon other sectors of society began requesting inoculation, since there was growing scepticism about the drugs used to treat yellow fever patients and the plans to improve sanitation in Rio de Janeiro. After Freire's republican friends seized power in 1889, the Domingos Freire Institute was created, with functions similar to those conferred on the Bacteriology Institute of São Paulo, a state-run health department set up in 1891. These were the first institutional results of the impact of microbiology on Brazil's public health system.[8]

Carried by the abundant influx of migrants to Brazil after the abolition of slavery in May 1888, yellow fever spread to numerous inland towns, strengthening the assumption that it was caused by a microorganism that could travel by train or ship via people or objects. According to a source published in 1898, 13,000 people had been vaccinated by that point in the capital city and the states of Rio de Janeiro, Minas Gerais and São Paulo, and the vaccine had been used as far afield as the British and Spanish Caribbean and other European colonies.[9]

New contributions to yellow fever research by the Italian bacteriologist Giuseppe Sanarelli heightened the competition to discover the real germ and the right cure. Sanarelli was invited to run the Institute for Experimental Hygiene, inaugurated in March 1896 in Montevideo, Uruguay. At a well-attended conference held at the Institute in June 1897, he announced the discovery of *Bacillus icteroides*. Months later, he started field tests with a curative serum in São Paulo.[10] The Rio press begged the Brazilian government to determine whether the true agent of yellow fever had been discovered. Improving sanitation in the Brazilian capital was considered urgent, mostly in order to combat yellow fever, but the uncertainty surrounding the aetiology and prevention of the disease hampered the progress of the social forces interested in cleaning up the city.

Freire's vaccine and microbe fell into disuse after his death on 21 August 1899. The National Academy of Medicine[11] passed a motion to pay homage to him as a 'great servant of humanity', and in the very same session a new member of the academy was appointed: Oswaldo Gonçalves Cruz. Aged just 27 and recently returned from the Pasteur Institute in Paris, he had been put in charge by the federal government of a new laboratory on the Manguinhos farm on the outskirts of Rio de Janeiro, with the goal of manufacturing a serum and vaccine for bubonic plague. Under the leadership of Gonçalves Cruz, a change in the approach to yellow fever was about to propel a new generation of bacteriologists to the front line of public health in Brazil.

Sea change in the approach to yellow fever

Two events lie behind this change in approach: Cuban scientist Carlos Finlay's theory, proposed in 1880–81, that yellow fever was mosquito borne and transmitted by *Culex fasciatus*, a theory conclusively confirmed twenty years later by the US army Yellow Fever Commission headed by Walter Reed.[12] The Americans only conceded defeat to Finlay after occupying Cuba in 1898 and having to face their patent inability to deal with the disease there. Equally important was the presence on the island of Herbert Edward Durham and Walter Myers of the newly founded Liverpool School of Tropical Diseases. In June 1900, soon after Ronald Ross and the Italian team headed by Giovanni Grassi demonstrated that both bird and human malaria were transmitted by *Culex* and *Anopheles* mosquitoes, Durham and Myers travelled via Cuba to the Amazon region to investigate yellow fever.[13] Their hypothesis was that the disease was also transmitted by mosquitoes.

In August, soon after they left Cuba, American physician Jesse William Lazear, a colleague of Reed's on the Yellow Fever Commission, began experiments with mosquitoes supplied by Finlay, while his fellow researchers James Carrol and Aristides Agramonte continued work on what were by then high priority studies of the alleged yellow fever bacillus. In September, Lazear died after he was bitten by mosquitoes infected by yellow fever. Walter Reed hurriedly wrote a preliminary note and began a series of better controlled experiments to prove that the mosquito was the host of the yellow fever 'parasite', that the disease was not transmitted by air, and that fomites were not contagious.

In 1901, the Reed Commission presented its results, William Gorgas inaugurated a mosquito campaign in Havana, and entomologist Frederick Vincent Theobald of the British Museum included the *Culex* species associated with yellow fever in the new genus *Stegomyia*, as *S. fasciata*. The Reed Commission's findings were verified elsewhere; Rio de Janeiro was visited by researchers from Hamburg's Institute for Maritime and Tropical Diseases and, for longer stays, by members of the Pasteur Institute in Paris.[14] The yellow fever campaigns organised by Oswaldo Cruz in Rio de Janeiro (1903–7) and Belém (1909), by Gorgas in Havana and Panama, and by the British and French in parts of West Africa were all based on the idea that the unknown yellow fever agent had only two hosts: humans and a single mosquito species, rechristened *Aedes aegypti* in the 1920s.

The Reed commission left unsolved the hypothesis that the yellow fever agent was a 'filterable virus', and analogies drawn between malaria and yellow fever prompted many researchers to believe it was protozoan. In 1905, Schaudinn and Hoffmann announced the discovery of the syphilis agent, *Spirochaeta pallida* (*Treponema pallidum*). *Spirochaetae* were then seen by some researchers as protozoa. Shortly before this discovery, Schaudinn[15] formulated the hypothesis that a *Spirochaetae* small enough to pass through the finest bacteria filters was the cause of yellow fever. Three years later, Arthur Marston Stimson of the US Public Health Service found *Spirochaeta interrogans* in a victim of the disease. This theory gained much ground during the First World War, when Japanese bacteriologist Ryokichi Inada and his collaborators named *S. icterohaemorrhagiae* the agent of Weil's disease, or haemor-rhagic jaundice, known today as leptospirosis. In 1918, in Guayaquil, Ecuador, Hideyo Noguchi, a bacteriologist with the Rockefeller Insti-tute, described a spirochete as the agent of yellow fever. He established a new genus, *Leptospira*, which encompassed both Inada's agent and this *Leptospira icteroides*, with which he developed a vaccine and a serum for yellow fever.[16]

The Rockefeller Foundation had decided, since 1914, to eradicate yellow fever using the key theory: they would destroy the breeding grounds for *Stegomyia fasciata*, but only in a few endemic centres along the coast, from which the disease was presumed to spread to inland settlements.[17] The campaign began in Guayaquil in November 1918, and by 1922 the Rockefeller Foundation's International Health Board con-sidered the east coast of South America virtually free of the disease. This left Brazil as the main endemic area in the hemisphere. The Foundation's sensitive negotiations with President Artur Bernardes (who was elected in 1922) regarding yellow fever intervention in Brazil were fuelled by an epidemic in the north-eastern part of the country. People there turned to the serum and vaccine produced in Noguchi's laboratory.[18]

On 1 May 1923, the Brazilian government authorised the National Department of Public Health to accept the cooperation of the Inter-national Health Board, despite heated patriotic objections to its inten-tion to take over a field where Brazilian health experts had proven expertise.[19] In November 1923, members of the Rockefeller Founda-tion's anti-yellow fever campaign team set sail from New York, accom-panied by Noguchi, who would stay in Salvador, Bahia, until February 1924. Noguchi's intention was to demonstrate his discoveries to Brazil-ians so as to neutralise criticism voiced by well-known Cuban yellow fever specialists. In a letter to Frederick F. Russell, director general of the International Health Board, Henry Rose Carter assessed Noguchi's time in Brazil as an 'outright success.'[20] As one of the masterminds of the project to eradicate yellow fever worldwide, Carter had taken part in the mission headed by Gorgas in 1916 to map out key centres on the American continent. In the same letter, he wrote that: 'Noguchi showed consummate tact – and tact founded on good feeling – when he had the Brazilians find their own Leptospirae.'[21] Russell endorsed this appraisal in a letter to Noguchi: 'Your success will help our yellow fever campaign in Brazil more than anything else that could have happened.'[22]

New developments in the approach to yellow fever

In 1920, Juan Guiteras Gener, a collaborator of Finlay, succeeded Gorgas as the head of a Rockefeller Foundation commission entrusted with ascertaining whether the measures adopted against yellow fever in the Americas would be viable in West Africa. Studies in the region on *Leptospira icteroides* and attempts to identify authentic clinical cases of yellow fever met with failure. Doctors at the time firmly believed that black people were resistant to yellow fever. The stories that Guiteras heard in Africa and his own statistical inferences prompted him to draw a correlation between the low number of whites and the limited range of the disease, which he thought was dying out on the African continent. Since yellow fever had supposedly originated in the Americas, and since it was almost under control there, Guiteras assumed that it would also die out on the other side of the Atlantic.[23]

In the early 1920s, Carter began investigating the origins of yellow fever, research which was published in book form posthumously.[24] Backed by an arsenal of historical documentation, Carter endorsed the theory defended by Brazilian Emilio Goeldi, former director of the Pará Museum of Natural History and Ethnography, according to which *Stegomyia fasciata*, and therefore yellow fever, were African in origin.[25]

In 1925, a second Rockefeller Foundation commission, headed by Henry Beeuwkes, was sent to Lagos, Nigeria. For two years they examined many cases of yellow fever, but failed to isolate Noguchi's microorganism or to establish a clear epidemiological profile of the disease. This fuelled suspicions that African yellow fever was different from its American counterpart.[26]

In Africa, the colonial authorities often requested Noguchi's serum and vaccine. In 1926, his work began to be questioned by laboratories versed in the techniques of immunology. Two groups, one headed by Max Theiler and Andrew Watson Sellards and the other by Wilhelm Schüffner and Achmad Mochtar, noted that the reactions of *L. icteroides* and *L. icterohemorrhagiae* were identical.[27] This entailed a complex research programme. If *L. icteroides* did not cause yellow fever, that meant that cases of leptospirosis were being misdiagnosed, as

Rockefeller staff in the Americas were using Noguchi's theory to confirm what were frequently unclear diagnoses. At the same time, some specialists believed infectious jaundice to be the yellow fever of temperate zones, and in the opinion of Sellards,[28] the idea that the cycle of the yellow fever agent was confined to man and mosquito required serious scrutiny.

In May 1927, Beeuwkes had purchased some rhesus and crown monkeys from India and marmoset monkeys (saguis) from Brazil. He then set off for Lagos with Adrian Stokes, who had taken part in the first commission sent to Africa in 1920 and who was one of the first researchers in Europe to verify Inada's discoveries. In Kpeve, near Accra, they drew blood samples from patients with mild infections, one of whom was a 28-year-old African male named Asibi. Days later, monkeys and guinea pigs were inoculated with blood from groups of human cases, as it was hard to tell if any one individual had the disease. Some monkeys died, with changes suggestive of yellow fever. In a report dated 14 July 1927, the search narrowed: a rhesus monkey (*Macaca mulata*) inoculated with material from Asibi showed promising signs of the disease. However, there were still many unresolved issues on both sides of the equation. There were few reliable tools for diagnosing human yellow fever, especially mild cases, and very little was known about incubation of the virus in monkeys, whose normal and pathological histology was poorly understood. Furthermore, how could the few strains obtained be preserved? A whole new set of problems was raised by these microorganisms, invisible to the most powerful microscopes and only detectable in the lesions produced as they moved relentlessly from one organism to another.

The Americans and Britons collaborating with them needed a clearcut human case affected by the virus. Human experimentation did indeed take place, but it was involuntary and dramatic: after accidentally becoming infected, Stokes died on 19 September 1927, an incident that promptly accelerated the pace of work. The following year, a preliminary note and then a more comprehensive article were published by Stokes (credited posthumously), Bauer and Hudson,[29] showing that the infection was transmitted from monkey to monkey and from monkey to man by blood injection or by *Aedes aegypti* bite. Bauer also reported on the transmission of yellow fever by three other mosquito species.[30]

In November 1927, Noguchi disembarked in Accra. His observations took him in a totally different direction, which, if proven, would corroborate the idea that American and African yellow fever were in fact distinct but related diseases, like *Leptospira icteroides* and *icterohaemorrhagiae*. He was preparing to return to New York when he was hospitalised with yellow fever and died on 21 May 1928. William Alexander Young, director of the British hospital in Accra, did all he could to preserve evidence of Noguchi's work. Eight days later, however, he too died of yellow fever.[31]

Viral aetiology and a change of strategy

In that same ill-fated month of May 1927, Rio de Janeiro experienced the outbreak of an epidemic[32] demolishing any hopes that it would be an easy task to eradicate yellow fever. The newly discovered evidence from West Africa inspired a flurry of experimental studies and intense exchanges of information among Europe, the Americas and Africa. In the 1920s, yet another characteristic of the virus, which was already linked to sixty-four other diseases, was identified: it depends on living cells to reproduce.[33] New biochemical techniques for manipulating viruses were being developed in the field of virology, which was then emerging from its Pasteurian cocoon.

Diagnosing yellow fever meant interpreting often misleading clinical signs or relying on observations of lesions after death. A new diagnostic technique came into widespread use after 1930, thanks to Max Theiler's discovery that when white mice received intracerebral inoculation, they died of encephalitis and suffered lesions to their central nervous system. In this culture medium new breeds of virus were obtained, with properties not observed in human or animal hosts. The retrospective diagnostic routine performed by hospital pathologists was replaced by a technique that could be used by non-specialised personnel in regions where dissecting corpses was a grievous sin. It involved the viscerotome, an instrument with a handle and blade that could be used to remove a fragment of liver from people who had died of suspect fevers. Viscerotomy posts were set up around Brazil, and systematic research began on the distribution of yellow fever immunity using mice, which revealed the problem to be much broader than imagined.[34]

In 1930, Frederick Lowe Soper was put in charge of totally reorganising Brazil's yellow fever service, taking advantage of new techniques for visualising the disease and also of the revolution of 1930, which brought Getúlio Vargas to power[35] and led to a political environment that was more favourable to the vertical control of both vectors and humans. In order to eradicate *Aedes aegypti* completely, all buildings were numbered and inspected and urban areas were divided up so that one inspector could cover each area in one week. Inspection staff was now part of the service's strictly hierarchical structure for supervising both the population and the work of yellow fever service personnel.[36]

Soper and his Brazilian collaborators[37] verified that in Latin American forests the virus was also transmitted by vectors other than *Aedes aegypti* and that it had other vertebrate hosts besides people. In those vast, sparsely inhabited regions, yellow fever attacked mostly adults who ventured into the jungle.[38] After it was noted that mosquitoes were abundant in the crowns of trees,[39] new collection methodologies made it possible to identify other species associated with the transmission of yellow fever – especially of the genus *Haemagogus* – and other arboviruses.[40] Protection tests, also used on wild animals, helped to identify the virus's vertebrate hosts, such as howler monkeys (genus *Alouata*).

Serological research on the African continent also led to a more precise definition of yellow fever's endemic zone. In addition to *Aedes aegypti*, at least sixteen species proved capable of transmitting the yellow fever virus there. The enzootic cycle in African tropical forests, from monkey to monkey, is sustained mainly by *Aedes africanus*.[41]

In the Americas, the last urban epidemic was reported in 1942, in Sena Madureira, Acre, until urban yellow fever reappeared in 2008 in San Lorenzo, Paraguay.[42] However, the extensive presence of sylvatic (jungle) yellow fever – from Panama to Argentina and from Peru to Brazil – showed that it could adapt to a wide variety of ecologies.

By 1940, the Yellow Fever Service, now run solely by Brazilians, had succeeded in eliminating *Aedes aegypti* over wide stretches of Brazil. After DDT was introduced in 1947, the eradication programme was accelerated. The Pan American Health Organization (PAHO) approved a yellow fever eradication plan for the whole continent in October 1947, the year Soper became head of its executive agency, the Pan American Sanitary Bureau (PASB). Eleven years later, on 2 October 1958, the Fifteenth Pan American Sanitary Conference declared Brazil, the Canal

Zone, and nine additional countries (Belize, Bolivia, Ecuador, French Guiana, Nicaragua, Panama, Paraguay, Peru and Uruguay) free of the urban vector.[43]

Progress towards a new vaccine

Sylvatic yellow fever made vaccine development imperative.[44] In 1928, Max Theiler and Andrew Sellards showed that an injection with serum and virus produced active immunity in monkeys, but serum vaccination was deemed risky after human testing in Rio de Janeiro and Bahia. In 1928–29, Edward Hindle in England and Henrique Aragão and Lemos Monteiro at the Oswaldo Cruz and Butantã Institutes in Brazil made a vaccine from monkey livers and spleens using chemical methods to attenuate the pathogen's virulence. Aragão's vaccine was administered to some 25,000 people in the Brazilian capital.

An alternative to using tissue from live animals materialised in 1931, when it was observed that several membranes of embryonated eggs were susceptible to infection by different viruses. As mentioned, encephalitis developed in white mice inoculated intracerebrally. The virus 'fixed' in this fashion behaved differently from the virus that provoked lesions in organs like the liver. After several passages through mouse brains, the 'neurotropic' virus lost its ability to cause visceral lesions in monkeys, although it still attacked the central nervous system. In 1931, immunisation experiments were conducted at the Rockefeller Institute for Medical Research in New York using the neurotropic virus combined with human immune serum. This vaccine was used to control infections in laboratories. The New York researchers had two goals: modifying the virus by changing the conditions under which it was cultured, so that the resultant strain would display fewer adverse effects and greater immunising power; and obtaining sera richer in antibodies – so-called hyperimmune sera – to better protect people from the risk of the vaccine itself.

In 1936, Lloyd, Theiler and Ricci successfully cultured a virus derived from Asibi, the African patient mentioned earlier, in embryonic mouse tissue. His blood had been injected into a rhesus monkey on 30 June 1927, and over the subsequent six-and-a-half years, the virus had passed through mosquitoes and other monkeys. The letters following the experiment numbers indicated the culture media being tested.

One route yielded 17D, from the same origin but modified through successive cultures in different media, until arriving at in vitro passage through embryonic chick tissue from which the central nervous system had been removed. Using subculture 214, many parallel series were begun, some in embryonated eggs. In 1937, the process yielded what Brazilians called the 'friendly' virus, which protected rhesus monkeys in subsequent inoculations with virulent material and no longer caused encephalitis when injected into their brains (although it still did so in mice).

In March 1937, a laboratory to produce the vaccine opened on the campus of the Oswaldo Cruz Institute. By the end of that year, in municipalities of Minas Gerais experiencing sylvatic yellow fever, 38,077 people were vaccinated. Another 49,000 received coverage during a single week in January 1938. The vaccine was used in Colombia, where production began in January 1939.[45] In 1938, in the south and southeast of Brazil, a wide-ranging sylvatic epidemic prompted the immunisation of 1,059,328 people, primarily in rural settlements.[46]

The vaccine had to be kept at a low temperature, all the more complicated at a time when refrigerators were still rare. To ensure it had survived the trip, each vaccination unit used mice. The first dose from each vial was used for intracerebral inoculation of a group of mice, while the last dose was used on a second group, both of which were observed for twenty-one days. Ending up with an inactive virus or one with a low titre were not the only risks: the yellow fever virus killed mice after the third day.[47]

The move from laboratory to large-scale vaccination was not seamless.[48] At the Oswaldo Cruz Institute laboratory, Hugh Smith and Henrique de Azevedo Penna made important changes to the technique developed in New York to boost vaccine yield. The virus was cultured in live chick embryos, in fertile eggs. On the fifth day, the embryos were extracted, minced and mixed with normal human serum, and filtered. In 1939, certain vaccine batches achieved an immunisation rate of only 20 per cent.[49] The vaccine's decreased antigenic strength was blamed on the many transfers of the virus. The maximum number of subcultures was then set at 255 and the minimum at 210.[50] Vaccination resumed but a new problem cropped up: catarrhal jaundice. A study among those vaccinated in Espírito Santo, Brazil, in 1939–40 identified 1,000 cases and twenty-two deaths.[51] The technique was modified, eliminating the human serum suspected of transmitting another virus, later identified as hepatitis B. In November 1940, vaccination resumed again with a new 17D strain, but the next year a third serious problem surfaced: cases of encephalitis among the immunised due to a mutation of the 'friendly' virus itself.[52] The seed lot system was then introduced, later adopted worldwide in the manufacture of other vaccines.[53]

The problems at the laboratory in Rio de Janeiro seemed to be under control, but not at the New York laboratory, which was still using human serum. It had to move quickly to large-scale production, and the change in technique would require a number of tests. Output was around 56,000 doses in January 1941 and nearly eight million by December, shortly after the USA entered the Second World War. Fearing a biological attack from Japan, in January 1942 the US government decided to vaccinate its entire army.[54] That March, over 28,000 cases of jaundice were detected among newly vaccinated soldiers in California, resulting in sixty-two deaths.[55] Later research with veterans showed that about 330,000 had been infected with hepatitis, the largest hepatitis epidemic recorded in the annals of public health.[56]

The clinical studies performed in Brazil by USA and native specialists after immunisation with the vaccine manufactured on a large scale after 1937 were surprisingly sophisticated compared to those conducted previously for yellow fever vaccines (and maybe vaccines in general),[57] but historians have not yet fully investigated the reactions prompted by such widespread vaccination at this time. Angelo Moreira da Costa Lima, a researcher at the Oswaldo Cruz Institute, accused the Rockefeller Foundation of using Brazilians as human guinea pigs;[58] however, response to his criticism was limited. As part of a well-oiled vertical structure, vaccination teams mobilised the support of mayors, priests, physicians, pharmacists and large landowners in inland towns and farms before setting out to vaccinate local people, who were mostly rural workers subject to long-standing systems of oligarchic domination.[59] It seems that they were willing to receive the yellow fever vaccine, although it would be wise to procure more substantial evidence about consent procedures. Were local leaders and doctors also willing to be vaccinated? How did they behave when they heard about vaccination hazards? We should not forget that in 1904 there was a violent uprising against smallpox vaccination in the Brazilian capital.[60] Yellow fever vaccination, however, benefited from rural sanitation work conducted in the 1930s to 1940s on behalf of vulnerable people. Yet there were often violent reactions to the viscerotomies conducted in inland parts of the country by physicians and laypersons, demonstrating a culture clash between the mentality and knowledge of coastal doctors and the outlook of rural Catholics, for whom death rites were extremely important.

In the 1950s, the Oswaldo Cruz Institute laboratory was meeting the yellow fever vaccine needs of South America and, less regularly, those of Africa, Europe and Asia. Although *Aedes aegypti* was eliminated from various parts of the continent, South America continued to be swept by outbreaks of sylvatic yellow fever. In 1967, *Aedes aegypti* re-emerged in northern Brazil (Pará) and gradually regained its initial territory. A network of viscerotomy posts was re-established in 1979 and a five-year vaccination cycle was implemented in regions exposed to sylvatic yellow fever[61] aimed at people drawn to the Amazon and west-central Brazil thanks to huge settlement, mining and public works projects. The seriousness of the threat was underscored when American actor Jason Robards caught yellow fever while filming *Fitzcarraldo* with director Werner Herzog in the Amazon rainforest.[62] Warning that the disease could re-urbanise, a number of specialists argued that a continental response to the resurgence of *Aedes aegypti* was needed.

The reinfestation of Brazilian cities produced not the feared urban yellow fever but Brazil's first dengue outbreak, which occurred in the northern state of Roraima in 1982. Dengue fever had emerged as an imminent danger with the Cuban epidemics of 1977 and 1981. It became a chronic problem in many Brazilian cities and has been an important research field for entomologists and public health workers since. (As I put the final touches on this chapter, Chikungunya and Zika viruses, transmitted by the same mosquito, emerge as new threat in Brazil.)

Waves of yellow fever in endemic areas in the Afro-American belt and fear of an epidemic in, thus far, unaffected areas of the Far East led to an international symposium in Belém, Brazil, in April 1980, to review aspects of the disease in the light of virology, molecular biology and genetics.[63] The Rio de Janeiro laboratory produced 80 per cent of the world's output of the yellow fever vaccine. The following sections examine its relationship to other vaccines in the context of transformations in global health, Brazilian society, and in the institution that is still Brazil's main vaccine producer.

The Oswaldo Cruz Foundation and immunisation programmes

The laboratory established by the city of Rio de Janeiro in 1900 to manufacture bubonic plague serum and vaccine became the Oswaldo Cruz Institute (IOC) in 1908, primarily in recognition of the successful campaign against yellow fever that Cruz had led in the city, then capital of Brazil. Work at the Institute expanded on three fronts: biological products manufacture, research and teaching. Research carried out into human, animal, and to a lesser extent plant diseases fostered relationships with clients and research communities, reinforcing the Institute's social network. The expansion of frontiers also had geopolitical implications, as it did for the institutes operating in European colonies.

Hired by railway companies, hydroelectric power plants, agricultural and livestock raising enterprises, and extractive industries, Oswaldo Cruz Institute researchers journeyed through the Brazilian hinterlands to study and combat diseases such as malaria. They encountered pathologies about which little or nothing was known, along with biological material that greatly broadened the horizons of tropical medicine in Brazil. The 1909 discovery of Chagas disease – the next human trypanosomiasis to be identified after sleeping sickness – turned protozoology and entomology into central research areas at the Institute. Between the two world wars, it manufactured over thirty products; these largely obviated the need to import immunotherapeutics.[64]

In 1970, during the harshest period of the military regime that took power in 1964, the Oswaldo Cruz Institute was reorganised as the Oswaldo Cruz Foundation (Fiocruz).[65] At this time, modern fermentation methods developed after the Second World War had still not been implemented at the Foundation. With the exception of yellow fever and smallpox vaccines, which were essential for public health, its other products were of dubious quality and did not address the preventable diseases on the agenda of international health organisations.

In the 1960s and 1970s, there were some important synergies between yellow fever and smallpox vaccines. Sixty-four laboratories worldwide, including the foundation named after Oswaldo Cruz, were certified to manufacture the millions of doses required every year for the global campaign, launched in 1967 and ended ten years later. Henrique de Azevedo Penna, who was responsible for the yellow fever vaccine at the Institute, put one of his assistants in charge of modernising the smallpox vaccine, which until then had been produced using live calves, a technique employed since the nineteenth century. Thomas Milton Rivers had made smallpox vaccines in embryonated eggs in the USA, though he failed to obtain good levels of immunity. Penna began culturing the smallpox virus in one membrane of embryonated eggs, without making the mistake of subjecting the virus to more than five passages.[66] Both processes coexisted until the end of the smallpox campaign, which was eradicated from Brazil in 1971.

The campaign boosted confidence in the potential of immunisation programmes to eliminate transmittable diseases. In 1968, while student and workers' movements shook major cities in Brazil and elsewhere, the PAHO held a seminar in Montevideo to discuss why vaccination programmes were obtaining such limited results in the Americas. The problems highlighted included poor planning and decision-making and badly inactivated, preserved and distributed vaccines produced using outdated processes.[67]

In September 1973, Brazil launched its National Immunisation Programme, aimed at controlling measles, tuberculosis, diphtheria, tetanus, pertussis (whooping cough) and polio.[68] In May 1974, the Expanded Programme on Immunization (EPI) was approved by the World Health Assembly, with the aim of reducing morbidity and mortality rates related to these six diseases, and stimulating national and regional self-sufficiency in vaccine production and quality control. Of great importance to the programmes launched at this time was the PAHO's Revolving Fund, created in 1977. Through the joint procurement of vaccination supplies, which meant larger volumes and therefore improved bargaining power with suppliers, the fund effectively enabled drastic price reductions and improved quality.[69] The percentage of vaccination coverage for the selected diseases rose considerably and the programme began to target the eradication of polio, measles and neonatal tetanus.[70]

In the 1970s, there was a growing gap in Brazil between public health, which came under the aegis of the Ministry of Health, and individual health care, which was within the jurisdiction of the welfare system. Health became big business, a trend that went hand in hand with the underfunding of public services.[71] Indicators pointed to a decline in the living standard of those who did not share the benefits of economic growth. The gross domestic product was growing at over 10 per cent a year.[72] Economic policy prioritised durable consumer goods, energy, and transport and communication industries, combining foreign borrowing, tax breaks for major national and foreign investors, wage squeezes, and political and trade union repression. There was a marked concentration of wealth, the public sector and state companies expanded, family and subsistence farming declined, and export-oriented agribusiness flourished. Huge numbers of rural workers migrated to the poverty-stricken outskirts of big cities or to the major worksites and colonisation projects designed to expand land occupation in the Amazon and central-west region.

The Geisel administration (1974–79) launched the Second National Development Plan containing measures designed to strengthen the nation's scientific resources and bring more technology to Brazil, rather than just foreign capital. But by the late 1970s, the signs of economic decline, which would shortly worsen, were already discernible. Foreign debt was growing out of control, inflation started spiralling and industrial growth declined. At the beginning of 1974, a serious meningitis epidemic erupted involving both type C and type A of the *Neisseria meningitidis* bacteria. The Ministry of Health decided to vaccinate everyone in Brazil, something that not even the smallpox campaign had achieved. The vaccine Brazil needed was produced by the Mérieux Institute in France. In March 1975, air shuttle service between the Mérieux factory in Marcy-l'Étoile and Brazil began. In São Paulo, 700 teams vaccinated ten million people in just five days. 'Hundreds of volunteers … with these new needleless syringes … vaccinate, so to speak, *à tour de bras* … men, women and children … The efficacy of the organisation set up by the Brazilians is outstanding!' Charles Mérieux declared.[73]

A new lease of life for the Oswaldo Cruz Foundation

On 5 August 1975, while the campaign against meningitis was underway, President Geisel announced the revival of the Oswaldo Cruz Foundation. The primary objective was to modernise vaccine production through technology transfer. Fiocruz vaccines were produced by a few researchers in laboratories in different buildings of the former Oswaldo Cruz Institute. The only ones delivered on an industrial scale were for smallpox and yellow fever. The yellow fever laboratory formed the core of a new production centre, and Vinícius da Fonseca, the new president of Fiocruz (1975–79), took advantage of the meningitis outbreak to obtain resources, allies and up-to-date technologies.

Brazil's massive orders of the meningitis vaccine helped to convince Charles Mérieux to donate what was required for Brazil to become self-sufficient in a fermentation technique that could be used for other bacterial vaccines. This project was related to global processes that had a major impact on the strategies and organisations of public institutions and businesses in the chemical, pharmaceuticals and biotechnology industry, and on disease prevention policies adopted by states and international health agencies.[74]

In Chapter 6 of this book, Blume analyses how the public and private vaccine production industries in Europe and the USA changed in the 1970s in response to multiple factors: the advent of new biotechnologies; the imposition of intellectual property rights; increased technical difficulties and economic costs incurred in production; increasingly strict surveillance and standardisation of the use of vaccines; and the risk of side effects and related financial consequences. Many companies decided to leave the vaccine market, while others joined via mergers and other market concentration processes.

Under pressure from the French state to scale up its operations, the Pasteur Institute in Paris – the original model for the Oswaldo Cruz Foundation – created the Institut Pasteur Production in 1973.[75] Three years later, a partnership was cemented with Sanofi, a pharmaceuticals subsidiary of Elf-Aquitaine, a French state-owned petrochemicals company. The negotiations divided Institut Pasteur Production into two: one area for vaccines (Pasteur Vaccins) and another for diagnosis reagents (Diagnostics Pasteur).[76] In 1985, Pasteur Vaccins merged with the Mérieux Institute, which had sold part of its shares to Rhône-Poulenc, one of the largest chemical and pharmaceutical companies in France.[77]

Mérieux saw investment in Fiocruz as part of a plan to expand activities on animal and human vaccines around Latin America with his partner, Rhône-Poulenc. In 1975, a contract for the donation of equipment and technical services was signed between the Mérieux and

Oswaldo Cruz foundations, with a view to creating a pilot plant for bivalent meningococcal vaccines at Fiocruz. The plant was opened in June 1976, one month after the restructuring of Fiocruz, with the creation of Bio-Manguinhos to produce vaccines and other biological products, and Far-Manguinhos for chemotherapeutics. Akira Homma, a Brazilian veterinarian working at Bayer in Germany, was hired as director of Bio-Manguinhos. In 1977, still within the ambit of the French-Brazilian cooperation agreement, a Centre for Medical Virology was set up at the Oswaldo Cruz Institute (since 1970 one of Fiocruz's key units).

General João Batista Figueiredo (1979–84) became Brazil's last military president in a period marked by severe economic crisis and the crumbling of the authoritarian regime. With recessive economic policies and rising oil prices, the 1980s came to be known as the 'lost decade' for Brazil. This did not prevent the physical restructuring and intellectual repopulation of Fiocruz. The newly established areas of immunology, biochemistry and molecular biology enhanced its expertise in vaccine and drug innovation.

New alliances took shape between the Brazilian Ministry of Mines and Energy and Japan, which had an interest in Brazil's mineral resources; though no less important was the fact that Akira Homma, director of Bio-Manguinhos, was of Japanese descent. He would later run the Ministry of Health's National Programme for Self-Sufficiency in Immunological Products. Between 1980 and 1984, the Japanese government invested around five million dollars in Fiocruz, supplied equipment, and trained technical staff from Bio-Manguinhos, who subsequently set up the measles vaccine laboratory.[78] The transfer of technology for the Sabin polio vaccine was also covered by the agreement with Japan. This effort helped to control the disease in Brazil. Almost 92,000 vaccination stations were set up for the programme, mostly in schools, and 320,000 workers were involved, most of whom were volunteers. On 12 December 1994, Brazil received a certificate from the WHO attesting to the elimination of wild poliovirus (the last case on the continent was in 1991 in Peru).

For the large-scale immunisation programmes to work, epidemiological surveillance and vaccine quality control had to be improved. In 1981, the National Institute for Quality Control in Health (INCQS), the largest entity of its kind in Latin America, was inaugurated at

Fiocruz.[79] When it failed samples of DPT produced by Syntex, the US multinational stopped production of immunological products in Brazil in reprisal. The closure of other laboratories exacerbated the shortage of vaccines and serums in the country.[80] Stricter quality control, the vaccine sector's lack of funding even in developed countries, the formation of monopsonies like the PAHO's Revolving Fund, Unicef's public tenders, and centralised procurement by the Brazilian government discouraged investment by big international laboratories in the local production of vaccines. An added factor were the huge claims filed against vaccine laboratories in wealthy countries by victims of adverse vaccine events. In this context, Brazil launched its Programme for National Self-Sufficiency in Immunological Products, aimed at modernising the country's public laboratories.[81]

In Chapter 7, Blume studies the Dutch and Swedish response to similar circumstances, which was to privatise their public laboratories. Meanwhile, Carrillo's analysis of the Mexican case shows it to have much in common with Brazil. In Mexico, the state had produced and regulated the use of immunological products since the late nineteenth century. In 1977–78, all of the Mexican public institutes and laboratories that produced vaccines and reagents were merged into a single government entity, the Dirección General de Producción de Biológicos y Reactivos, which became the country's sole producer of such products. With this move, Carrillo says, Mexico became self-sufficient in the field, and by the end of the 1980s was exporting biological products to several Central and South American countries. It lost this self-sufficiency, however, after the government decided to privatise the industry, resulting in the creation in 1999 of Laboratorios de Biológicos y Reactivos de México (Biomex), albeit maintaining a majority shareholding. I now examine how these broader processes interfered with the production and distribution of the yellow fever vaccine in Brazil.

Changes in the vaccine and in yellow fever control tactics

At the international symposium in Belém in 1980, one of the problems discussed was the lack of thermal stability in the yellow fever vaccine, which made distribution dependent on a chain of often impracticable low temperature conditions. Obsolete equipment also hampered larger-scale production. The vaccine consisted of a virus attenuated in chick embryo juice, and medical literature showed that eggs provoke allergic reactions. Moreover, it had been found that yellow fever vaccines manufactured in Brazil and other countries were contaminated with viruses of the avian leukosis group.[82] The approval of a programme to modernise yellow fever vaccines[83] coincided with Bio-Manguinhos' cooperation agreement with the Japanese. The yellow fever laboratory received more sophisticated equipment, facilities, and protocols, boosting its production capacity four-fold. A stabiliser was developed for the vaccine based on the measles vaccine technology.[84] Replacement of embryonated eggs with in vitro cell culture was attempted,[85] but the inoculant consumption was very high and the cost prohibitive: a seed lot, which could feed production in embryonated eggs for ten years, would be exhausted in cell culture in less than one year.[86]

Bio-Manguinhos' most important partner in this innovative endeavour was Canada's International Development Research Centre. Both institutions took part in the modernisation of Nigeria's production laboratory at the height of an epidemic crisis. Fears about the potential urbanisation of yellow fever were rekindled by a new wave of sylvatic yellow fever in Brazil. The number of reported cases rose from three in 1997 to eighty-five in 2000, though we know this is but the tip of the iceberg, with actual mortality rates about 50 per cent higher than reported cases. In the long-standing competition between strategies to combat the urban vector versus vaccination, the second method won out this time. In 1994, the yellow fever vaccine was adopted by Brazil's National Immunisation Programme. Four years later, routine vaccination of children became part of the Expanded Immunisation Programme. Vaccination grew over 600 per cent, soaring from 2,587,788 doses in 1996 to 16,125,871 in 1999.[87]

On 16 October 1999, a 5-year-old girl from Goiânia, Brazil, died days after receiving a dose administered along with the MMR vaccine. Four months later, on 27 February 2000, a 22-year-old woman died in Americana eleven days after being vaccinated with the yellow fever antigen alone. An international committee of experts analysed the two incidents. Passive surveillance of adverse events, introduced in 1998, had recorded 244 incidents, most not serious, out of 34,693,189 doses administered through to March 2000.[88] Two more deaths were identified during retrospective searches. According to Ricardo Galler of the Oswaldo Cruz Foundation, if a selection mechanism had favoured replication of a mutant virus in the vaccine suspension, there would be no way to account for its lethal effect in only two individuals. It was the result of processes triggered after inoculation and linked to the vaccinal virus's interaction with as yet unknown organic peculiarities in the individuals.[89] The expert committee ruled that universal vaccination was no longer advisable but that the risk–benefit equation justified continued vaccination in risk areas, as long as a new protocol was designed for the surveillance of adverse events.[90]

On 23 February 2001, sylvatic yellow fever was confirmed near Belo Horizonte, the capital of Minas Gerais, leaving fifteen dead. Some three million doses of the vaccine were administered in the Belo Horizonte region. On 18 March, another death was linked to the vaccine. Other subsamples of the 17D strain had similar tragic consequences. Up to the present, news of adverse vaccination effects continues to emerge, alongside alarming reports of sylvatic yellow fever close to Latin American cities. Deaths by the disease occurring in early 2008 in San Lorenzo, Paraguay, show that urban yellow fever remains a potential threat.

Post-vaccination accidents have also lent urgency to attempts to clarify the mechanisms of viral virulence and the immune response of the invaded organism.[91] It is known that both the viscerotropism of the wild virus and the neurotropism of the attenuated virus are connected to the intrinsic or genetic properties of both the virus and the vertebrate host. There appear to be some differences between the South American and African types, although their precise nature is unclear. Furthermore, we now have evidence that human immunological response to the disease can be modified by prior exposure to other flaviviruses such as dengue. This cross-protection is actually one of the explanations for the surprising fact that yellow fever has not yet invaded the cities of the Americas.

Bio-Manguinhos is still the world's largest producer of the yellow fever vaccine, but critical changes are about to happen in production techniques based on different approaches still under development. One is infectious clone technology that makes it possible to manipulate the genome of the vaccine virus and engineer mutants capable of expressing heterologous antigens in humans, thereby triggering an immune reaction against more than one disease.[92] Adverse events associated with the live virus explain the current preference for vaccines made of inactivated virus. A vaccine developed by Monath's team, based on chemical methods, is now undergoing clinical trial,[93] while the vaccine developed at the Oswaldo Cruz Foundation using the Vero cell method and inactivation through high hydrostatic pressure is still in the preclinical phase.[94]

In January 2011, Bio-Manguinhos, the Fraunhofer Center for Molecular Biotechnology, and the US company iBio Inc. began another innovative process. The gene that encodes the main protein of the yellow fever virus, which is responsible for inducing an organism's immune response, is being introduced into leaf cells from *Nicotiana benthamina*, a tobacco species. As the plant develops, its leaves produce large amounts of the antigen that can be used in the vaccine. If this biofactory is successful, vaccine production will no longer require special embryonated eggs. These are, however, questions of great complexity that should be dealt with in a separate article.

Conclusion

Domingos Freire's vaccine came at a time when the production of scientific facts was still associated more with individuals than institutions. It was an important catalyst for the reception of Pasteurian medicine in Brazil. At the time, the vaccine was of great symbolic significance, bolstering the dual movements of slavery abolition and republicanism with the power of science. Although the vaccine was presented as a potential redeemer of the nation from the 'slavery' of yellow fever, it never supplanted the sanitisation projects in urban areas, least of all in Rio de Janeiro, then the capital city, where a major urban renewal project was implemented, paralleling Oswaldo Cruz's campaign against yellow fever (1903–7).

At the end of the period of monarchy (1808–89) and in the early republican years known as the First Republic (1889–1930), the Brazilian state was patriarchal, oligarchic, and mercantile, fostered by a society dominated by large-scale export agriculture and mercantile groups. The ruling classes were marked by a patrimonial bureaucracy which, while paying lip service to the ideas of scientific progress, actually demonstrated conservative attitudes and a dependency on the economic and cultural domination of the major world powers. Throughout this period, Britain, France, Germany, and the USA vied for supremacy over Brazil, with the USA finally prevailing in the interwar years. Vaccines and serums helped propel the institutionalisation of microbiology and tropical medicine in south-eastern Brazil, where the country's economic and political power was concentrated. This process was due not least to the efforts of actors and groups who managed to counteract state inertia. Of all the biomedical institutions created at the turn of the twentieth century, it was the one named after Oswaldo Cruz in Rio de Janeiro that took the lead. The yellow fever campaign was crucial for the Institute's capacity to overcome resistance from the oligarchs and trade groups that controlled the state and gain the support of the public and key opinion-forming groups in the country.

Hideyo Noguchi's vaccine and serum were produced in a far more integrated, interdependent global context, where scientific data was disseminated by teams of researchers and institutions subject to state policies and by international health organisations. Noguchi's vaccine and serum never stopped being a backup tool for the campaigns launched in the Americas and Africa, waged in the belief that yellow fever was transmitted by a single vector to just one vertebrate host in a few identifiable key centres. The history of leptospirosis as a globally acknowledged health problem was largely separate from the history of the disintegration of Noguchi's theory of yellow fever. His serum and vaccine seem to have been used most widely in Africa, where the vector eradication campaign did not take off as it did in the Americas. Despite the vast apparatus set in motion by the International Health Board on both sides of the Atlantic, there does not seem to have been much difference between the artisanal production methods for Noguchi's and Freire's immunological products. Both left the scene on the eve of a sea change in the approach to yellow fever.

Beginning in 1928, the development of a new vaccine, the only weapon possible against sylvatic yellow fever, required more complex production processes involving laboratories and specialists from the fields of microbiology, biochemistry, virology, and immunology. Successive vaccines were given to increasingly large numbers of people, surpassing one million by 1938.

The creators of the viral vaccines continued to test their products hastily on humans. Nevertheless, the clinical studies and observations performed by USA and Brazilian specialists in response to cases of low immunity or encephalitis and jaundice after immunisation with the vaccine manufactured after 1937 were very sophisticated. Obviously, the control procedures were far from ideal if we take as a benchmark the standards adopted after the Second World War for research ethics and human experimentation. The 1930 revolution marked the beginning of a period of national developmentalism that prevailed until the 1980s. Throughout successive periods of authoritarian and democratic political rule, industrialisation grew apace, while the state adopted a successful strategy of national development derived from a strong alliance between the industrial bourgeoisie and the state apparatus.

Developmentalist economic policies mostly benefited urban groups who were protected by labour laws and the increasingly comprehensive health care and welfare system. The main target of the yellow fever vaccine was rural populations, and it became an important component of national agencies tackling endemic diseases in the interior. Mediating the relationship between city and countryside, the vaccine was valuable in the expansion of internal frontiers, a process symbolised by the inauguration of the new capital city, Brasilia, on 21 April 1960 during the administration of Juscelino Kubitschek (1956–61). It was during this period that the elimination of *Aedes aegypti* from Brazil and other countries in the Americas was also announced. The yellow fever vaccine was an important facilitator of the large-scale enterprises in agriculture, livestock farming, mining, energy, and infrastructure that were pursued after the 1964 coup d'état.

The yellow fever laboratory served as a cornerstone for important transformations in other vaccines at Fiocruz, which is still the largest supplier in the country and a key player in the health policies adopted since the creation of Brazil's Unified Health Service (SUS), a sort of national health system, an outcome of the new 'Citizen's Constitution' passed in 1988, in which health care was defined as a right of citizens and a duty of the state.

The vaccines and therapeutic agents produced by Fiocruz explain to a large extent the strategic role it plays in SUS. Its future depends on successful connections between these industrial activities and on the ability of Fiocruz research areas to respond to the challenges of innovation in the increasingly competitive world of Big Science, which commands astronomical budgets, increasingly complex national and international networks and teams, and equipment, techniques, and laboratories that must be constantly upgraded. Although new types of vaccines are on the horizon, not least for parasitic diseases, the procedures involved are increasingly complex and new paradigms are emerging at the interface between technical/scientific and socioeconomic issues concerning yellow fever and other diseases, involving vaccinology, molecular biology, genetics, entomology, ecology, and public health.

Notes

1 My reflections on the Brazilian state are based on Luiz Carlos Bresser-Pereira, 'Public Bureaucracy and Ruling Classes in Brazil', *Revista de Sociologia e Política*, 28:3 (2007), pp. 9–30.

2 R. Jorge, *La fièvre jaune et la campagne sanitaire a Rio de Janeiro (1928–1929)* (Paris: Office International d'Hygiene Publique, 1930), p. 7.

3 For a detailed analysis of this process and references to works published at the time, see J. L. Benchimol, *Dos micróbios aos mosquitos. Febre amarela e a revolução pasteuriana no Brasil* (Rio de Janeiro: Editora da UFPR Janeiro/ Editora da Fundação Oswaldo Cruz, 1999), pp. 345–82.

4 Freire's trip and related documentation are analysed in Benchimol, *Dos micróbios aos mosquitos*.

5 'On The Vaccine of Yellow Fever', *Medical News*, 51 (17 September 1887), pp. 330–4.

6 United States Marine Hospital Service, *Report on the Etiology and Prevention of Yellow Fever by George M. Sternberg* (Washington: Government Printing Office, 1890).

7 G. Sternberg, 'Rapport sur la prophylaxie de la fièvre jaune par l'inoculation', *Annales de l'Institut Pasteur*, 4:4 (25 April 1890), p. 253.

8 For more on these institutions, see N. Stepan, *Beginnings of Brazilian Science: Oswaldo Cruz, Medical Research and Policy, 1890–1920* (New York: Science History Publications, 1981); J. L. Benchimol 'Pasteur, la santé publique et la recherche biomédicale au Brésil', in N. T. Lima and M.-H. Marchand (eds), *Louis Pasteur & Oswaldo Cruz* (Rio de Janeiro: Editora Fiocruz/Banco BNP Paribas Brasil SA, 2005), pp. 215–73; also J. L. Benchimol and M. R. Sá, 'Insects, People and Disease: Adolpho Lutz and Tropical Medicine', in J. L. Benchimol and M. R. Sá (eds), *Adolpho Lutz, Obra Completa*, vol. II, book 1: *Yellow Fever, Malaria & Protozoology* (Rio de Janeiro: Ed. Fiocruz, 2005), pp. 245–457.

9 Freire's statistical apparatus is analysed in Benchimol, *Dos micróbios aos mosquitos*.

10 *Ibid.*, pp. 345–82.

11 'Sessão de 24 de Agosto de 1899', *Annaes da Academia de Medicina do Rio de Janeiro*, III, vols 65–6 (Rio de Janeiro: Imprensa Nacional, 1899–1900), pp. 518–21.

12 N. Stepan, 'The Interplay between Socio-economic Factors and Medical Science: Yellow Fever Research, Cuba and the United States', *Social Studies of Science*, 8 (1978), pp. 397–423; F. Delaporte, *Histoire de la fièvre jaune* (Paris: Payot, 1989).

13 J. L. Benchimol, 'Bacteriologia e medicina tropical britânicas: uma incursão a partir da Amazônia (1900–1901)', *Boletim Museu Parense Emílio Goeldi. Ciencias Humanas*, 5:2 (May–August 2010), pp. 315–44.

14 I. Löwy, 'La mission de l'Institut Pasteur à Rio de Janeiro: 1901–1905', in M. Morange, *L'Institut Pasteur, contribution à son histoire* (Paris: La Découverte, 1991), pp. 195–279 and in Benchimol and Sá, 'Insects, People and Disease'.

15 F. Schaudinn, 'Generations und Wirtswechsel bei Trypanosoma und Spirochaete', *Arbeiten aus dem Kaiserl. Gesundheitsamte*, 20:3 (1904), pp. 566–73.

16 I. R. Plesset, *Noguchi and His Patrons* (Cranbury, NJ: Associated University Presses, 1980); J. L. Benchimol, M. R. Sá, K. Kodama, Márcio Magalhães de Andrade, Vivian da SilvaCunha, *Cherry Trees and Coffee Farms: Medical Scientific Relations between Brazil and Japan and the Saga of Hideyo Noguchi* (Rio de Janeiro: Bom Texto, 2009), pp. 511–647.

17 M. Cueto (ed.), *Missionaries of Science: The Rockefeller Foundation & Latin America* (Bloomington and Indianapolis: Indiana University Press, 1994); M. Cueto, 'The Cycles of Eradication: The Rockefeller Foundation and Latin American Public Health, 1918–1940', in P. Weindling (ed.), *International Health Organisations and Movements, 1918–1939* (Cambridge: Cambridge University Press, 1995), pp. 222–43.

18 The correspondence relating to shipments of the vaccine is analysed in Benchimol *et al.*, *Cherry Trees and Coffee Farms*, pp. 231–51.

19 S. C. Williams, 'Nationalism and Public Health: The Convergence of Rockefeller Foundation Technique and Brazilian Federal Authority During the Time of Yellow Fever, 1925–1930', in Cueto (ed.), *Missionaries of Science*, pp. 23–51, on pp. 14–15.

20 H. R. Carter to Frederick Russell, 22 February 1924. RF, box 84, RG 5, IHB/D, S 1 – correspondence, SS 1, General, 1924. F-1207. Yellow Fever Commission, Noguchi, H. January–March 1924. The Rockefeller Archive Center.

21 *Ibid.*

22 F. Russell to Hideyo Noguchi, 24 February 1927. Coll. RF, RG 5, IHB, S-1, SS-1 Box 120 F-1634. The Rockefeller Archive Center.

23 J. Guiteras Gener, 'Expedición al África y estudios de fiebre amarilla', *Anales de la Academia de Ciencias Médicas, Físicas e Naturales de la Habana*, 57 (1920–1921), pp. 265–87, on pp. 272–80.

24 H. R. Carter, *Yellow Fever: An Epidemiological and Historical Study of its Place and Origin* (Baltimore, MD: Williams & Wilkins, 1931).

25 E. Goeldi, *Os mosquitos no Pará* (Pará: Estabelecimento Graphico C. Wiegandt, 1905).

26 Benchimol *et al.*, *Cherry Trees and Coffee Farms*, pp. 511–647.

27 M. Theiler and A. W. Sellards, 'The Relationship of *L. Icterohaemorrhagiae* and *L. icteroides*', *The American Journal of Tropical Medicine*, 6:6 (1926), pp. 383–402; A. W. Sellards and M. Theiler, 'Pfeiffer Reaction and Protection Tests in Leptospiral Jaundice (Weil's Disease) with Leptospira Icterohaemorrhagiae and Leptospira icteroides', *American Journal of Tropical Medicine*, 7 (1927), pp. 369–81; W. Schüffner and A. Mochtar, 'Versuche zur Aufteilung von Leptospiren-stämmen, mit einleitenden Bemerkungen über den Verlauf von Agglutination und Lysis', *Centralblatt für Bakteriologie, Parasitekunde und Infektionskrankheiten*, 101:8 (1927), pp. 405–13; W. Schüffner and A. Mochtar, 'Gelbfieber und Weilsche Krankheit', *Archiv für Schiffs-und Tropen-Hygiene*, 31 (1927), pp. 149–65.

28 A. W. Sellards, 'The Pfeiffer Reaction with Leptospira in Yellow Fever', *American Journal of Tropical Medicine*, 1–7:2 (1927), pp. 71–95.

29 A. Stokes, J. H. Bauer and N. P. Hudson, 'Experimental Transmission of Yellow Fever to Laboratory Animals', *American Journal of Tropical Medicine*, 8 (1928), pp. 103–64; A. Stokes, J. H. Bauer and N. P. Hudson, 'Transmission of Yellow Fever to *Macacus rhesus*, a Preliminary Note', *Journal of the American Medical Association*, 90 (1928b), pp. 253–4.

30 J. H. Bauer, 'Transmission of Yellow Fever by Mosquitoes other than *Aedes aegypti*', *American Journal of Tropical Medicine*, 8:1 (July 1928), pp. 261–82.

31 Plesset, *Noguchi and his Patrons*; Benchimol *et al.*, *Cherry Trees and Coffee Farms*.

32 C. Fraga, *A febre amarella no Brasil. Notas e documentos de uma grande campanha sanitária* (Rio de Janeiro: Off. Graph. da Insp. de Demographia Sanitária, 1930).

33 S. S. Hughes, *The Virus: A History of the Concept* (London: Heinemann Educational Books/New York, Science History Publications, 1977), pp. 93–108.

34 F. L. Soper, 'The Geographical Distribution of Immunity to Yellow Fever in Man in South America', *American Journal of Tropical Medicine*, 17:4 (July 1937), pp. 457–511; W. A. Sawyer, J. H. Bauer and L. Whitman, 'The Distribution of Yellow Fever Immunity in North America, Central America,

The West Indies, Europe, Asia and Australia, with Special Reference to the Specificity of the Protection Test', *American Journal of Tropical Medicine*, 17 (March 1937), pp. 137–61.

35 Getúlio Vargas seized power in Brazil on 3 November 1930. He led the provisional government, was elected president by Parliament in 1934, and was a dictator during the Estado Novo period (1937–45). These were years of profound change in Brazil; the decentralised structure of the previous regime was replaced by strong state control.

36 F. L. Soper, B. D. Wilson, S. Lima and W. S. Antunes, *The Organization of Nationwide Anti-Aedes aegypti Neasures in Brazil* (New York: The Rockefeller Foundation, 1943); I. Löwy, *Virus, moustiques et modernité: la fièvre jaune au Brésil entre science et politique* (Paris: Éditions Contemporaines, 2001).

37 F. L. Soper, H. Penna, E. Cardoso, J. Serafim Jr, M. Frobisher Jr and J. Pinheiro, 'Yellow Fever Without *Aedes aegypti*: Study of a Rural Epidemic in the Valle do Chanaan, Espírito Santo, 1932', *American Journal of Hygiene*, 18 (1933), pp. 555–87.

38 F. L. Soper, 'Progressos realizados nos estudos e combate da febre amarela entre a IX e a X Conferências Sanitárias Panamericanas 1934–1938', *Separata dos Archivos de Hygiene*, 9:1 (February 1939), pp. 3–25, on p. 5; F. L. Soper, *Summary of Activities of the Yellow Fever Service of Ministry of Education of Brazil* (Rio de Janeiro: Imprensa Nacional, 1939), pp. 6–7.

39 F. L Soper and D. B. Wilson, 'Species Eradication: Practical Goal of Species Reduction in the Control of Mosquito-Borne Disease', *Journal of National Malaria Society*, 1 (1942), pp. 5–24.

40 R. A. G. B. Consoli and R. L. de Oliveira, *Principais mosquitos de importância sanitária no Brasil* (Rio de Janeiro: Editora Fiocruz, 1994). pp. 102–34.

41 T. P. Monath, 'Yellow Fever: Victor, Victoria? Conqueror, Conquest? Epidemics and Research in the Last Forty Years and Prospects for the Future', *American Journal of Tropical Medicine and Hygiene*, 45:1 (1991), pp. 1–43, on pp. 31–5; J. Meegan, 'International Aspects of Yellow Fever Prevention', in *Simpósio Internacional sobre Febre Amarela e Dengue, Cinquentenário da introdução da cepa 17D no Brasil* (Rio de Janeiro: Fundação Oswaldo Cruz/Bio-Manguinhos, 15–19 May 1988), pp. 219–31, on p. 219; A. Nasidi, 'Yellow Fever Control: the Nigerian Experience', in *Simpósio Internacional sobre Febre Amarela e Dengue*, pp. 40–64, on pp. 41–2.

42 P. L. Tauil, 'Aspectos críticos do controle da febre amarela no Brasil', *Revista de Saúde Pública*, 44:3 (2010), pp. 555–8; T. P. Monath, 'Review of the Risks and Benefits of Yellow Fever Vaccination Including Some New Analyses', *Expert Review of Vaccines*, 11:4 (2012), pp. 427–48, on p. 437.

43 O. Franco, *História da febre amarela no Brasil* (Rio de Janeiro: Ministério da Saúde, 1969), pp. 144–5.

44 The history of this vaccine is analysed in detail in J. L. Benchimol (ed.), *Febre amarela: a doença e a vacina, uma história inacabada* (Rio de Janeiro: Bio-Manguinhos/Editora Fiocruz, 2001). For reasons of space, I do not refer here to the literature produced by specialists involved in developing the new vaccine. See also Löwy, *Virus, moustiques et modernité* and F. L. Soper, 'Vacinação contra a febre amarela no Brasil, de 1930 a 1937', *Separata dos Archivos de Hygiene*, 7:2 (November 1937), pp. 379–90.

45 H. Groot, 'Sessenta anõs de vacuna antiamarílica', *Biomedica*, 19:4 (1999), pp. 269–71.

46 Soper, *Summary of Activities of the Yellow Fever Service*, pp. 13–17.

47 J. F. da Cunha, interview (Rio de Janeiro: Fiocruz/Casa de Oswaldo Cruz/ Departamento de Arquivo e Documentação, 1987–1988), tape 02.

48 F. L. Soper, 'Febre amarela panamericana, 1938–1942', in *Collected Papers on Yellow Fever*, VII (New York: International Health Division of The Rockefeller Foundation, 1945), pp. 1–12; I. Löwy, 'Le premier scandale du sang contaminé, 1937–1942: le virus de l'hépatite et la vaccination de la fièvre jaune' (Rio de Janeiro: Casa de Oswaldo Cruz, 2000), mimeo; I. Löwy, *Virus, moustiques et modernité*; Benchimol, *Febre amarela: a doença e a vacina*.

49 A. N. Bica, 'Desenvolvimento da cepa 17D e requisitos para a produção da vacina contra a febre amarela', in *Simpósio Internacional sobre Febre Amarela e Dengue*, pp. 155–65, on p. 164.

50 F. L. Soper, H. H. Smith and H. A. Penna, 'Yellow Fever Vaccination: Field Results as Measured by the Mouse Protection Test and Epidemiological Observations', Third International Congress for Microbiology, New York, 2–9 September 1939. *Report of the Proceedings* (New York, 1940), pp. 351–3.

51 J. P. Fox, C. Manso, H. Penna and M. Pará, 'Observations on the Occurrence of Icterus in Brazil Following Vaccination Against Yellow Fever', *American Journal of Hygiene*, 36 (1942), pp. 68–116.

52 J. P. Fox, E. H. Lenette, C. Manso and J. R. S. Aguiar, 'Encephalitis in Man Following Vaccination with 17D Yellow Fever Virus', *American Journal of Hygiene*, 36 (1942), pp. 117–42.

53 J P. Fox, S. L. Kossobudzki and J. Fonseca da Cunha, 'Field Studies on Immune Response to 17D Yellow Fever Virus: Relation to Virus Substrain, Dose and Route of Inoculation', *American Journal of Hygiene*, 38:2 (September 1943), pp. 113–38.

54 M. Furmanski, 'Unlicensed Vaccines and Bioweapon Defense in World War II', *Journal of the American Medical Association*, 282:9 (1 September

1999), pp. 822–3, on p. 822; S. H. Harris, *Factories of Death: Japanese Biological Warfare, 1932–1945 and the American Cover-Up* (New York: Routledge, 1994).

55 W. A. Sawyer, K. F. Meyer, M. D. Eaton, J. H. Bauer, P. Putnam and F. F. Schwentker, 'Jaundice in Army Personnel in the Western Region of the United States and its Relation to Vaccination against Yellow Fever', *American Journal of Hygiene*, 39:3 (May 1944), pp. 337–430, 40:1 (July 1944), pp. 35–107; Löwy, 'Le premier scandale du sang contaminé', pp. 10–15.

56 L. B. Seeff, G. W. Beebe, J. H. Hoofnagle, J. E. Norman, Z. Buskell-Bales, J. G. Waggoner, N. Kaplowitz, R, S. Koff, J. L. Petrini Jr, E. R. Schiff, J. Shorey and M. M. Stanley, 'A Serologic Follow-Up of the 1942 Epidemic of Post-Vaccination Hepatitis in the United States Army', *New England Journal of Medicine*, 316:16 (16 April 1987), pp. 965–70; J. E. Norman, G. W. Beebe, J. H. Hoofnagle and L. B. Seeff, 'Mortality Follow-up of the 1942 Epidemic of Hepatitis B in the US Army', *Hepatology*, 18 (1993), pp. 790–7.

57 On this issue see R. de M. Martins, 'Estudos clínicos som vacinas realizados no âmbito da Fundação Oswaldo Cruz: memória, avaliações e lições' (PhD dissertation, Instituto Oswaldo Cruz, 2014).

58 A. M da Costa Lima, 'Considerações sobre a propagação da febre amarela e a vacinação contra esta doença', *Revista Médico Cirúrgica do Brasil*, 46 (March 1938), pp. 371–82.

59 By November 1941, 2,084,668 individuals had been vaccinated in Brazil, most of rural origin. 'Ligeiros dados sobre os 25 anos de atividade da Fundação Rockefeller no Brasil no período de 1916 a 1941'. Centro de Pesquisa e Documentação de História Contemporânea de Brasil (Rio de Janeiro), CPDOC, GC 35.02.15/h, p. 12. Typed doc. 13 pp.

60 Discussion of this important episode in the history of Brazilian public health can be found in J. L. Benchimol, 'Reforma urbana e revolta da vacina na cidade do Rio de Janeiro', and in J. Ferreira and L. de A. Neves, *O Brasil republicano. Economia e sociedade, poder e política, cultura e representações*, vol. 1 (Rio de Janeiro: Editora Civilização Brasileira, 2003), pp. 231–86.

61 Pan American Health Organization (PAHO) and World Health Organization (WHO), *A Symposium on Yellow Fever* (Belem, 18–22 April 1980), p. 13.

62 'Doença Perene. A febre amarela existe na selva amazônica', *Veja*, 659 (22 April, 1981), p. 78.

63 PAHO and WHO, *A Symposium on Yellow Fever*.

64 On the history of Oswaldo Cruz Institute see N. Stepan, *Gênese e evolução da ciência brasileira*; J. L. Benchimol, *Manguinhos do sonho à vida: a ciência na Belle Époque* (Rio de Janeiro: Fiocruz/COC, 1990).

65 The Oswaldo Cruz Institute Foundation, renamed Oswaldo Cruz Foundation (Fiocruz) in 1974, aggregated institutions that operated under the Ministry of Health, among them the National School of Public Health. The Oswaldo Cruz Institute became one of Fiocruz's key units.

66 J. F. da Cunha, Interview (Rio de Janeiro: Fiocruz/Casa de OswaldoCruz/ Departamento de Arquivo e Documentação, 1987–88). Eighth interview, 3 March 1988.

67 Organización Panamericana de la Salud, Seminario sobre Métodos e Administración en Programas de Vacunación, 10–16 November 1968 (Montevideo: 1969).

68 Brasil, Ministério da Saúde, *Programa Nacional de Imunizações – PNI* (Brasília: Ministério da Saúde, 1973).

69 A. Homma, Interview, 7 March 2001. Rio de Janeiro, Fiocruz/Casa de Oswaldo Cruz/Departamento de Arquivo e Documentação, tape 3, side A.

70 Organización Panamericana de la Salud, 'Pro Saluti Novi Mundi: Historia de la OPS', *Boletín de La Oficina Sanitaria Panamericana*, 113:4 and 6 (November–December 1992), p. 528; C. G. de Macedo, *Notas para uma história recente da saúde pública na América Latina* (Brasília: Escritório de Representação da Organização Pan-Americana de Saúde no Brasil, 1997), p. 45.

71 H. Cordeiro, *A indústria de saúde no Brasil* (Rio de Janeiro: Graal, 1980).

72 E. Diniz, 'Empresariado, regime autoritário e modernização capitalista: 1964–85', in M. C. D'Araújo, G. Soares and C. Castro (eds), *21 Anos de regime militar: balanços e perspectivas* (Rio de Janeiro: Fundação Getúlio Vargas, 1994), pp. 198–231.

73 C. Mérieux, *Le virus de la découverte* (Paris: Éditions Robert Laffont, 1988), pp. 158–60.

74 C. A. G. Gadelha, 'Biotecnologia em saúde: um estudo da mudança tecnológica na indústria farmacêutica e das perspectivas de seu desenvolvimento no Brasil' (MA dissertation, Universidade Estadual de Campinas, 1990).

75 S. G. M. dos Santos, 'Estado, ciência e autonomia: da institucionalização à recuperação de Manguinhos' (MA dissertation, Universidade Federal do Rio de Janeiro, 1999), p. 67.

76 Santos, 'Estado, ciência e autonomia', pp. 166–7. See also C. A. G. Gadelha and J. G. Temporão, *A indústria de vacinas no Brasil: desafios e perspectivas. Relatório técnico de pesquisa* (Rio de Janeiro: BNDES, July 1999), p. 168.

77 Mérieux, *Le virus de la découverte*, pp. 148, 150.

78 M. da L. F. Leal, Interview, 4 February 2001 (Rio de Janeiro, Fiocruz/Casa de Oswaldo Cruz/ Departamento de Arquivo e Documentação), tape 1, side A.

79 J. A. Z. Bermudez, 'Vacinas: grupo de trabalho de controle de qualidade de imunobiológicos', in Encontro Nacional de Controle de Doenças. Doenças Evitáveis por Imunização, *Anais* (Brasília: Centro de Documentação do Ministério da Saúde, 1983), pp. 115–23.

80 Gadelha and Temporão, *A indústria de vacinas no Brasil*, p. 27.

81 Brasil, *Programa Nacional de Imunizações 30 anos*; P. M. Buss, J. G. Temporão and J. da R. Carvalheiro, *Vacinas, soros e imunizações no Brasil* (Rio de Janeiro: Fiocruz, 2005).

82 PAHO and WHO, *A Symposium on Yellow Fever*.

83 Pan American Health Organization and World Health Organization, *Meeting to Develop Guidelines and Protocols for the Production of Yellow Fever Vaccine in Cell Cultures* (Washington, DC: 21–3 February1984).

84 O. de S. Lopes, 'Desenvolvimento da vacina contra a febre amarela em cultura de tecido: resultado de produção em cultura de células', in Simpósio Internacional sobre Febre Amarela e Dengue, pp. 253–59.

85 S. B. Halstead, 'Development of Yellow Fever Tissue Culture Vaccine', in *Simpósio Internacional sobre Febre Amarela e Dengue*, pp. 235–8, on pp. 236–7.

86 Leal, *Interview*.

87 Brasil, Ministério da Saúde, FUNASA, *Eventos adversos sérios associados com a vacina 17D contra a febre amarela* (May 2000).

88 Brasil, *Eventos adversos*.

89 R. Galler, K. V. Pugachev, C. L. S. Santos, S. W. Ocran, A. V. Jabor, S. G. Rodrigues, R. S. Marchevsky, M. S. Freire, L. F. C. Almeida, A. C. R. Cruz, A. M. Y. Yamamura, I. M. Rocco, E. S. T. Rosa, L. T. M. Souza, P. F. Vasconcelos, F. Guirakhoo and T. P. Monath, 'Phenotypic and Molecular Analyses of Yellow Fever 17DD Vaccine Viruses Associated with Serious Adverse Events in Brasil', *Virology*, 290:2 (2001), pp. 309–19.

90 Brasil, *Eventos adversos*.

91 An excellent review of studies regarding these mechanisms can be found in R. de M. Martins, 'Estudos clínicos com vacinas ...'

92 T. P. Monath, 'Yellow Fever Vaccines: The Success of Empiricism, Pitfalls of Application, and Transition to Molecular Vaccinology', in S. A. Plotkin and B. Fantini (eds), *Vaccinia, Vaccination, Vaccinology: Jenner, Pasteur and their Successors* (Paris: Elsevier, 1996), pp. 57–182, on pp. 178–9.

93 T. P. Monath, C. K. Lee, J. G. Julander, A. Brown, D. W. Beasley, D. M. Watts, E. Hayman, P. Guertin, J. Makowiecki, J. Crowell, P. Levesque, G. C. Bowick, M. Morin, E Fowler and D. W. Trent, 'Inactivated Yellow Fever 17D Vaccine: Development and Nonclinical Safety, Immunogenicity and Protective Activity', *Vaccine*, 28:22 (14 May 2010), pp. 3827–40.

94 L. P. Gaspar, Y. S. Mendes, A. M. Yamamura, L. F. Almeida, E. Caride, R.
    B. Gonçalves, J. L. Silva, A. C. Oliveira, R. Galler and M. S. Freire, 'Pressure-
    Inactivated Yellow Fever 17DD Virus: Implications for Vaccine Develop-
    ment', *Journal of Virological Methods*, 150:1–2 (June 2008), pp. 57–62.

8

A distinctive nation: vaccine policy and production in Japan

Julia Yongue

Introduction

Public health authorities in every nation have devised distinctive policies to deal with the prevention and spread of infectious diseases, what Jeffrey Baker has referred to as a national 'style' of vaccination.[1] While Japan's climate and geography as an island nation in the Far East have had a direct impact on the prevalence of certain infectious diseases, preventive vaccination policies, which were influenced by numerous factors ranging from changing societal expectations and pressure from parent, patient and physician groups to new scientific discoveries, may have had an even greater impact on the formation of Japan's distinctive approach to immunisation and production.[2]

One reason for Japan's distinctive vaccination policies is the long history of outside influences on its institutional framework. German, and more recently, American contacts have had a profound effect on Japan's most fundamental regulatory institutions as well as other features such as regulators' preference for full self-sufficiency in vaccines and domestically developed strains. Another area where Japan remains distinctive is regulators' approach to risk. This can be illustrated by two policy choices: approval of fewer vaccines than in other developed nations and extreme caution vis-à-vis the introduction of combination vaccines. In 1983, the US routine vaccine schedule was identical in number (eight vaccines) to that of Japan; however, in the mid-1980s the situation began to diverge considerably. By 2011, the number listed in the former had doubled while Japan's list remained virtually unmodified (Table 8.1).

Table 8.1 Vaccine schedules in Japan and the United States, 2011

Japan	United States
Diphtheria	Diphtheria
Pertussis	Pertussis
Tetanus	Tetanus
Polio (OPV)	Polio (IPV)
Measles	Measles
Rubella (offered only to adolescent girls before 1994)	Mumps
Japanese encephalitis	Rubella
BCG	Hepatitis B
*Influenza (individuals over 65)	Rotavirus
	Pneumococcal
	Varicella
	Hepatitis A (children; recommended for high risk groups)
	Hib
	Meningococcal (for high risk groups)
	Influenza (children/yearly)
	HPV

*Type II vaccination.
Source: Infectious Disease Surveillance Center (Japan)
http://idsc.nih.go.jp/vaccine/dschedule/lmm11EN.pdf#search=%27Japanese
+vaccine+schedule+2011%27.
Centers for Disease Control and Prevention (USA)
www.cdc.gov/Mmwr/preview/mmwrhtml/mm6005a6.htm.

Although the number of routine vaccines has proliferated in western nations, particularly since the 1980s, in Japan, a country whose population is one of the world's healthiest and the leader in life expectancy, the number has actually decreased since the end of the Second World War.[3] Given the assumption that disease prevention through vaccination is basic to maintaining good health, this paradox merits closer investigation. Japan's divergence from widely accepted international norms of vaccination, particularly the rejection of the commercially successful combination vaccines, provides another paradox, given the country's otherwise full integration into the system of global capitalism and active participation in all the major institutions of world health.

Through examples of Japanese vaccination policy choices primarily from the early post-war period to the 2000s, this chapter illustrates the ways that Japanese policy makers took a different policy approach from other nations and explores the reasons why. As analysed throughout this volume, the collective consciousness of citizens, which was formed by the history of vaccine-induced adverse events, differs in every nation. In Japan, apart from some widely publicised cases of adverse vaccine-induced reactions, the topic of vaccination generated relatively little public interest. However, the H1N1 epidemic in 2009 marked a true turning point. This outbreak received extensive media coverage and heightened general awareness of the dangers of infectious diseases.

A measles epidemic in 2007 resulting in nationwide school and university closures, an alarming rise of rubella cases in recent years and reports of adverse reactions to the HPV (human papillomavirus) vaccine also piqued citizens' interest in public health issues, while also sensitising them to the importance of making informed vaccination choices.[4] This chapter traces the formation of the collective consciousness in Japan by examining some of the most distinctive features in Japan's vaccination history and the ways in which health authorities have dealt with outbreaks and prevention.

The historical legacy

From an early date, the state played the key role in the formation of Japan's distinct approach to dealing with the spread of infectious disease. In the 1630s, the Tokugawa government (1603–1868) officially closed the country to contact with the outside world for some 250 years. This was not simply a momentous political decision. By limiting foreign exchanges, administrators had also unwittingly enacted the first nationwide public health policy. The fact that Japan remained a 'closed nation', or *sakoku* in Japanese, for so many years also had a limiting effect on the incursion of infectious diseases from abroad. After the start of the Meiji period (1868–1912) one of the first large-scale public health threats was cholera, which began to spread nationwide after the imposition of the so-called 'unequal treaties' forcing the 'opening of the nation', or *kaikoku*, and Japan's official entry into the global economy. As shown in this chapter, Japanese policy makers have followed a similar pattern of artificially 'opening' and 'closing' the nation, not to foreigners, but to new vaccines as well as new forms of vaccine delivery, namely combination vaccines. The metaphors of the country's 'closing' and 'opening' are used again in this chapter in the more modern context of Japan's vaccination policy.

Transfers of knowledge and institutions were also of vital importance to Japan's history of vaccination. Japan continued to open its doors throughout the Meiji period by dispatching scientists to foreign universities, particularly in Germany, which created enduring professor-student relationships. By the late Meiji period, the number of dispatches gradually diminished due to the need for their assistance at home at newly opened universities and research institutions. During the Taishō period (1912–26), connections with Germany became strained due to Japan's position in the First World War. Despite this, scientific activities continued as bacteriologists turned their attention to the causes of diseases endemic to Japan. One of the first important findings was that of Inada Ryōkichi and Idō Yutaka, whose research was first published in Japan in 1915. They identified the causative agent of Weil's disease, the vaccine for which would be listed on Japan's first vaccination schedule.[5] Noguchi Hideyo's work on infectious diseases is also widely recognised, particularly in Japan where his image began to appear on the 1000-yen note in 2004.[6]

While Kitasato Shibasaburō is perhaps Japan's most prominent bacteriologist, there were many others, including his student Shiga Kiyoshi, who returned to Japan in 1924 with a BCG strain from the Pasteur Institute. Like Kitasato, Shiga left Japan to do research in Germany where he worked with Paul Ehrlich as did Hata Sahachirō, another researcher at Kitasato's institute and developer of arsphenamine 606, the first medicine in the world for the treatment of syphilis and first synthetic chemical. In 1897, Shiga discovered the bacillus causing dysentery, *Shigella dysenteriae*, while working at Kitasato's newly opened Institute for the Study of Infectious Diseases. Kitasato, a scientist who truly embodied a European approach through his involvement not only in research on infectious diseases but also in the commercial production and sale of sera, was rare among Japan's early scientists. Kitasato can be credited for bringing to Japan an institute-based model of sera and vaccine research combined with commercial production. Even today, institutes are the principal suppliers of vaccines in Japan, as opposed to most other countries, where virtually all of the vaccine-producing institutes and laboratories have closed and been replaced by large, multinational pharmaceutical companies.

Organisational foundations

The institutionalisation of Japan's model for vaccine production got underway in 1893 with the establishment of the Institute of Infectious Diseases (IID), what the historian of Japanese science and technology James Bartholomew has referred to as 'the most important research facility built [in Japan] before World War I'.[7] The IID played a major role not only in scientific research on sera and vaccines but also in contributions to the formation of science and technology in Japan. Kitasato, who oversaw its activities until it was placed under the Ministry of Education, made a vital contribution to the institutionalisation of a research-based Japanese vaccine production model as a private sector activity.

Known in Japan as the 'father of bacteriology', Kitasato received his medical degree from the University of Tokyo in 1883. Before entering government, he went to study at the University of Berlin where, as an assistant of Robert Koch, he produced a pure culture of tetanus bacilli.[8] Kitasato, who revered his mentor throughout his lifetime, based the IID's operational model on that of the Koch Institute.[9] Like its German counterpart, the IID performed three functions: (1) research, (2) production and sale of sera and vaccines, and (3) treatment. While in Berlin, Kitasato worked alongside Emil von Behring and succeeded in developing serum therapy for the treatment of tetanus.

Kitasato was aided in his efforts to found an institute similar to those in Germany and France by several prominent and politically powerful figures. First and foremost was Nagayo Sensai, the first chief of the Bureau of Hygiene at the Ministry of Home Affairs, the equivalent of today's MHLW (Ministry of Health, Labour and Welfare), followed by two other influential politicians, Gotō Shinpei, Nagayo's successor, and in later years, Hasegawa Tai, who helped Kitasato to obtain state funding. Nagayo felt that Kitasato's leadership was essential to the success of the institute; however, since he knew that Kitasato had a number of powerful enemies, he proceeded with his plans with caution.[10]

Kitasato initially founded a small research laboratory in 1892, thanks to financial backing from Fukuzawa Yukichi, a moderniser and the founder of one of Japan's most reputable private institutions, Keio University, Morimura Ichizaemon, an entrepreneur, and the Great Japan Hygiene Society. Like Nagayo, Fukuzawa had studied western science at Tekijuku under Ogata Kōan, the key propagator of the Jennerian vaccination technique in Japan. Fukuzawa provided Kitasato not only with funding but also a plot of land for his activities. The scale of Kitasato's first operation was inadequate, and efforts were made to procure funds from the government to expand production. This move caused the first round of tensions between Kitasato and his academic rival at Tokyo Imperial University (later the University of Tokyo), Ogata Masanori.[11] In the end, the IID was awarded the necessary funds, thus ensuring its financial stability. Having been officially placed under the jurisdiction of the Ministry of Home Affairs in 1899 as a national institute, IID became the largest vaccine and sera producer in Japan and the first in the world to employ serum therapy to combat cholera, tetanus and diphtheria.[12]

In 1912 the second round of tensions erupted over the jurisdiction of the IID, this time between Kitasato and the Japanese government led by Prime Minister Ōkuma Shigenobu. According to the government's proposal, the IID was to be situated in Tokyo Imperial University and placed under the jurisdiction of the Ministry of Education. Though it was agreed that Kitasato would remain executive director, he vehemently opposed the new arrangement. Thus shortly after the government's plan was approved, Kitasato resigned along with his entire staff and opened his own private vaccine-producing research institution. Thanks to his foresight in procuring a production licence shortly before his resignation, research activities could be financed through sales of sera and vaccines. The dispute led to the establishment of the Kitasato Institute as a wholly private entity.

In 1947 during the US occupation, IID underwent yet another major organisational change. The end result was the creation of a new national institute of infectious diseases with an organisational model similar to that of the National Institutes of Health (NIH) in the United States. Although the Supreme Commander for Allied Powers (SCAP) in accordance with the recommendation of Brigadier Army General Crawford Sams of the Public Health and Welfare Section (PHW) officially approved its establishment, key Japanese, in particular, Nanbara Shigeru, law professor and president of Tokyo Imperial University and Tamiya Takeo, head of IID at the end of the war, were also intimately involved with its creation behind the scenes. Based on proposals drawn up by Nanbara, SCAP founded the NIH, later the National Institute of Infectious Diseases (NIID), whose new jurisdiction would become the Ministry of Health and Welfare (MHW). IID (now the Institute of Medical Science, University of Tokyo) remained intact, initially as a research and inspection facility, though many of the staff later migrated to NIID.

NIID's early activities included: (1) research on the causes, treatment, and prevention of infectious diseases, (2) inspections of vaccine quality, (3) development, production and distribution of certain vaccines with limited demand such as the rabies vaccine, and (4) pilot production and distribution of vaccines and sera.

Placed under the MHW (Ministry of Health, Labour and Welfare since 2002), the American and Japanese-inspired institution provided the organisational foundations for post-war research on infectious diseases and vaccines in Japan. In addition to NIID, another entirely new and autonomous institution, the Biologicals Production Association (now the Association of Biological Manufacturers of Japan) was established the same year, 1947.[13]

Foreign influences on Japan's vaccination policy approach

Like the institutions mentioned here, the Preventive Vaccine Law (PVL) was also in a sense a western import, as it was Sams of PHW who officially implemented it. At that time, the need for a new policy framework for disease prevention was great: with the turmoil caused by returning soldiers and citizens from abroad, coupled with unsanitary domestic conditions, infectious diseases were rampant.[14] This was particularly true in Tokyo, where repeated aerial raids in the final days of the war left many destitute and homeless.[15] The measures taken to stop the spread of disease were draconian. According to Watanabe Mikio, PVL, introduced in 1947, was unprecedented anywhere in the world for its severity.[16] Vaccination was made mandatory without exception and onerous fines were imposed on those who violated it.[17]

Japan's first routine schedule comprised smallpox, diphtheria, para-typhoid, pertussis, tuberculosis, typhus, plague, scarlet fever, influenza and Weil's disease vaccines. Like the transfer of penicillin production technology from the United States, which was carried out in part to control the spread of sexually transmitted diseases among the troops stationed in Japan, the introduction of mandatory vaccination was also partly motivated by American self-interest.[18] Japanese nationals working directly with SCAP were the first to be vaccinated. Further, according to Watanabe, self-sufficiency in vaccines was encouraged not to promote industrial development in Japan but to respond to criticism in the United States of the financial burden of stationing troops and adminis-trative personnel in Japan.[19]

Though SCAP officials' efforts to provide safe and effective vaccines were well intentioned, adverse incidents occurred. The most famous incident was the 1948 Kyoto-Shimane Diphtheria Tragedy, which resulted in an exceptionally high death toll of eighty-three. Despite this, no reports of widespread public dissent vis-à-vis PVL exist and little news of this incident was reported in the media due to strin-gent censorship. According to Wake Masayoshi, while the issue was discussed in Japanese Diet sessions, SCAP officials hindered the dis-semination of such information to the general public.[20] Following the incident, Sams halted the sale of all Japanese vaccines and sera and began inspections of some forty-one facilities nationwide. Of these, ten facilities were granted permission to engage in produc-tion. It is noteworthy that Sams believed that vaccine production should be carried out solely by the private sector and opted not to allow IID to manufacture vaccines on account of its status as a public entity.

In addition, as was the case for the transfer of penicillin production technology, a specialist from the board of health of the state of Michigan came to Japan to provide direct assistance and supervision in vaccine production at the ten selected facilities. Thanks to these endeavours, the quality of the vaccine produced in Japan improved to the extent that these manufacturers were able to export vaccines to aid in the Korean War (1950–53).[21]

The lessons of the Kyoto-Shimane Diphtheria Tragedy may have left a mark in the collective memories of some public health admin-istrators; however, because the incident received so little mention in the press, it was never able to serve as a platform for a wider national debate on PVL or the risks associated with vaccination. While responsibility for the tragedy could easily be placed on the severity of SCAP's vaccination policies, evidence suggests a certain degree of complicity on the part of Japanese health policy makers. Indeed, rather than amending the policy of *mandatory* vaccination, it stayed in place until 1994, while the penalty of a fine was not officially removed until 1977.[22]

According to Chris Aldous, while Sams and others may have seen their reforms as revolutionary, there was also a certain degree of continuity in Japan's health policy approach. The foundations of some of the institutions of hygiene, particularly those established at the community level, had already been put in place, in some cases since the Meiji period, but had been severely weakened during the war.[23] While PVL has undergone numerous revisions since its introduction during the occupation, it continues to be the bedrock of all Japanese vaccination policy. The following provides another example of foreign influences on Japan's approach to vaccination policy-making in the 1960s and beyond.

The polio vaccine: emergency measures

The history of polio vaccine manufacturing in Japan began in 1958 when an investigating committee for infectious disease prevention recommended domestic production of IPV (inactivated polio vaccine) and research on OPV (oral polio vaccine). This came in the wake of a large-scale polio outbreak in 1960 with some 5,606 reported cases and 317 deaths.[24] When the number of cases reported in the first half of 1961 surpassed those of the previous year, health authorities decided to take the emergency measure of importing OPV from the United States and Canada and later also from the Soviet Union, even though domestic clinical trials had not yet commenced. In the meantime, standards for IPV manufacturing were set in October 1960, and six establishments – Biken (Research Foundation for Microbial Diseases of Osaka University), Kaketsuken (Chemo-Sero-Therapeutic Research Institute), Takeda Pharmaceutical Company, Chiba Kessen (no longer in operation today), Kitasato (Kitasato Institute) and Denka Seiken – received production licences. As a result of their efforts, by

1962 the number of new outbreaks dropped to 289 and in 1963 to 131.[25] In July 1962, the six private entities joined forces by forming a single producer, Japan Poliomyelitis Research Institute (JPRI), to manufacture OPV domestically. This enabled Japan to meet domestic demand by 1964 and later achieve full self-sufficiency in the polio vaccine.

According to an interview with Abe Shinobu, Executive Director of the JPRI, on 20 February 2014, the idea of having a sole supplier of the polio vaccine was not that of the institute or the government but of Albert Sabin. Sabin based his recommendation on Japan's relatively small geographical size and the need to ensure high quality standards. He personally contributed to Japanese polio production by donating one of his strains to the JPRI in March 1963. The same strain is still in use today.[26] Given the risk of OPV-derived paralysis (5.8 million to one for infants), scientists at JPRI began research on IPV production using the Sabin strain in 1976.[27] They succeeded in producing the world's first Sabin IPV, known as s-IPV. Because the vaccine had not been tested for use in a combination vaccine, collaborative research began to develop an s-IPV-DTP vaccine.[28] Initially, five DTP-producing establishments were involved in the project; however, by 2005 only Biken and Kaketsuken remained.

The polio vaccine example illustrates three characteristic features of Japan's vaccine policy approach. First, unlike in the United States, Japanese health authorities encouraged a sole supplier of the polio (and BCG) vaccine to guarantee a higher safety level since contamination problems could be better dealt with at a single rather than multiple locations. Second, unlike most other developed nations, Japan made no use of combination vaccines using the polio component until late 2012. Third, Japanese health authorities continued to promote the use of OPV due to its good record of safety and superior immunity over IPV, despite over a decade of widespread use of IPV in many countries.[29] Also, by using the oral vaccine, regulators were able to avert another risk: injection-associated infections.[30]

The decision to switch from OPV to IPV in 2012 sparked wide attention in the media and strong public criticism of Japanese regulators for several reasons. First, it left the average Japanese with the impression that Japan was a 'backward nation' in terms of vaccination policies.[31] Like the Hib vaccine, the decision came much later than in many other developed countries; the United States had switched to IPV over a decade earlier. Second, the debate over the polio vaccine also brought to light an inconsistency between Japan's domestic stance on vaccination and its global one. Although Japanese representatives had for many years supported WHO's position on promoting the use of IPV in countries where polio had been eradicated, domestic health authorities continued to keep OPV on the domestic routine vaccination schedule.[32] Finally, because the switch away from OPV could not be made immediately, some believed that health authorities were jeopardising public health and even took it upon themselves to import IPV directly.[33] Perhaps in response to strong public criticism, the health ministry made the rare move of approving the foreign vaccine, IMOVAX Polio, manufactured by Sanofi Pasteur.

Thus in September 2012, health authorities added a foreign vaccine, cIPV, to Japan's routine vaccination schedule then just two months later, approved the combination vaccine, DTaP+sIPV (Table 8.2). One

Table 8.2 Approvals of Japan's first combination vaccine with a polio component

Name of vaccine	Manufacturer	Type	Application	Date	Launch
IMOVAX Polio	Sanofi Pasteur	cIPV	23 Feb. 2012	26 Apr. 2012	Sept. 2012
Tetrabik Subcutaneous injection syringe	Biken	DTaP+ sIPV	27 Dec. 2012	27 Jul. 2012	Nov. 2012
Quattrovac Subcutaneous injection syringe	Kaketsuken	DTaP+ sIPV	27 Jan. 2012	27 Jul. 2012	Nov. 2012

Source: Based on information provided in an interview with Dr Abe Shinobu, Executive Director, laboratory division at Japan Poliomyelititis Research Institute, Tokyo, 20 February 2014.

can see a similarity in the situation in the 1960s, when the Japanese government resorted to importing the polio vaccine from overseas until a domestic substitute was available.

Current changes in Japan's vaccination policy approach

To clearly elucidate more recent changes, it is useful to divide the period examined in this section into two phases: (1) the closing of the country (*sakoku*) to new vaccines from 1989 to 2006, and (2) the reopening (*kaikoku*) from 2007 to the present. The main catalyst for closing the country was a series of adverse events associated with the MMR combination vaccine, which began shortly after its launch in April 1989. It is of note that commercial production in Japan was only realised in 1986, which is much later than in some other countries, particularly the United States where use commenced more than a decade earlier in 1973. According to Tezuka Yōsuke, the particularly long delay was due to patent ownership issues.[34]

With grants from the Ministry of Education in 1968, research institutions began developing their own mumps vaccines. Four establishments, Biken (approved in 1981), Kitasato (1981), Takeda (1982) and Kaketsuken (1985), were granted approval, each using a different strain and process.[35] By the early 1980s, three establishments, Kitasato, Takeda and Biken, had each developed an MMR vaccine that was ready for launch. Rather than allowing all of the establishments to market different competing MMR products, Japanese health authorities decided to approve a single standardised version, what might be called a 'national MMR vaccine'. Authorities then selected one vaccine from each establishment and combined them. Thus in 1989, Japan's first MMR combination was introduced using Kitasato's measles, Biken's mumps and Takeda's rubella vaccines. Biken took an early lead in mumps research and developed two vaccines using different strains: Urabe AM-9 and Hoshino. According to Okuno Yoshiomi, in 1978, the Urabe strain had already been tested on some 10,000 persons in Japan and South Korea and had an excellent record of safety.[36] It is likely that regulators selected Biken's Okabe strain based on this data rather than reports in 1987 and 1988 of a small number of adverse events in Canada, followed by the Canadian health authorities' decision to suspend production.[37]

From a regulatory standpoint, Japan's system of routine (mandatory) and non-routine vaccines complicated the provision of the MMR vaccine. According to the 1976 revision PVL, the measles vaccine became part of Japan's routine vaccination schedule, which meant that patients could receive it free of charge. On the other hand, the rubella vaccine was routine only for adolescent girls, while the mumps vaccine could be administered upon request for an additional fee. Although the parent/guardian could opt to receive both the rubella and mumps vaccines each as a single-dose injection, use of the combination MMR vaccine was initially promoted by the government for its superior coverage and was encouraged by many physicians.[38] Indeed, according to Tezuka, after the launch of MMR, some medical institutions *only* offered the MMR vaccine, making it a de facto routine vaccination in some parts of the country.[39]

As shown in Table 8.3, after the 1989 introduction of the MMR vaccine, adverse events soon ensued. MHW officials initially kept information regarding a possible correlation between the mumps vaccine and the incidence of adverse events confidential, a point that would later become a source of public suspicion and mistrust.[40]

Table 8.3 Adverse events following the introduction of MMR in 1989[41]

Important dates	Vaccination-related developments
1 April	Start of MMR vaccine
June	Results of survey by Japan Medical Association, Maebashi, Gunma Prefecture showed a high incidence of aseptic meningitis.
19 September	MHW announcement of 1 : 100,000 to 200,000 incidence ratio of aseptic meningitis and decision 'to continue to promote the use of MMR' despite the rise in adverse events.
25 October	MHW announcement of 1 : several thousand to 30,000 incidence ratio of aseptic meningitis and decision 'to proceed with MMR vaccination with caution.'
20 December	MHW announcement of 1: several thousand incidence ratio of aseptic meningitis and decision 'to administer MMR only when requested by the parent/guardian.'

In September 1989, health authorities received reports of six cases of adverse reactions to the mumps vaccine; however, since the incidents were not life-threatening and caused no long-term harm, they continued to promote its use. In Japan, the central government allots funds to municipal and prefectural governments for the purpose of purchasing and administering vaccinations; however, it is the latter that actually implements and executes vaccination programmes at the local level. Under this system, which provides a certain degree of local autonomy, some municipal and prefectural governments took the decision to suspend the use of MMR based on their own surveys, yet others continued their vaccination programmes using MMR in accordance with the government's recommendation, despite reports of incidents.[42] Regulators' general reaction to the incidents differed significantly from the DTP vaccine, which was added to the routine schedule of mandatory vaccinations in 1969 but temporarily withdrawn for three months in 1975 following reports of adverse events. In the case of MMR, it was not until April 1993 that officials finally decided to withdraw it completely.

In 1991, MHW officials began an investigation to determine the source of the problem but were unable to obtain any conclusive results. Then in October of the same year, they decided to allow individual vaccine producers to manufacture their own MMR vaccines, a decision that was likely taken due to suspicions regarding Biken's Okabe AM-9 strain.[43] In April 1992, health authorities announced a revision of their adverse event ratio to 1:1000, but did not withdraw the MMR vaccine. In April 1993, the results of another investigation provided evidence that the mumps strains of the other establishments were less effective than Biken's Okabe AM-9 strain. With such puzzling and in some cases conflicting results, regulators simply decided to withdraw the MMR vaccine altogether. Several days after the withdrawal of the MMR vaccine, it was revealed that Biken had 'illegally' modified its vaccine production process.[44] It was also found that Biken had combined its approved mumps vaccine with another one that had been manufactured according to a modified process. According to Ueno Hideo, a plaintiff in the trial that followed, *combining* the two mumps vaccines was the most likely cause of the adverse events.[45] Whatever the true cause, the revelation shed public doubt on the safety of vaccination in general, and more specifically on Japan's use of combination vaccines in the long term.

Litigation ensued. The court of first instance ruled against the manufacturer and a settlement was made between the victims' families and Biken, a decision that the latter did not appeal. The Tokyo Supreme Court determined that the state was at fault for not fulfilling its obligation to provide proper guidance and supervision, yet no formal government apology was ever issued. According to Ueno, from the perspective of a parent of one of the victims, while justice was in part served, a number of important questions remained unanswered: (1) Was modifying the production process the *only* cause of the problem? (2) Who was responsible for introducing the strain? (3) Who makes the decision to suspend a vaccine when adverse events occur? (4) Why were health authorities so slow in taking action to withdraw the MMR and reinstate vaccination using the single-injection measles vaccine?.[46]

Ueno's fourth question, concerning decision-makers' choice in the type of vaccine administered, is particularly difficult to answer since there are no records available. In an invited commentary, one vaccine expert, Stanley Plotkin, wrote that the Japanese government's motives for not importing the Jeryl Lynn strain, using a strain known to cause a higher incidence of adverse reactions, and completely eliminating the mumps vaccine from the routine schedule despite scientific evidence collected by Japanese scientists of a high incidence of deafness resulting from the mumps, are indicative of 'protectionism in favour of indigenous manufacturers'.[47] Whatever the real motives, regulators have not changed their stance on the MMR vaccine, although a modified version, the MR vaccine (measles-rubella), was introduced in 2005.

Between 1989 when the first adverse events occurred to 2006, a new *sakoku* began as Japan closed its doors to new vaccines. During this period, policy-makers' approach to new vaccine approval was one of extreme caution. Apart from the hepatitis A vaccine (non-routine), health authorities did not introduce any truly 'new' vaccines. As Table 8.2 shows, until 2012 when health authorities approved vaccines with the IPV polio component, no combination vaccines were in use apart from DTaP and MR. In contrast, from the late 1980s, health authorities in the United States approved and favourably endorsed combination vaccines, which began to proliferate particularly after the launch of the Hib vaccine and the switch to IPV, both in 1987.

Table 8.4 Vaccines approved for use in Japan and
the United States (1985–2006)[48]

Approval year	Japan	United States
1985	Hepatitis B (1)	
1987	Live attenuated varicella	Hib
		IPV
1988	Pneumococcal (2)	
	Recombinant Hepatitis B	
	MMR (3)	
1991		aP (acellular pertussis) (5)
1992		DTaP
		Japanese encephalitis (6)
1993		DTaP-Hib
1994		Plague
1995	Hepatitis A	Varicella (7)
1996		Hib-Hepatitis B
		Inactivated Hepatitis A
2000		PCV for children (8)
2001		Hepatitis A/B combination
2002		DTaP-IPV-B
2003		Live intranasal influenza
		DTP for adults
2005	MR (4)	MMR-Varicella
		Meningococcal (conjugate)
2006		Rotavirus

(1) Approved in the USA, 1982.
(2) Approved in the USA, 1977.
(3) Approved in the USA, 1971 and launched in Japan in 1989.
(4) MR is MMR without the mumps vaccine. It was reapproved as a
two-vaccine combination following adverse reactions to the mumps vaccine.
(5) Approved in Japan in 1981 and exported to the USA.[49]
(6) Developed in Japan and approved in 1976.
(7) Technology transfer from Japan.
(8) 7-Valent Pneumococcal Vaccine for Children.

In the backdrop of the MMR vaccine trial were many others such as those involving the influenza and polio vaccines, which are not covered in this chapter, that called into question government responsibility.[50] In 1994, PVL underwent a major revision: Japanese health authorities changed their long-standing policy of mandatory mass vaccination. Mandatory vaccination became voluntary, that is, according to the wording of the revised law: all citizens '*must* make reasonable efforts to vaccinate', although vaccination itself would not be mandatory. Mass vaccination programmes that had previously taken place in schools were also discontinued. Thus the revision transferred the burden of choice and responsibility from the state to the individual.[51] Unlike in other countries with a similar system, Japanese health authorities have not implemented any coercive vaccination measures since inoculation rates remain in the 90 per cent range for all the routine vaccines, although they are low – 30–40 per cent – for non-routine vaccinations, many of which are routine in other countries.[52] Also, since 1994, physicians are obliged to provide information on the risk of vaccine-associated adverse events and obtain informed consent before vaccinating.

The second phase, or opening (*kaikoku*) of the country to vaccines got underway around 2006, with the government's issuing of the *Vaccine Industry Vision: Supporting Measures to Prevent Infection while Aiming to Respond to Societal Expectations of Industry* (hereafter Vaccine Vision) in 2007. This voluminous six-section policy statement marked the culmination of two years of regular discussion. To build a consensus among all those involved, MHLW officials invited a wide range of participants. Attendees included representatives from academia, regulatory and business organisations such as the International Federation of Pharmaceutical Manufacturers and Associations (IFPMA) and the Food and Drug Administration (FDA), physicians, foreign and domestic industry representatives, among others.[53] The document clarified the government's new stance and was symbolic of a larger, more fundamental change in Japan's health care system. The Vision's encouragement of vaccination, including what some would consider 'non-essential', gives a clear signal that Japanese health authorities have begun incorporating more *preventive* policy measures into a system that had traditionally focused almost exclusively *curative* care. By so doing, regulators have also indirectly addressed other urgent issues, namely the country's demographic dilemma: a growing elderly population coupled with a shrinking birth rate as well as rising health care expenditures. The dialogue that the Vaccine Vision opened among government, health specialists and industry was a first for Japan, though similar discussions had already begun elsewhere in the 1980s.[54]

The first three chapters of the Vaccine Vision statement provide a general overview of the domestic vaccine industry and outline global growth and consolidation trends. By comparing the evolution of the global industry with the Japanese situation, the document sheds light on two fundamental features of the vaccine supply model: production almost exclusively by small-scale institutes and full vaccine self-sufficiency. According to the document's authors, while there are definite disadvantages to having an industry comprised of small research-based institutes, full self-sufficiency (98.5 per cent) is a beneficial and globally unique feature of Japan's vaccine supply model.[55] Chapter 4 examines the needs and expectations of society and considers the introduction of evidence-based methodologies such as QALY analyses, which had never before been applied to vaccine policy-making in Japan.[56]

The final two chapters describe the government's plans to foster domestic vaccine industry growth. Chapter 5 contains a section entitled 'Basic Stance on an Industrial Policy for the Vaccine Industry', urging Japanese producers to develop new vaccines, both to bring greater benefits to society and improve international competitiveness. The final chapter posits an 'Action Plan', laying out the new roles of industry and government, including a government pledge to provide financial support for new vaccine development and the expansion or improvement of plants while also encouraging collaborative partnerships with foreign multinationals. The Vaccine Vision defined policy makers' new openness to vaccines on many levels, as illustrated by the new approvals made since its publication and special subsidies allotted to municipal and prefectural governments to encourage their use nationwide.[57]

Japan's decision to approve the Hib vaccine for childhood bacterial meningitis in 2007 is particularly noteworthy since it occurred much later than in most other countries (Table 8.5). WHO representatives have advocated that infants be immunised against the disease, and by

Table 8.5 US–Japan comparison of vaccine approvals (2007–11)

Vaccine	Japanese approval	US approval
Hib (haemophilus influenzae type B)	January 2007	1985
HPV (human papillomavirus)	October 2009	2006 (Gardasil)
PCV (pneumococcal conjugate)	October 2009	2002
Rotavirus	October 2011	1998 (RotaShield)

Source: cdc.gov and mhlw.go.jp.

2006 health authorities in some 100 countries had approved the Hib vaccine, ninety of which listed it in their routine vaccination schedules.[58] Despite international consensus, most Japanese vaccine experts long maintained that incidence of the disease is much lower in Japan making approval unnecessary. In 1998, Kamiya and others challenged this assumption with the publication of a study showing Hib to be the leading cause of childhood bacterial meningitis in Japan.[59] After collecting new data in domestic trials, Sanofi Pasteur (then Pasteur, Mériex Connaught), which established a joint venture with a Japanese firm in 1997, applied for approval and finally succeeded in launching ActHib in 2007 as the first foreign paediatric vaccine ever approved in Japan.

Given Japan's closed stance toward new vaccine approvals and policy of full self-sufficiency, few multinationals such as GSK even attempted to penetrate the domestic vaccine industry. Merck, however, through its fully owned subsidiary Banyu Pharmaceutical Company, has endeavoured to make inroads for many years with limited success. Merck (MSD) succeeded in 1988 in launching Recombivax HB, the world's first recombinant hepatitis B vaccine; however, sales failed to reach the levels seen in other overseas markets. Health authorities approved Merck's application after representatives submitted new trial data collected in Japan, ironically on the same day as another domestic manufacturer, Kaketsuken. Though hepatitis B was once considered a 'national disease' in Japan, the incidence today is low making the recombinant hepatitis B vaccine (HBV) a type of travel vaccine whose cost is high and demand relatively low. Because HBV was never made routine, sales of the vaccine have never achieved the levels attained by the company in other countries. Other domestic entrants (Mitsubishi Kasei, Meiji Dairies) also launched HBV vaccines but later withdrew due to limited demand.

A major hurdle that foreign multinationals face is costly and time-consuming clinical trials. Both Merck and Sanofi Pasteur were required to conduct new trials in Japan despite a substantial amount of data already collected in other countries and regions. Despite the progress made at the International Conference on Harmonisation of Technical Requirements for Registration of Pharmaceuticals for Human Use (ICH), since the 1980s, including the implementation of a special measure, ICH-E5 or *Ethnic Factors in the Acceptability of Foreign Clinical Data*, Japanese regulators' reluctance to accept foreign data has remained a contentious issue.[60]

Perhaps more frustrating to foreign vaccine manufacturers, however, is Japan's strict quality control standards. Though Sanofi Pasteur's Hib vaccine received approval in 2007, the first shipments did not reach most medical institutions until December 2008. Even in 2009, there was still a two-month waiting list due to shortages. The delays were not caused by reservations regarding safety. The vaccine had received a favourable endorsement from the Japan Medical Association,[61] and was gaining wider recognition among parents.[62] According to an article in *Weekly Aera* (the equivalent of *Newsweek* or *Time*), in March 2009, an infant in Kyoto died from meningitis caused by the Hib virus. The infant's parents, a gynaecologist and a paediatrician, were on a waiting list for the vaccine. In the article, the couple endorsed vaccination as the best way to prevent future problems.[63] The main reason for the supply shortage was defective packing, specifically the glass vials, which did not present any health risks whatsoever but caused grave suspicions among health authorities.[64] According to Japanese inspectors, some contained black specks and thus had to be recalled.[65] Foreign multinationals have automated vial inspections using laser detectors; however, in Japan, personnel manually examine each individual vial before shipment to prevent recalls.[66] The French were finally able to remedy their defect problems by introducing a similar manual inspection system for all vials exported to Japan.

Conclusion

Foreign influences have played a major role in the formation of Japan's distinctive approach to vaccination policy, including the cornerstone, PVL. The institutional framework, including Japan's mainly institute/ laboratory-based vaccine production system, though introduced in the Meiji period by Kitasato, was redefined and reinforced by Sams and others during the occupation period. Other foreign influences include Japan's introduction of the Sabin strain (and BCG), which is still in use today in the s-OPV and s-IPV vaccines. While in many ways influenced by foreign factors, Japan has opted not to follow the global trend of promoting the use of combination vaccines. This decision followed adverse events caused by the MMR vaccine, and until 2012 only two combination vaccines, DtaP and MR were available for use.

Japan's current business model for vaccine production is in many ways closer to the European institutes, whose model Kitasato observed and introduced to Japan in the nineteenth century, than it is to today's multinationals. Another significant difference between the two is that earnings at Japanese institutes are mainly reinvested in research and development activities rather than used as dividends. While healthy competition exists among all of them, there is ample evidence of cooperation to achieve common national goals (the development of a 'national' MMR vaccine), a feature that is rare among the highly competitive multinationals. Tradition has also played an important role in Japan's distinctiveness as a vaccine-producing nation not only in terms of strain selection (Okabe AM-9 versus the Jeryl Lynn strains) but also in the choice of its producers to remain private (Kitasato).

Japan makes an interesting case for its many differences. While parents in many countries have criticised their health authorities for a surfeit of vaccinations, in the more recent past their counterparts in Japan have complained of the opposite. Under pressure to respond to society's demands, policy makers have recently made more 'new-to-Japan' vaccines available. Since Japan's *kaikoku* or opening up to vaccines in 2007, national distinctions have gradually begun to fade as the country's vaccine supply model converges with the mainstream model of other countries. Whether limiting access to vaccines through policy-making by creating a modern-day *sakoku* has been beneficial or detrimental to public health conditions in Japan is unclear, and goes to the heart of the fundamental debate over vaccination itself and the role that the state should play.

Notes

1 J. P. Baker, 'Immunization the American Way: 4 Childhood Vaccines', *American Journal of Public Health*, 90 (February 2000), p. 199.
2 M. Akazawa, J. Yongue, S. Ikeda and T. Satō, 'Considering Economic Analyses in the Revision of the Preventive Vaccine Law: A New Direction for Health policy-making in Japan?' *Health Policy*, 118 (2014), pp. 127–34.
3 'Japan: Universal Health Care at 50 years', *The Lancet* (11 August 2011), www.thelancet.com/series/japan (accessed 16 September 2015).
4 On 22 January 2014, the Centers for Disease Control and Prevention issued a 'Level 2 Alert' for travellers to Japan due to a rubella outbreak (14,357 cases since early 2013, compared to 2,353 cases in 2012). Also see' Nationwide Rubella Epidemic – Japan, 2013', www.cdc.gov/mmwr/ preview/mmwrhtml/mm6223a1.htm (accessed 31 July 2014); www. nc.cdc.gov/travel/notices/alert/rubella-japan (accessed 25 February 2014). See extensive Japanese media coverage of the HPV vaccine due to the increase in adverse events (1,968 cases since approval), which surpassed those of other developed nations. 'Health Ministry Withdraws Recommendation for Cervical Cancer Vaccine', *Asahi Shimbun* (English version) (15 June 2013), https://ajw.asahi.com/article/behind_news/social_affairs/AJ201306150057 (accessed 25 February 2014).
5 Y. Kobayashi, 'Discovery of the Causative Organism of Weil's Disease: Historical View', *Journal of Infection Chemotherapy*, 7:1 (2001), pp. 10–15.
6 Noguchi did not benefit from a government scholarship as Kitasato and others did, and left to study in the United States under Simon Flexner rather than Germany. Best known for his 1911 discovery of the agent causing syphilis and his extensive work on tropical diseases, Noguchi also directly contributed to the development of new vaccines such as those for snakebite.
7 J. R. Bartholomew, *The Formation of Science in Japan: Building a Research Tradition* (New Haven, CT: Yale University Press, 1989), p. 100.
8 C. Gradmann (translation by Elborg Forster), *Laboratory Disease: Robert Koch's Medical Bacteriology* (Baltimore, MD: Johns Hopkins University Press, 2009), p. 122.
9 For information regarding the close relationship between Kitasato and Koch, see Mariko Ogawa, 'Robert Koch's 74 Days in Japan', *Kleine Reihe 27*

(Mori Ogai-Gendenkstätte der Humboldt-Universität zu Berlin, 2003). http://edoc.hu-berlin.de/series/kleine-reihe/27/PDF/27.pdf#search='sh rine+kitasato+koch' (accessed 25 February 2014).

10　T. Kodaka, *Densenbyō Kenkyūsho: Kindai Igaku Kaitaku no Michinori* (The Institute for Infectious Diseases: Forging a Path to Modern Medicine) (Tokyo: Gakkai Shuppan Sentā, 30 November 1992), p. 43.

11　Bartholomew, *The Formation of Science in Japan*, p. 101.

12　*Ibid.*, p. 122; M. Miyajima, *Kitasato Shibasaburō den* (Biography of Kitasato Shibasaburō) (Tokyo, 1933), p. 115.

13　S. Yamazaki and I. Kurane (eds), *Nihon no Wakuchin Kaihatsu to Hinshitsu Kanri no Rekishiteki Kenshō* (Japanese Vaccine: An Investigation of the History of Development and Quality Control) (Tokyo: Iyaku jyānaru, 2014), pp. 26–8.

14　Editing Committee of the 50-Year History of the Ministry of Health and Welfare (eds), p. 1070. Other examples of Japanese discoveries include the causative agent for tularaemia (by Ohara Hachirō, research published in 1925), scrub typhus (Nagayo Mataro, Tamiya Takeo, 1924) and vibrio parahaemolyticus food-borne infection (Fujino Tsunesaburō, 1950).

15　Supreme Commander for Allied Powers, General Headquarters, *Summation of Non-Military Activities in Japan and Korea, 1945–1948*, no. 1, section 1 (1945), 1–2 (Tokyo: National Diet Library).

16　M. Watanabe, 'Wagakuni no yobōsesshu seido nitsui no rekishiteki ichikōsatsu' (A *historical consideration* about the Preventive Vaccination Law Constituted in 1948), *Minozoku eisei*, 73–6 (2007), p. 244.

17　Pharmaceutical and Medical Device Regulatory Science Society of Japan (eds), *Drug-Induced Suffering in Japan: A Review from Regulatory and Social Perspectives* (English title of bilingual volume) (Tokyo: Yakuji Nippō, 2013), p. 11. The 3,000–yen fine was costly given that a national civil servants' monthly salary was 13,000 yen.

18　J. Yongue, *The Introduction of American Mass Production Technology to Japan during the Occupation: The case of penicillin*, in P. Donzé and S. Nishimura (eds), Organizing Global Technology Flows (New York and London: 2014), pp. 213–29.

19　Watanabe, 'Wagakuni no yobōsesshu seido nitsui no rekishiteki ichikōsatsu', p. 249.

20　M. Wake, 'Cause Analysis of the 1948 Diphtheria Tragedy', *Bulletin of Social Medicine*, 23 (2005). Also see M. Kurokawa and R. Murata, 'On the Toxicity of the "Toxoid" Preparation Responsible for the Kyoto Catastrophe in 1948', *Japanese Journal of Medical Science & Biology*, 14 (1961), pp. 249–56. Both articles were published over a decade after the occupation ended.

21 S. Yamazaki and I. Kurane (eds), *Nihon no Wakuchin Kaihatsu to Hinshitsu Kanri no Rekishiteki Kenshō* (Japanese Vaccine: An Investigation of the History of Development and Quality Control) (Tokyo: Iyaku jyānaru, 2014), p. 31.

22 The threat of a large fine served as a deterrent as there are no records of actual collection.

23 C. Aldous, 'Transforming Public Health?: A Critical Review of Progress Made Against Enteric Diseases During the American-led Occupation of Japan (1945–52)', *Nihon Igaku Zasshi*, 54:1 (March 2008), pp. 9–16.

24 M. Hirayama, 'Porio Wakuchin no Kinkyūdōnyū no Keii to sonogono Porio' (Hirayama's English title: 'Progress on Urgent Introduction of Live Polio Vaccine in Japan and Poliomyelitis Thereafter), *Journal of the Japan Society for Paediatric Infectious Diseases* (in Japanese), 19:2 (2007), pp. 189–96, on p. 193.

25 Hirayama, 'Porio Wakuchin no Kinkyūdōnyū no Keii to sonogono Porio', p. 193.

26 Interview with Dr Abe Shinobu, Executive Director, laboratory division at Japan Poliomyelititis Research Institute, Tokyo, on 20 February 2014.

27 A. Otani, K. Mise and K. Tanaka, *Wakuchin to yobōsesshu nosubete: Minaosareru sono miryoku* (Introduction to Vaccines and Vaccination Remarkable Effects Recently Recognized) (Tokyo: Kanehara Shuppan, 2013), p. 40.

28 S. Yamazaki and S. Abe, 'Nihon niokeru fukatsuka porio wakuchin (sIPV) Kaihatsu no keii to genjō' ('Development of Sabin strain-derived inactivated poliovirus in Japan'), *BIO clinica*, 26:13 (2011), pp. 45–51.

29 US health authorities switched to IPV over a decade earlier on 1 January 2000.

30 Otani, Mise and Tanaka, *Wakuchin to yobōsesshu no subete: Minaosareru sono miroku*, pp. 59–60.

31 K. Kobayashi, 'Wakuchin no Kōshinkoku, Nihon' (Japan, Backward Nation for Vaccines), *Journal of the Japan Society for Pediatric Infectious Diseases* (in Japanese), 20:4 (2008), p. 445–6. See also, R. Shimazawa and M. Ikeda, 'The Vaccine Gap between Japan and the UK', *Health Policy*, 107 (2012), pp. 312–7; A. Saitoh and N. Okabe, 'Current Issues with the Immunization Program in Japan: Can we Fill the "Vaccine Gap"?', *Vaccine*, 30:32 (2012), pp. 4752–6.

32 M. Hosoda, H. Inoue, Y. Miyazawa, E. Kusumi and K. Shibuya, 'Vaccine-Associated Paralytic Poliomyelitis in Japan', *The Lancet*, 379:9815 (11 February 2012), p. 520.

33 *Ibid.*

34 Y. Tezuka, *Sengō gyōsei no kōzō to dikenma: Yōbōsesshu gyōsei no hensen* (The Structural Dilemma of Post-war Public Administration: Changes in Preventive Vaccination Policy) (Tokyo: Fujiwara Shoten 2010), p. 238.

35 Y. Okuno *et al.*, 'Uirusubyō no yobō chiryō ni kansuru kenkyū no ayumi' (Research on the History of Prevention and Treatment of Viral Diseases), *Virus 28* (commemorative issue, 1978). www.jstage.jst.go.jp/article/jsv1958/28/Special/28_Special_73/_pdf (accessed 27 October 2015).

36 *Ibid.*

37 See *Canada Diseases Weekly*, 13–35 (5 September 1987) and 14–46 (11 November 1988).

38 According to H. Ueno, whose daughter was vaccinated in 1991, during her hospital visit, the infant's grandmother requested separate inoculations but due to the physician's strong insistence, she reluctantly agreed to use MMR. 'MMR Wakuchin no Jittai' (The actual conditions surrounding the adverse effects of the MMR vaccine), in Pharmaceutical and Medical Device Regulatory Science Society, *Shitte okitai Yakugai no Kyōkun* (*Lessons to Learn About the Harmful Effects of Medicines*) (Tokyo: Yakuji Nippōsha, 2012).

39 Tezuka, *Sengō gyōsei no kōzō to direnma*, p. 238.

40 M. C. Andreae, G. L. Freed and S. L. Katz, 'Safety Concern Regarding Combination Vaccines: Experience in Japan', *Vaccine*, 22 (2004), pp. 3911–16, on pp. 3913.

41 H. Ueno, 'MMR Wakuchin no Jittai' (The Status of the MMR Vaccine), in Pharmaceutical and Medical Device Regulatory Science Society, *Shitte okitai Yakugai no Kyōkun* (Lessons to Learn About the Harmful Effects of Medicines), (Tokyo: Yakuji Nippōsha, 2012), p. 113.

42 The municipality of Kokubunji decided in October to switch from MMR to measles and only administered MMR when there was a 'strong request from the parent/guardian'. Osaka, Shiga Prefecture, Kyoto and Nara Prefectures took measures to discourage the use of MMR, while Wakayama and Hyogo continued administer it.

43 Tezuka, *Sengō gyōsei no kōzō to direnma*, p. 243.

44 *Ibid.*, p. 244.

45 Ueno, *MMR Wakuchin no Jittai* (The Status of the MMR Vaccine), pp. 116–17.

46 *Ibid.*, p. 122.

47 S. A. Plotkin, 'Commentary: Is Japan Deaf to the Mumps Vaccination?' *Pediatric Infectious Disease Journal*, 28 (2009), p. 176.

48 MHLW, *Wakuchin Sangyō Bijon Kanseishō Taisaku wo sasae, shakaiteki kitai ni kotaeru sangyōzō wo mezashite*, p. 23.

49 Y. Sato and H. Sato, 'Development of Acellular Pertussis Vaccines', *Biologicals*, 27 (1999), pp. 61–2. Also S. Yakazaki and I. Kurane (eds), 'Nihon no Wakuchin: Kaihatsu to Hinshitsu Kanri no Rekishi Kenshō', pp. 62–7. Based on the findings of Sato Yūji at the Japanese National Institutes of Health, a 'national project' with collaboration by paediatricians, health authorities and scientists at the six production establishments got underway to develop a safer pertussis vaccine. Sato's acellular pertussis vaccine is now administered worldwide and is particularly recognised in China, where it is known as the 'Sato vaccine'. Sato's personal experiences in developing the pertussis vaccine are described in: Y. Sato, 'Nihon de Kaihatsu sareta seisei hakunichi seki wakuchin no kisokenkyu, kaihatsukatei oyobi donyugo no ugoki (Basic Research and Development of Purified Pertussis Vaccine in Japan, the Vaccine and Thereafter), *Shonikansen Meneki*, 20:3 (2008), on pp. 347–58.

50 The following two volumes (1778 pages) contain the proceedings of the influenza and polio vaccine trials. K. Nakadaira, M. Ōno, T. Hirota, Y. Yamakawa, M. Akiyama and T. Kōno (eds), *Nihon saibashorui zenshū, Tokyō yobōsesshukasoshō* (Complete Collection of Japanese Court Records, Tokyo Preventive Vaccination Trials) (Tokyo: Shinzansha, 2005).

51 H. Nakatani, T. Sano and T. Iuchi, 'Development of Vaccination Policy in Japan: Current Issues and Policy Directions', *Japanese Journal of Infectious Diseases*, 55 (2002), pp. 101–11, on p. 103.

52 According to T. Nakayama, 'Vaccine Chronicle in Japan', p. 788, rates in 2010 for all routine vaccinations (BCG, DTaP, OPV, MR) were between 90 and 95 percent (80 per cent for JEV), but only 30 to 40 per cent for non-routine vaccinations. For more detailed statistical information, see the WHO website: http://apps.who.int/immunization_monitoring/globalsummary/countries?countrycriteria%5Bcountry%5D%5B%5D=JPN&commit=OK (accessed 25 February 2014).

53 For a full list of the participants and their affiliations, see Ministry of Health, Labour and Welfare, *Wakuchin Sangyō Bijon Kanseishō Taisaku wo sasae, shakaiteki kitai ni kotaeru sangyōzō wo mezashite* (Vaccine Industry Vision: Supporting Measures to Prevent Infection while Aiming to Respond to Societal Expectations of Industry) (MHLW, March 2007), pp. 2–3.

54 Institute of Medicine Division of Health Promotion and Disease Prevention (eds), *Vaccine Supply and Innovation* (Washington DC: National Academy Press, 1985), p. vi.

55 Ministry of Health, Labour and Welfare, *Wakuchin Sangyō Bijon Kanseishō Taisaku wo sasae, shakaiteki kitai ni kotaeru sangyōzō wo mezashite*, p. 31; p. 15.

56 Akazawa, Yongue, Ikeda and Satō, 'Considering Economic Analyses in the Revision of the Preventive Vaccine Law', pp. 127–34.

57 *Ibid.*

58 www.who.int/immunization/policy/Immunization_routine_table1.pdf (accessed 25 February 2014).

59 H. Kamiya, S. Uehara, T. Kato, K. Shiraki, T. Togashi, T. Morishima, Y. Gotō, O. Satō and S. Standaert, 'Childhood Bacterial Meningitis in Japan', *Pediatric Infectious Disease Journal*, 17:9 (September 1998), pp. 183–5.

60 J. Yongue, 'Shin'yaku Kaihatsu wo meguru kigyō to gyōsei' (Corporate Development of New Drugs and Drug Policy) in A. Kudō and M. Ihara (eds), *Kigyō to Gendai no Shihonshugi* (*Enterprises and Modern Capitalism*; Kyoto: Minerva Shobō, 2008), pp. 166–91 and W. H. Kuo, 'Japan and Taiwan in the Wake of Bio-Globalization: Drugs, Race and Standards' (PhD dissertation, Massachusetts Institute of Technology, September 2005). See also, www.fda.gov/downloads/Drugs/GuidanceComplianceRegulatoryInformation/Guidances/ucm073120.pdf (accessed on 21 July 2014).

61 This has not always been the case. Physicians have been able to influence policy by refusing to administer vaccinations. Tezuka, *Sengyō Gyōsei no Kozō to Direnma*, pp. 178–82.

62 www.mhlw.go.jp/shingi/2008/12/dl/s1225-141.pdf#search= 'サノフィ国家検定' (accessed on 5 March 2012).

63 'The "Two-Month Wait" and Barrier of Having to Bear the Cost Yourself: The Ban on the Hib Vaccine is Finally Lifted' (Nikagetsu machi to jibara no kabe: yatto kaikin sareta hib wakuchin), *Weekly Aera* (9 March 2009), p. 76.

64 Interview with former head of Pasteur Mérieux Connaught Daiichi in Lyon, France on 17 June 2011.

65 This point was made during numerous interviews with current and previous managers at Sanofi Pasteur. The same problem of black specks is mentioned in Roy Vagelos and Louis Galambos, *Medicine, Science, and Merck*, (Cambridge University Press, 2004), p. 190.

66 Interview with Professor Ueda Shigeharu (executive director of Biken or the Institute for Microbial Diseases, Osaka University) and Professor Nojima Hiroshi on 4 August 2011 at the University of Osaka and observations I made during a visit to the Biken factory in Kagawa, Shikoku on 15 November 2011.

III

Vaccination, the individual and society

9

The MMR debate in the United Kingdom: vaccine scares, statesmanship and the media

Andrea Stöckl and Anna Smajdor

Introduction

In 1998, British surgeon and researcher Andrew Wakefield published a paper in the British journal *The Lancet,* suggesting that there was a link between the triple vaccine against measles, mumps and rubella (MMR) and the development of childhood autism.[1] This publication inflamed an already existing debate on the role of childhood vaccination in the UK and contributed to a substantial decline in vaccination uptake in the UK in the early 2000s.[2] The impact of this decline was still being felt in 2012 and 2013 when a measles epidemic broke out in the Welsh city of Swansea, in which one person died and 1,200 young adults were diagnosed with measles.

This chapter situates the British MMR controversy within the broader historical context of public debates over science and government policy in the years 1998–2003. We focus on the role of political leaders as models for the general public for dealing with what is broadly understood as modern risk society.[3] In addition to previous research on the MMR debate in the UK, which locate it in the controversies on science in society and the impact of the media on decision-making processes, we adopt a socio-historical approach that allows us to contextualise the MMR debate in its relationship to the decision making processes of public figures, and here in particular Tony Blair.[4] Through an analysis of media reports from the time, we show how a series of scandals and controversies through the early 2000s were tackled by the British government with an explicit, and sometimes aggressive, pro-science rationalism that tended to polarise public opinion. We argue that analysing the significance of a politician's health care decision and its impact on a national debate can shed new light on researching the emotional aspects of public health – an aspect that is often overlooked.

The single shot MMR vaccine was introduced in the UK in 1988; uptake reached a peak in 1995 when 92 per cent of children who had reached the age of two were vaccinated. By 1997, this rate had declined to 79 per cent.[5] Although concerns about MMR and autism originated in the UK, they began to spread to other countries including Australia and New Zealand.[6] Parents who were reluctant to have their children vaccinated were able to cite the purported link between the vaccine and autism as their rationale.[7] There was also concern about the safety of the MMR vaccine in other European countries such as the Netherlands, Sweden and France (discussed in this book).[8] However, the specifically British response to Wakefield's study is of interest for two key reasons: First, because the controversy arose at a time of particular tension over the role of government in science. Second, because of the unique way in which Prime Minister, Blair, his wife Cherie and son Leo, became personally embroiled in the debate.

We draw on policy documents concerned with the role of science in British society and use qualitative content analysis to research the debates in selected newspapers between 1998 and 2003.[9] We searched the archives of two major newspapers, the *Guardian* and the *Daily Mail*, for debates on MMR, Andrew Wakefield and the decision-making process of the then prime minister. We defined the search terms as 'Wakefield' and 'MMR', and 'Blair' and 'MMR'. We chose these two newspapers because we deemed them as representative for the British newspaper readership and thus for a certain public debate. We used websites such as www.nrs.co.uk or www.abc.org.uk to help us understand the impact of the newspapers.

The UK has a relatively stable newspaper market and readership. Research on the influence of the newspapers on public opinion shaping in the UK has been well established. Several research projects have analysed the influence of the media on the swine flu epidemic and the HPV vaccination.[10] Newspaper distribution and readership has been researched extensively and we thus follow the analysis of Shona Hilton and team who have researched the readership of British newspapers by age and social class.[11] We also examine the role that the British Broadcasting Company (BBC) played in these debates. Before doing so, we wanted to situate these debates in a historical context in order to show that these controversies did not arise out of the blue but are indeed to be contextualised in the political climate of the time.

The role of Andrew Wakefield's paper and public health in the UK context, 1998–2003

In February 1998 Andrew Wakefield and several colleagues published a paper in *The Lancet* under the title 'Ileal-lymphoid-nodular Hyperplasia, Non-specific Colitis, and Pervasive Developmental Disorder in Children'.[12] In this paper, now retracted by *The Lancet*, Wakefield and his co-authors argue that their preliminary research had shown that 'onset of behavioural symptoms was associated by the parents, with measles, mumps, and rubella vaccination in eight of the 12 children who were studied'.[13] Wakefield and his team had recruited twelve children who were referred to his pediatric gastroenterology unit with 'a history of normal development followed by loss of acquired skills, including language, together with diarrhoea and abdominal pain'.[14] In spite of its low number of participants, Wakefield's findings were classified for publication as an 'early report' in *The Lancet*.

Openness and transparency in keeping the public informed had become a political priority following the BSE scandal a decade earlier.[15] A policy of openness also harmonised with a new type of public participation in health matters, in which individuals were increasingly expected to take responsibility for their own health and well-being. Prevention of disease rather than curing disease was the new agenda of public health planning. At the same time public awareness about the risks of new technologies and medical interventions had increased. These changes in responsibility for health and well-being urged by the state coincided with the emergence of a number of scares such as HIV/ AIDS, BSE and the planned introduction of genetically modified (GM) foods.[16] The new public health message was that being a modern, forward-looking British citizen meant protecting oneself against health risks by keeping up with government and medical information and recommendations. Yet at the same time it was becoming apparent that this protection was precarious; to follow government advice could itself be seen as risky, especially if it was tainted by political interest, if it was seen as deceptive, or perhaps just mistaken.

The MMR debate emerged at a time when public trust in government pronouncements on science and risk had already been severely tested. During the 1990s, the UK had been embroiled in uncertainty and anxiety over a possible connection between BSE in cattle and what has come to be known as variant Creutzfeld Jakob Disease (vCJD). Fearing a crisis of public confidence, and its possible effects on the farming industry, the government reassured the public that it was impossible to contract the disease from eating beef. In 1990, a statement was issued by Chief Medical Officer, Sir Donald Acheson, saying that after reviewing all the scientific and medical evidence, he was confident that 'beef can be eaten safely by everyone, both adults and children, including patients in hospital'.[17] The message was reinforced when the then Agricultural Minister in the Tory cabinet, John Gummer, attempted to feed his 4-year-old daughter a beefburger while being photographed by the press.[18] As the sociologist of science, Sheila Jasanoff, says, the BSE controversy of 1996 can be seen as an unprecedented illustration of 'expertise and democracy, technological risk and policy uncertainty' coming together in one event.[19] The policy system grappled with a worst case scenario, as Jasanoff puts it, because there was a disease of uncertain origin which was transmissible and its incidence 'might have been, but was not, curtailed by timely governmental action'.[20]

Are there historical links?

As noted, an analysis of public and parliamentary debates shows that concerns over the trustworthiness of governments' pronouncements on matters of risk and science did not originate with the Wakefield controversy – rather, Wakefield's paper exacerbated existing anxieties which can be traced back to various sources, including the BSE crisis. In the early 1990s, there was little data to establish whether BSE was linked to vCJD but the government had hastened to reassure the public by claiming to know with scientific certainty that there was no link.[21] When this was proved wrong, it set the scene for a more cautious approach to the claims set out in Wakefield's paper. Perhaps because of this, the methodological limitations of Wakefield's paper did not prevent his claims from being taken seriously. His paper was based on anecdotal evidence of twelve cases linking the MMR vaccine with autism. Scientists and politicians did not want to repeat the mistakes of the BSE crisis.

Some scholars argue that the MMR debate was a transposition of mistrust which resulted directly from the mismanaged BSE crisis.[22] Sheila Jasanoff has argued that a particular characteristic of the UK public is to place its faith in politicians' statements based on how reliable or trustworthy they are perceived to be, rather than on the enquiry into the factual accuracy of their claims. This, she suggests, is fundamentally different from the USA where transparency and objectivity are taken to be the necessary basis for ensuring trust in government decision-making.[23]

Gummer's attempt to make his daughter consume beef in the full glare of the media spotlight can be seen as an attempt to capitalise on this British tendency. Assuming himself to be perceived as reliable and trustworthy, he recognised that his gesture would convey a powerful message to the public – more so than merely citing scientific evidence. However, as it became clear that the scientific evidence *was* starting to suggest a link between beef consumption and vCJD, Gummer's public gesture returned to haunt him: it 'turned him into a figure of fun and led to a lasting public mistrust of government pronouncement on food scares – notably Blair's reassurances on genetically-modified food'.[24]

The peculiarly British way of placing trust which Jasanoff identifies is perhaps unavoidably associated with a deeper and more emotional sense of outrage when this trust is shown to have been betrayed or misplaced. It could be that this partly explains the periodic scandals in the UK when people start to disbelieve government pronouncements and assurances. There is a long history of contention when it comes to innovations in science and technology in general in the UK, especially with regard to medical innovations and immunisation policies.[25] Notable here is the smallpox vaccination controversy in the late nineteenth century and the diphtheria-tetanus-pertussis (DTP) vaccine debate, which took place from roughly 1974 to 1986.[26]

The DTP vaccine had been in use for more than twenty years when reports emerged from the Hospital for Sick Children at Great Ormond Street in 1974 suggesting that children who had been given the vaccine had developed neurological complications. The media took this up and a storm of publicity followed.[27] As with the MMR debate that would erupt twenty years later, a pivotal medical figure, Gordon Stewart, initiated the concern by citing research that he had carried out involving children of parents who had concerns about the vaccine. The Department of Health initiated a public campaign in order to pursuade parents to have their children vaccinated. The daughter of the then health minister was vaccinated, as was Prince William, 'amidst great publicity'.[28] Again, this seems to corroborate Jasanoff's interpretation of the relationship between the British public and their politicians. The advice and actions of trusted individuals was taken to be an appropriate means of getting the public to accept risks and uncertainties, even where the data did not straightforwardly support the messages that were being conveyed.

The role of the media

As with the DTP controversy, the MMR debate was played out in the media, in broadsheets such as *The Times* and the *Guardian*, and tabloids such as the *Daily Mail*. The BBC also reported on the debate and opened discussion fora on its website so that the public could participate in the debate. This high level of media activity may – as with DTP – have contributed to the fall in vaccination rates from 92 per cent before the controversy to 80 per cent in 2004 in England.[29]

The MMR controversy reached its peak in 2002 when the vaccination status of Tony Blair's son, Leo, became a focus of attention. Interestingly, as media analysts point out, the MMR controversy was not only reported by science correspondents: it became part of the national news agenda rather than a minor story in the science pages. The areas that were linked were the safety of the triple jab, the role of the Prime Minister and his son's vaccination status, and the 'expert parent' (i.e. the parent who is well-informed about the scientific background to the MMR jab).[30]

Wakefield and his team published their paper in February 1998. By 25 March 1998 the *Guardian*, a left-leaning newspaper predominantly read by a young, metropolitan readership, was responding to Wakefield's claims. The *Guardian's* perspective was that the MMR vaccination fears were not justified and that the most recent paper by Wakefield and his team should be viewed with scepticism. Throughout 1998 and

1999, the *Guardian* kept a critical stance towards Wakefield's publication. Their argument was that the practices of science and the pressure to publish as many papers as possible had led to an increase in bad research and publications and that Wakefield's controversial paper was one such instance. Sarah Boseley, the *Guardian*'s health editor, especially took on this line of argument by saying that doctors, who are also researchers, faced a dilemma and were 'damned if they published, damned if they don't' (27 February 1998).

The *Guardian* kept up this line of reporting throughout those early years of the debate; rather than reporting straight from the field by their health editor, though, their commentators wrote many opinion pieces. For instance, the political commentator Catherine Bennett argued that Britain would face an epidemic of irrational fear rather than a measles epidemic. She attributed this to the fault of the Department of Health which, she argued, treated the parents as 'cattle' rather than people with a valuable opinion (*Guardian*, 5 September 1998). Throughout 1999, the *Guardian*'s reports discussed the perspectives of the parents while at the same time pointing out that Wakefield's paper was 'suspect science'. However, direct reporting of parents' viewpoints rarely appeared in these early articles. If there was a bias, it was clearly towards the faulty science rather than towards the fears of the parents. The few parents who did write opinion pieces were mostly the *Guardian*'s own commentators, such as Jay Rayner whose usual remit was to write about food and restaurants. Rayner's opinion in September 2003 was that 'the failure by parents to inoculate their children against such a vicious illness is, undoubtedly, a middle-class disease, passed on at the school gates'.

The reporting style of the *Guardian* on MMR changed radically after the birth of the Tony Blair's son Leo on 20 May 2000. Two days after his birth, the *Guardian* published an article called 'Decisions, Decisions' in which the commentator argued that bringing up Leo would be 'political as well as critical', especially considering the fact that 'every parent faces a dilemma over immunisation' and that the Blairs would have to also make a decision about vaccinating Leo (*Guardian*, 22 May 2000). Little did the journalist know how prophetic this article would be. The debate on the vaccination status of the Blairs' son became extremely heated. The level of immunisation in early 2001 dropped sharply; the alternatives to the MMR jabs were not considered safe, and the Blairs refused to disclose whether they had opted for the MMR vaccine for their son.

Shortly before Christmas 2001, the *Guardian* published several articles criticising Tony Blair over his refusal to state whether Leo had or had not received the MMR vaccine. On 22 December, the political editor, rather than the health editor, wrote an opinion piece arguing that Blair should be urged to 'set jab row example'. Given that the government was advising parents to have their children immunised with the MMR vaccine, and that uptake was declining amid parents' anxieties about the risks, Blair was in the perfect position to lead by example. Why miss the opportunity to demonstrate his conviction that the vaccine was safe? On 20 December 2001, Catherine Bennett urged Blair to disclose whether baby Leo had had the jab or not. Her comments were critical of Cherie Blair in particular, whose penchant for consulting alternative medicine gurus was cited (20 December 2001). However, Bennett also understood the reasons why Cherie Blair did not want to 'come clean'; after all, she argued, she was a private citizen who has the right to privacy; she 'is not responsible for public health policy'.

The issue of privacy was discussed in several other publications as well, but in Bennett's article from 20 December, privacy issue was the leading concern. The Blair family reacted to these publications and on 21 December 2001, the *Guardian* reported that he had asked the media to 'leave them alone'. Blair specifically referred to the 'horrors' of John Gummer who had fed his daughter with a beefburger when the BSE debate was at its height. The *Guardian* reported that Blair insisted that his family had a right to privacy in health-care matters. On 21 December, the newspaper reported that Blair had 'given in' and that they could finally reveal that 'Leo Blair has been given the controversial triple vaccination'. The *Observer*, which is the *Guardian*'s Sunday paper, reported that Blair had found the intrusion into his private life and the suggestion that he would not give the jab to his son as 'offensive beyond belief'. Blair justified his non-disclosure as a choice he had made to protect his family from this intrusion because once he would start commenting on one, 'it is hard to see how we can justify not commenting on them all' (*Observer*, 23 December 2001).

The theme of privacy returned the following day in a report by the then chief political correspondent of the *Guardian*, who reported that Blair's efforts to 'quell the public demand to know whether his son had been given the controversial MMR jab appeared to have failed yesterday after politicians and patient groups intensified calls for him to give a definitive answer'. The political correspondent, however, noted that even though Blair had 'hurried out' a statement on the previous night, he had left enough ambiguity to 'claim that he had protected the principle of his children's privacy' (*Guardian*, 24 December 2001).

The debate went on for another day or two over this Christmas period, with the publication of another article on Blair's behaviour, entitled 'Jab dilemma that pricked consciences' and again written by another chief political correspondent. The *Guardian* editorial on 24 December 2001 also suggested that there is a right to Leo's privacy. However, the article suggested in a subheading, that this privacy had come 'at a price for public health'. The last opinion paper, published on 30 December 2001 in the *Observer*, was by Richard Ingrams, the editor of the satirical magazine *Private Eye*. He commented on the fact that we still could not know for sure whether Leo had been given the MMR, however, we could for sure say that his parents were rather 'swarmy, barmy' because they believed in Ayurveda medicine and in rebirthing rituals (30 December 2001).

After this heated debate around Christmas time of 2001, the debate picked up again in spring 2002. Sarah Boseley again reported on the likely outbreak of measles in 2002 because of the MMR scare. In general, the theme of reporting switched to drawing parallels with the 1970s whooping cough (pertussis) debate. The reporting focused on the perceived failure of the public health authorities to inform the public appropriately. The lead comment in the *Guardian* from 7 February 2002, argued that 'this is no longer a question of calculating risk on all the available scientific evidence … it has become a test for this government about how to handle a crisis in public confidence' (*Guardian*, 7 February 2002). The journalists who reported on the MMR vaccine crisis were again the health editors.

The debate intensified in the second week of February 2002, with the political commentator Andrew Rawnsley asking: 'Who can we believe these days?' He wondered how to survive in a world in which public trust in medical authority 'had gone'. Rawnsley argued that because of this mistrust, the Prime Minister would have to make a full statement on whether he had given the triple jab to his son a year earlier. He argued that it was not a question of whether the MMR jab was safe or not, but a bigger question of whether the public would trust the Prime Minister with anything at all. 'This crisis of confidence is the latest example of the wider crisis of confidence in all the figures to whom society used to look for leadership and judgment', Rawnsley concluded (10 February 2002). A week later, the deputy editor of the political magazine *New Statesman*, Christina Odone, wrote a comment in the *Guardian* lamenting that 'the white coats are looking grubbier after one too many scandals'. Odone here drew on previous debates, and explicitly on the BSE debate, to argue that 'BSE, MMR and a catalogue of blunders have jerked the science gurus off their pedestals' (17 February 2002).

The sacking of Wakefield from the Royal Free Hospital and his move to the USA sparked another discussion. This time it was about disputes within the medical scientific community. Sarah Boseley reported that, 'Doctors turn on each other as MMR debate rages again' (1 November 2003). Simon Murch, one of the co-authors of the paper published with Andrew Wakefield, had published an open letter to *The Lancet* warning of a measles epidemic, stating that he could no longer detect the link between the MMR jab and an autism epidemic. This was picked up by the *Guardian*. The debate thus shifted from focusing on Blair and his family back to discussing the reliability of science in itself. In February 2003, John Grace linked the 'peer trouble' of the Wakefield paper to previous science scandals and fabrication of data, such as the chemicals in the GM crop debate. Grace discussed the increase in the malpractice and explained it as competition for funding and in the academic job market (*Guardian*, 11 February 2003). The debate in the *Guardian* had thus come full circle.

The BBC and the *Daily Mail*

The BBC is a public serving broadcasting statutory corporation and has the duty to inform the British public impartially, especially on science topics.[31] On 19 June 2002, the BBC reported on research by a team of epidemiologists who had compared 180 countries and found the MMR vaccine to be 'safe'.[32] The 'Talking Point' website on which it discussed the findings included some contributions from the public who still doubted the research and claimed anecdotal evidence that linked the vaccine to autism in their children.

It seemed that, for the British public, 'scientific research' had been tainted 'with the concerns and agendas of corporate finance'.[33] In this environment, the publication of reassuring scientific data was not – and perhaps never could be – enough to allay their suspicions. Parallels can be seen here with the Alder Hey scandal, in which it was discovered that tissue and organs from dead children had been taken and stored without the knowledge or consent of the parents. There was a public outcry, leading to radical changes in the law – and this was mostly driven by parental advocacy groups.[34] Experiential and anecdotal knowledge in the Alder Hey scandal assumed an importance equal to, or superior to that of scientific research and similar power shifts were evident in the MMR debate. Parents who had a child who developed autism after the MMR vaccine were given a media platform to recount their experiences: people reported overnight changes in the behaviour of their children following the MMR vaccination.

In 2005, a Cochrane review concluded that there was no significant association between the MMR immunisation and autism, asthma, leukaemia and other childhood disorders.[35] However, the *Daily Mail*, whose readership is mostly politically right-leaning, claimed that this report was 'baloney'.[36] The science editor of the *Daily Mail* argued that 'the MMR scandal is getting worse. Urgent questions about the vaccine's safety remain unanswered. The doctor who raised those questions is being subjected to what appears to be a witch-hunt. The parents' recourse through the courts has been blocked. Now they have to put up with being told yet again that the evidence of their own eyes is fraudulent'.[37] This prompted a reply in the *British Medical Journal* in which the author of a comment: 'Why can't the *Daily Mail* eat humble pie over MMR' suggested that the *Daily Mail* science editor, who has one of the best paid jobs in the British media, was captivated by 'Andrew Wakefield's self-professed status as a maverick and crusader against the establishment'.[38]

The role of the patients and parents

If one looks at research on parental attitudes carried out at the time of the crisis, an interesting diverse picture emerges. For instance, media researchers Speers and Lewis point out that the MMR debate in the media made use of the role of the expert patient, which in this case had been turned into the expert *parent*. Parents who were interviewed on their opinion of the MMR functioned as 'experts' who would 'provide a common sense, anecdotal expertise to support Wakefield's claims'.[39] This role was criticised on the grounds that the public lacked knowledge of basic science and rudimentary statistics to contribute effectively to the debate. The research by Speers and Lewis shows that the anecdotal views of the 'expert parent' were being pitted against those of what would in general be defined as classical, orthodox science. The argument here is not one of the hierarchy of scientific knowledge versus experiential knowledge of the parents, but these findings show that a subtle erosion of the public value of science had started to impact decision-making processes on the personal, rather than on the political level. Increasingly, media outlets presented both voices as a meeting of equals, rather than privileging the scientific view.

A historic precedent was the DTP controversy twenty years earlier in which parents had also played a major role. The Association of Parents of Vaccine-Damaged Children had presented cases to the media and they advocated for compensation in Parliament.[40] Similarly, in the MMR case, a group of parents called JABS (Justice, Awareness and Basic Support) who believed that their children had been damaged by the vaccine was founded in 1994.[41] This group was endorsed by the *Daily Mail* which held an anti-vaccination perspective throughout the debate. The *Daily Mail* reported that JABS at one stage had around 2,000 members whose parents believed that their children had been harmed by the triple vaccine.[42] Endorsement by the right-wing-leaning media of parents who were against the orthodox scientific view and who used this as a political platform thus had a historical antecedent.

In the meantime, back in the early 2000s, a rather high number of parents who refused to get their children vaccinated could be found in urban areas, with London and Brighton and Hove having the highest number of unvaccinated children.[43] Brighton and Hove is a town in the commuting vicinity for London. Research in Brighton and Hove again showed a different picture because a high number of parents who had been involved in anti-vaccination groups were more trusting of the government than was expected.[44] Yet, if one looks more closely at the research outcomes, it confirms our argument in the introduction to this chapter: an individualisation of implementing public health messages had happened. The main frame of reference in the decision-making process of these young parents was their own family history of vaccination, their experiences of the process of giving birth, and their immediate social environment such as other young mothers and friends. Yet, several mothers who had chosen 'natural birth' methods had later on also rejected the national vaccination programmes. The experience of being vulnerable also influenced decision-making processes: mothers whose parents did not live in their immediate environment or who could not provide them with support felt more vulnerable in general towards what they perceived as a hostile society and thus opted for the vaccination.

Poltorak's research also showed that the BSE and other previous scandals were no longer in the historical consciousness of the parents and were not perceived as having an impact on the decision-making processes. Parents were aware of the BSE scandal but were not worried by it and did not seem to have lost trust in the government. What they were worried about was being able to trust their own decision making.[45] Trust in science was thus a theme that came up frequently: there was a significant number of parents who did not want their children to be inoculated with the MMR vaccine who also held deep mistrust towards science in general. They found that 'both MMR acceptors and MMR refusers showed a high degree of ambivalence about the safety of MMR.'[46] In general, however, the parents who were refusers distrusted the government in their capacity to estimate risk, but trusted their general practitioners and other medical professionals with whom they had a personal relationship.[47]

Brownlie and Howson show that it was not only parents who were mistrustful of official health advice, but also health practitioners and general practitioners themselves (i.e. primary care doctors).[48] Their research suggested that health practitioners and GPs engaged critically with 'the processes of governmentality' in health care, so they employed 'critical trust' but were also tied to a self-regulation process of their professional bodies. Just like parents, health practitioners also had to make a leap of faith and trust their professional information-giving bodies that the information was right. They argue that trust in the health-care relationship at the time of the MMR crisis was tainted because 'the state in the UK plays a key role in the governance of child

immunization, it does so from a distance ... if this key role is not seen
as legitimate and trustworthy, then not only will patients distrust health
interventions, but professionals will lack a workable framework for
engaging with patients and each other.'[49]

Tony Blair, politics and science

In the section on the role of the media in the MMR controversy, we
argued that Tony Blair's non-disclosure of his private decision to vaccinate his son became a public affair. In this section, we discuss why the
political role of the then prime minister had been so crucial in this
debate. In 1997, Tony Blair, the leader of New Labour won the elections
and introduced a new style of government to British politics. Blair's
politics were described as 'presidential' because his style had authoritarian undertones in his personal, popular and political leadership. Political scientist Michael Foley describes Blair's leadership as a qualitative
shift in the British political process because the public persona and his
decision-making processes were not always tied to the democratic processes reached in the Houses of Parliament.[50] Foley cites Peter Liddell,
a *Times* columnist, who had described Blair's leadership as detached,
but also, as downgrading the collective and parliamentary aspects.
Blair's most important contribution to a change in leadership in politics
happened at the end of the 1990s and the beginning of the new millennium with his engagement in foreign politics. Under the Blair government, Britain supported the US-American war on terror and sent
British troops to support the invasion of Afghanistan in 2001 and the
invasion of Iraq in 2003. Blair's political style has been linked to a new
type of personalised political leadership which emerged at the end of
the twentieth century in western democracies. This style of politics has
seen an increase in the importance of the political leader over the collective of the party. The democratic decision-making process has been
reduced to one individual who influences public opinion and shapes
policy decisions.

Some political scientists attribute this development to an increasing
individualisation of society and of politics in general and politics would
be no exception.[51] Political analysts point out that Blair, prior to the
invasion of Afghanistan and subsequently Iran, was highly esteemed by
the British public: 'although voters gave the Blair government mixed

grades for its performance in office, Labour had a large lead over the Conservatives and the Liberal Democrats as the party best able to handle the election issues that voters considered most important'.[52] Blair had started his premiership with a lot of plans for stabilising the economy, levelling out the social inequalities in Britain, and forging strong links with European countries such as France and Germany. All this changed in 2001 when Britain decided to join the USA in its 'war on terror'. As Steven Philip Kramer put it, Blair seemed to succeed in his strategy until the invasion of Afghanistan alienated his European allies and changed the perception that the UK would act as a diplomatic bridge between Europe and the United States. As political analysts point out, the British willingness to participate in the military invasion was not an inevitable consequence of the so-called 'special relationship' between Great Britain and the USA, nor was there any pressure from Washington. Instead, Kramer suggests that the dominant reason for Blair's commitment to US policy was his 'intense and rather unique moral perspective on international politics'.[53] He had expressed this moral perspective already in a speech to the Economic Club of Chicago in 1999 when he referred to Saddam Hussein and Slobodan Milošević as dangerous and ruthless men who had endangered their own communities in vicious campaigns.

The participation of the UK in these overseas wars was highly controversial among the British public: in February 2003, an estimated 750,000 people took part in the march against the war in London alone, the BBC reported that in all of the UK, over a million people demonstrated against the participation in the war. Blair's foreign policy thus alienated many of the public who might otherwise have been regarded as natural Labour supporters and voters. Another way in which his government risked alienating the public was his espousal of science, and his characterisation of the British public as emotional and irrational where they expressed fear or mistrust of developments in science.

The Labour government was far more 'pro science' than the preceding Conservative one. Indeed, as Wilsdon and Wynne observe, science and scientific research occupied a very low status in the hierarchy of priorities in the 1980s, under the Conservative government.[54] The pro-science Labour government came into power at a pivotal point in the relationship between politicians, scientists and the British public. During the Conservatives' period in office, embryo research had become a possibility, and many people were excited about the new avenues for exploration that this might open. Scientists had assumed that the potential benefits of embryo research would guarantee the acceptance of such research both legally, and in terms of public and opinion. However, they were wrong. In February 1985, the Unborn Children (Protection) Bill – which would outlaw embryo research – received its second reading in Parliament, and received 238 to sixty-six votes. The scale and energy of opposition to embryo research came as a surprise to many scientists and their supporters. Scientists realised that they would need to fight in support of their cause. In short, it became clear that 'research has to be justified to the satisfaction of the lay community and its parliamentary representatives'.[55] The scientists who were newly mobilised to fight for their cause regarded themselves as fighters for scientific freedom, integrity and rationality, pitted against the ignorant, emotional and irrational public. They were successful in getting embryo research legalised, but a polarity arose in the debates on this issue, which persists to this day.

In this environment, where battle lines had already been drawn, the pro-science Labour government came to power. Unlike the Conservatives, Labour explicitly linked its political and ideological agenda with that of scientific advancement. There were eleven mentions of science in Labour's 2005 election manifesto; and none in the Conservatives'.[56] In 2006, Blair described Britain's path to the future as being 'lit by the brilliant light of science'.[57] This powerful conjunction of politics and science had significant effects on the status of science in the UK. The new presumption was that scientific freedom and progress should be restricted only reluctantly, and in the face of compelling evidence as to the negative consequences of failure to do so.[58] At the same time, extravagant claims were made about the medical, technological and economic benefits of biomedical research. A new mood of aggressive political optimism with regard to scientific advances emerged.[59]

However, there remained problems of trust and these tended to be increasingly polarised. Fears over GM food and MMR and other perceived dangers were portrayed by the Labour government as stemming from an emotional, irrational, risk-averse and under-educated public.[60] The public were not ready to accept every pronouncement made by the government or by government scientists and, as suggested, there are historical reasons to explain this. But independently of past events, the new alliance between science and politics may itself have served to further undermine the public's inclination to trust the information that they were being given. As noted earlier, 'tainted' science – where political or other ideological values are perceived to have infiltrated scientific data – provokes suspicion. A pro-science government may, ironically, result in a sceptical public. From this perspective, it is not surprising that the public's response to the concerns of the time (GM food, BSE, foot and mouth, MMR) revealed a degree of mistrust not only of scientists, but crucially also of politicians, and of the institutions which were set up to evaluate risks and reassure the public. In each case, the government enlisted scientists to bolster its position, to persuade the public that its strategy was appropriate, or that their fears were unfounded. Blair believed that those who objected to GM food crops were simply wrong – just as he believed those who objected to the wars in Afghanistan and Iraq were wrong. Rather than being a servant of democracy, whose function is to carry out the will of the people, Blair seems to have felt that his mission was to do what he knew to be right, regardless of public opposition.

Conclusion

This chapter has shown that public health campaigns and the way they are perceived are often linked to political debates that are not directly relevant to the clinical impact of a drug. There has been considerable research on the impact of the MMR controversy and why and how it happened. However, not a lot of research has actually looked at the actions of Blair's family and their decisions about vaccinations. We have shown that the MMR debate erupted in the UK at a time when public trust in science, research and medicine had sunk to an all-time low because of incidents such as the Alder Hey scandal. However, the behaviour of politicians influenced the private decision making of parents because of what politicians stand for: trust in medicine, trust in the state to look after its people and trust in their moral judgements. From a historical perspective, there are many parallels between the DTP and MMR debates: in both cases, combined vaccinations were linked to devastating neurological illnesses; in both cases a medical professional played a pivotal role in the medical debate; the media reporting offered a platform for the anti-vaccination discourse, and lay members of the public and parents played a major role in keeping the debate alive. We would like to argue that the historical setting of the MMR debate was particularly fraught with debates on the value of science, the public's engagement with science, the state and its duty towards its citizens, and Tony Blair's contested leadership style, but it cannot be understood without the debate on DTP that happened some decades earlier.

With the MMR debate, the British version of neo-liberal policy making had just started to have an effect on the changes in health-care delivery and the increasing role of personal responsibility that was calculated into the public's ideas on how to protect one's own health and that of the family. All of these elements contributed to an explosive assemblage, and the MMR controversy was the public arena in which all of these elements were played out. As Speers and Lewis put it, 'The Blair family's dilemma encapsulated many of the story's themes about parental concern, parental choice, and the degree of trust that can be placed in the official government line.'[61] We would thus like to suggest that even though the MMR debate can be seen within its historical context, it will also be significant for future controversies.

Notes

1 A. J. Wakefield, S. H. Murch, A. Anthony *et al.*, 'Retracted: Ileal-lymphoid-nodular Hyperplasia, Non-specific Colitis, and Pervasive Developmental Disorder in Children', *The Lancet*, 351 (1998), pp. 637–41.
2 See for instance the analysis of this time in the book by J. Fairhead and M. Leach, *Vaccine Anxieties. Global Science, Child Health and Society* (London: Earthscan, 2007) and the research papers by R. E. Casiday, T. Cresswell, D. Wilson and C. Panter-Brick, 'A Survey of UK Parental Attitudes to the MMR Vaccine and Trust in Medical Authority', *Vaccine*, 24 (2006), pp. 177–84, as well as J. Brownlie and A. Howson, ' "Leaps of Faith" and MMR: An Empirical Study of Trust', *Sociology*, 39 (2005), pp. 221–39, or M. Poltorak, M. Leach, J. Fairhead and J. Cassell, ' "MMR Talk" and Vaccination Choices: An Ethnographic Study in Brighton', *Social Science & Medicine*, 61 (2005), pp. 709–19, and finally J. Brownlie and A. Howson, ' "Between the Demands of Truth and Government": Health Practitioners, Trust and Immunisation Work', *Social Science & Medicine*, 62 (2006), pp. 433–43.

3 See U. Beck, *The Risk Society. Towards a New Modernity* (London: Sage Publications, 1992).

4 See especially the work of T. Speers and J. Lewis, 'Journalists and Jabs: Media Coverage of the MMR Vaccine', *Communication and Medicine*, 1 (2004), pp. 171–81.

5 For more information on statistics and numbers, see A. Pearce, C. Law, T. J. Cole *et al.*, 'Factors Associated with Uptake Of Measles, Mumps, and Rubella Vaccine (MMR) and Use of Single Antigen Vaccines in a Contemporary UK Cohort: Prospective Cohort Study', *British Medical Journal*, 336 (2008), pp. 754 ff.

6 www.abc.net.au/radionational/programs/rearvision/the-mmr-vaccine-scare/3121882 (accessed 30 May 2013).

7 See D. C. Burgess, M. A. Burgess and J. Leach, 'The MMR Vaccination and Autism Controversy in United Kingdom 1998–2005: Inevitable Community Outrage or a Failure of Risk Communication?' *Vaccine*, 24 (2006), pp. 3921–8.

8 For the situation in the Netherlands, see S. Blume and J. Tump, 'Evidence and Policymaking: The Introduction of MMR Vaccine in the Netherlands', *Social Science & Medicine*, 71 (2010), pp. 1049–55.

9 For an elaboration on content analysis as a method see K. Krippendorff, *Content Analysis. An Introduction to its Methodology* (Thousand Oaks: Sage, 2004).

10 S. Hilton, K. Hunt, M. Langan, H. Bedford and M. Petticrew, 'Newsprint Media Representations of the Introduction of the HPV Vaccination Programme for Cervical Cancer Prevention in the UK (2005–2008)', *Social Science & Medicine*, 70 (2010), pp. 942–50.

11 *Ibid.*

12 Wakefield *et al.*, p. 637.

13 *Ibid.*

14 *Ibid.*

15 C. Wilson, 'Intersecting Discourses: MMR Vaccine and BSE', *Science as Culture*, 13 (2004), pp. 75–88.

16 See Beck, 'Risk Society', and M. Leach and I. Scoones, 'Science and Citizenship in a Global Context', in M. Leach, I. Scoones and B. Wynne (eds), *Science and Citizens* (London: Zed Books, 2005).

17 http://news.bbc.co.uk/onthisday/hi/dates/stories/may/16/newsid_2913000/2913807.stm (accessed 30 September 2016).

18 http://news.bbc.co.uk/1/hi/uk/369625.stm (accessed 30 May 2013).

19 See S. Jasanoff, 'Civilization and Madness: the Great BSE Scare of 1996', *Public Understanding of Science*, 6 (1997), pp. 221–32, and 'Civilization and Madness: The Great BSE Scare of 1996', in M. Hissemoeller, R. Hoppe, W.

N. Dunn *et al.* (eds) *Knowledge, Power, and Participation in Environmental Policy Analysis* (New Brunswick, NJ: Transaction Publishers, 2001).

20 Jasanoff, 'Civilization and Madness', p. 252.

21 See Wilson, 'Intersecting Discourses.

22 *Ibid.*, p. 77.

23 Jasanoff, 'Civilization and Madness', p. 221.

24 http://news.bbc.co.uk/1/hi/uk/369625.stm (accessed 30 May 2013).

25 For a historical analysis see T. H. Engelhardt and A. M. Caplan, *Scientific Controversies. Case Studies in the Resolution and Closure of Disputes in Science and Technology* (Cambridge: Cambridge University Press, 1987), and for a more timely analysis see D. Brunton, *The Politics of Vaccination. Practice and Policy in England, Wales, Ireland and Scotland* (New York, NY: University of Rochester Press, 2008).

26 R. M. Wolfe and L. K. Sharp, 'Anti-Vaccinationists: Past and Present', *British Medical Journal*, 325 (2002), pp. 430–32.

27 Wolfe and Sharpe, 'Anti-Vaccinationists: Past and Present', p. 4004.

28 J. Baker, 'The Pertussis Vaccine Controversy in Great Britain, 1974–1986', *Vaccine*, 21 (2003), pp. 4003–10.

29 See Burgess, Burgess and Leach, 'The MMR Vaccination and Autism Controversy in United Kingdom 1998–2005', pp. 3921–8.

30 See J. Lewis, K. Wahl-Jorgensen and S. Inthorn, 'Images of Citizenship on Television News: Constructing a passive public', *Journalism Studies*, 5 (2004), pp. 153–64.

31 BBC Trust review of impartiality and accuracy of the BBC's coverage of science. www.bbc.co.uk/bbctrust/assets/files/pdf/our_work/science_impartiality/science_impartiality.pdf (accessed 30 March 2014).

32 http://news.bbc.co.uk/1/hi/talking_point/1802192.stm (accessed 30 May 2013).

33 L. O'Dell and C. Brownlow, 'Media Reports of Links Between MMR and Autism: a Discourse Analysis', *British Journal of Learning Disabilities*, 3 (2005), pp. 194–99.

34 B. Salter, *The New Politics of Medicine* (Basingstoke: Palgrave Macmillan, 2004).

35 V. Demicheli, T. Jefferson, A. Rivetti and D. Price, 'Vaccines for Measles, Mumps and Rubella in Children', *Cochrane Database of Systematic Reviews*, 2 (2005).

36 www.dailymail.co.uk/debate/columnists/article-367132/MMR-safe-Baloney-This-scandal-thats-getting-worse.html (accessed 29 May 2013).

37 *Ibid.*

38 M. Fitzpatrick, 'Why Can't the Daily Mail Eat Humble Pie over MMR?', *British Medical Journal*, 331 (2005), pp. 1148.

39 Speers and Lewis, 'Journalists and Jabs', p. 175.
40 J. Baker, 'The Pertussis Vaccine Controversy in Great Britain, 1974–1986'.
41 Jabs, 'The UK MMR Vaccination Briefing Note – November 2007', www. jabs.org.uk/the-uk-mmr-vaccination.html (accessed 30 September 2016).
42 www.dailymail.co.uk/health/article-14604/MMR-facts.html (accessed 29 May 2013).
43 Director of Public Health North London Great Authority, *Measles in London. Incidence and current action* (London: London Greater Authority, 2002).
44 Poltorak *et al.*, pp. 709–19.
45 *Ibid.*
46 Casiday *et al.*, 'A Survey of UK Parental Attitudes to the MMR Vaccine and Trust In Medical Authority', pp. 177–84, p. 182.
47 *Ibid.*
48 Brownlie and Howson, ' "Leaps of Faith" and MMR', pp. 221–39.
49 *Ibid.*
50 M. Foley, *The British Presidency* (Manchester: Manchester University Press, 2000).
51 For an analysis of this phenomenon see D. Garzia, 'The Personalization of Politics in Western Democracies: Causes and Consequences on Leader–Follower Relationships', *The Leadership Quarterly*, 22 (2011), pp. 697–709. For a more general sociological analysis see the work of Zygmunt Bauman such as Z. Bauman, *The Individualized Society* (Malden, MA: Polity Press, 2001).
52 H. D. Clarke, D. Sanders, M. C. Stewart and P. Whiteley, *Political Choice in Britain* (Oxford: Oxford University Press, 2004).
53 S. P. Kramer, 'Blair's Britain After Iraq', *Foreign Affairs*, 82 (2003), pp. 90–104.
54 J. Wilsdon, B. Wynne and J. Stilgoe, *The Public Value of Science* (London: Demos, 2005).
55 M. Mulkay, *The Embryo Research Debate* (Cambridge: Cambridge University Press, 1997).
56 Wilsdon *et al.*, 'The Public Value of Science'.
57 T. Blair (2002), 'Position Statements on Biotechnology', www.isaaa.org/kc/Publications/htm/articles/Position/speech1.htm.
58 Wilsdon *et al.*, 'The Public Value of Science'.
59 Parliamentary Office of Science and Technology (POST), *Public Dialogue on Science and Technology, Report No. 189* (November 2002).
60 D. Bruce, 'A Social Contract for Biotechnology: Shared Visions for Risky Technologies?' *Journal of Agriculture and Environmental Ethics*, 15 (2002), pp. 279–89.
61 Speers and Lewis, 'Journalists and Jabs', p. 176.

10

Pandemic flus and vaccination policies in Sweden

Britta Lundgren and Martin Holmberg

Introduction

During the summer of 2010, unexpected reports of narcolepsy in Swedish children and adolescents after vaccination with the pandemic influenza vaccine Pandemrix came to the attention of the Medical Products Agency (MPA). The main features of this condition are excessive daytime sleepiness, sudden loss of voluntary muscle tone (cataplexy) that may be triggered by strong emotions, vivid dreamlike images/hallucinations (hypnagogic hallucinations), and paralysis during sleep onset or when waking (sleep paralysis). Vaccination of the entire population had been recommended by the National Board of Health and Welfare as a preventive measure to stop the spread and mitigate the feared consequences of the A(H1N1) pandemic that began in the summer of 2009. Over 60 per cent of people living in Sweden were vaccinated during the fall of 2009 with a new vaccine. This was the single largest public health intervention in response to an outbreak in Swedish history.

Five different vaccines were developed during the pandemic and were approved by the European Medicines Agency (EMA) and the EU commission in a special fast-track procedure.[1] Sweden had signed a contract with one of the producers of the vaccine Pandemrix (GlaxoSmithKline). This vaccine contained a new formulation for the adjuvant, the component of a vaccine that enhances the immune response to the included antigen. Since the pandemic vaccines were approved under exceptional circumstances, information on possible side effects was limited. However, from the studies performed, the results showed that Pandemrix had very good efficiency, giving rise to protective antibodies to a higher degree than ordinary unadjuvanted influenza vaccines.

According to the MPA, between 200 and 300 cases of narcolepsy are estimated to have resulted from the Swedish mass vaccination programme; the exact number is uncertain, since the criteria for vaccine-associated narcolepsy are variable. Several independent research reports have been published in other countries, confirming the association of narcolepsy with Pandemrix.[2] This serious medical side effect was totally unexpected and has played a significant role in shaping public, medical, and authorities' opinions regarding flu epidemics and flu vaccines. Public trust in medical, social, and political authorities decreased. This is particularly evident in public debates in the traditional media as well as on blogs, websites, and Facebook groups. Although it is difficult to measure the exact uptake of seasonal flu vaccination in many regions, coverage has decreased since 2009.[3] Thus far, it has not affected the uptake of vaccines in the general child vaccination programme, as opposed to the case of the MMR vaccine following the 'Wakefield affair'.[4]

The mass vaccination programme and the resulting side effects point to the need for a historical and national perspective on the development of flu vaccination practices. This chapter discusses pandemic influenza as both an old and a contemporary problem, and places it within the framework of national and international flu vaccination practices. The chapter is based on earlier research on flu pandemics, on public documents, and on interviews carried out in March 2013 with parents of children with narcolepsy and officials working with pandemic planning at the Swedish national level.

Vaccinations and epidemics in Sweden

The history of immunisation programmes in Sweden began in the second half of the eighteenth century with the introduction of smallpox inoculations. During that entire century, smallpox was a serious and prevalent childhood disease in Sweden, as in other European countries. When inoculations began on a large scale in the 1860s, only physicians were licensed to perform them, and they were often resisted by a reluctant and sceptical public. Nevertheless, the incidence of smallpox decreased slowly during this period. How much the inoculations contributed to this decrease has been questioned, but the efforts were generally considered successful by the authorities. In contrast, the public sometimes blamed the recurring epidemics on the inoculations.[5]

When Jenner's new method of vaccination was published in 1798, it was quickly adopted in Sweden, beginning in 1801–2.[6] By this time, the public was more accepting, recognising the effectiveness of the vaccinations. Initially, anyone was free to administer them, but this changed after vocal criticism of unskilled vaccinators. After 1810, district physicians had to approve all vaccinators.

The limited number of approved vaccinators was a problem for mass implementation, and the low vaccine coverage of the population was a concern. A law on vaccination was adopted by Parliament in 1816, one of the most severe in Europe, making smallpox vaccination compulsory for children under the age of 2. The clergy and their assistants were appointed as vaccinators, breaking the monopoly of the medical profession and providing efficient vaccination organisation.[7]

The vaccination was very successful and incidents of the disease decreased dramatically during the nineteenth century, although there were still small regular outbreaks. But by the end of the century, there were hardly any smallpox deaths. There were a few isolated occurrences during the twentieth century, with the last one in 1963, affecting twenty-seven persons in the Stockholm area. This led to the voluntary mass vaccination of more than 300,000 people.[8] This mass vaccination resulted in a few serious adverse effects and special clinics for patients with vaccination complications were set up.[9] General smallpox vaccination continued on a compulsory basis, with liberal exemptions, until 1976.

Many epidemic diseases were drastically reduced during the first decades of the twentieth century. Smallpox, typhoid fever, and cholera had almost vanished by 1900 as a result of vaccination and sanitary reforms, although diphtheria, pertussis, and measles were still (diminishing) realities. Tuberculosis was still prevalent and polio became a growing threat during the first half of the twentieth century.[10] The three infectious diseases most feared during this period were tuberculosis, polio, and influenza, and they became increasingly urban phenomena as Sweden urbanised during the early twentieth century. Polio has been eliminated since the 1970s and tuberculosis is now a rare disease in Sweden, though influenza is as prevalent as it was a hundred years ago, a fact that is seldom acknowledged. Each year, up to 10 per cent of the population can be infected, and influenza-related complications cause hundreds of thousands of hospitalisations across Europe.

Following smallpox vaccination, tuberculosis and diphtheria vaccines were introduced during the 1940s, and included in the first general child vaccination programme of 1947, shortly followed by tetanus and pertussis vaccines. Midwives and paediatric nurses in the web of maternity and child clinics were appointed as the main vaccinators. The goal from the start of the programme was to inform pregnant women and vaccinate as many children as possible. In 1957, polio vaccination was added to the programme, with a Swedish-produced deactivated polio vaccine. Using this vaccine, polio was successfully eliminated in Sweden within a decade.

In 1970, the first measles vaccine was introduced, followed by the MMR triple vaccine in the early 1980s. Tuberculosis vaccination was taken off the general vaccination programme in 1975, and in 1979 the old pertussis vaccination was discontinued due to poor effectiveness and too many adverse effects. A new acellular pertussis vaccine was reintroduced in 1996, after the incidence of pertussis had begun to rise again during the 1980s.

In summary, Sweden rapidly introduced a general vaccination programme after the Second World War and had managed to adapt to changing situations, maintaining a high level of public trust in official vaccination policy.[11]

What kind of a problem is influenza?

The influenza A virus varies in terms of surface structure, giving rise to a large number of subtypes. The origins of all subtypes are aquatic birds, but several mammals, including humans, can be infected by some subtypes. The subtypes affecting humans often change in minor ways from year to year, but once in a while major new variants emerge that can cause pandemics.

In the industrialised countries that have undergone epidemiological transition,[12] where infectious diseases have been replaced by chronic diseases as the main causes of death, influenza still causes substantial mortality and morbidity, and returns every year. In fact, this mortality and morbidity is largely the effect of the combination of influenza with prevalent chronic conditions such as cardiovascular, respiratory, and metabolic diseases. It can be argued from this that influenza is not one single epidemic disease but a syndemic[13] of a viral disease together with several chronic conditions that are increasing in modern societies. Despite this, the authorities' response to seasonal influenza outbreaks has often been indecisive and ambiguous, with influenza-associated mortality often seen as inevitable.

Since the Second World War, vaccination has been considered the magic bullet to protect people from influenza, whether seasonal or pandemic. However, there remain significant problems associated with the current influenza vaccines that have not yet been solved, such as short-lived protection, narrow strain specificity, low effectiveness in protection against morbidity and probably also mortality, and potential neurological side effects such as Guillain-Barré syndrome and now also narcolepsy for some vaccines. There is no straightforward public health solution for dealing with seasonal or pandemic influenza. Neustadt and Fineberg,[14] in their review of the circumstances surrounding the decision to mass vaccinate the US population in 1976 as a result of the so-called Fort Dix incident, called it a 'slippery' disease. The five features they identified that combine to make influenza slippery are: the changing character of the influenza virus; the lack of effectiveness of influenza vaccines; that influenza symptoms are widely misunderstood; that influenza is not the only virus to give rise to influenza-like illness; and, finally, that the multitude of causes of flu-like illness makes it difficult to estimate the year-to-year impact of influenza on public health.

In order to match vaccines with currently circulating influenza strains, a WHO network of collaborating centres for influenza surveillance was created in 1948. A recommendation for the antigenic composition of the following year's influenza vaccine is made by the WHO and passed on to vaccine manufacturers. As of 1999, there have been two recommendations per year, one for the northern hemisphere and one for the southern hemisphere.[15] The WHO issues regularly updated influenza vaccine position papers, the most recent in 2012. Annual influenza vaccination has thus become a global concern for the WHO. However, many countries still have difficulties reaching the collectively decided goals for vaccine coverage. In many developing countries, influenza is not seen as a dominant public health problem; many other infectious diseases compete for attention and resources. Consequently, there is no global consensus on the public health importance of seasonal influenza and national vaccination programmes are not a top priority in many low- and middle-income countries.

The pandemics that appear irregularly a few times each century spread with increasing speed. Several studies have shown that global air travel is now a major driving factor in dissemination.[16] The annual influenza epidemics also have an international pattern of spread, where the same strains visit the southern and northern hemispheres during their cooler periods, while tropical and subtropical countries have a less seasonal pattern of appearance.[17]

Influenza pandemics have had an impact on public health, economy, and societal functions to different degrees throughout history, and since the Spanish flu of 1918 have been defined as a health threat by the medical profession. Since the beginning of the twenty-first century, they have also been declared a matter of national and international security, for health, societies, and states. This has fundamentally changed the way in which pandemics are perceived, with governments now anticipating severe pandemics of a magnitude similar to the Spanish flu. Most high- and middle-income countries have pandemic preparedness high on their agendas, strengthening emergency infrastructure and stockpiling antiviral pharmaceuticals and vaccines.

These global concerns have been formalised in the World Health Report 2007[18] and the new International Health Regulations adopted 2007, with increased obligations for member states to have adequate surveillance, reporting, and preparedness capacity for international health threats, including new influenza pandemics.

Historical perspectives on influenza

The history of influenza is long, but knowledge about the viral cause, the variability of the virus and the disease, the factors necessary for transmission, and the methods to stop its spread is more recent and still incomplete. The American historian George Dehner provides a historical perspective on the pandemic of 2009 and the recurring concerns with influenza pandemics.[19] Some descriptions of epidemics of respiratory disease from antiquity and medieval times could well have been influenza, and from the sixteenth century onward, influenza-like epidemics have been reasonably well described.

There have been an estimated thirty-one influenza pandemics since the first well described pandemic of 1580. From the end of the nineteenth century, five have impacted Sweden: Russian flu 1889–90, Spanish flu 1918–20, Asian flu 1957–58, Hong Kong flu 1968–70, and most recently A(H1N1) or swine flu 2009–10. How pandemics compare with each other in terms of severity is still a matter of debate; epidemiological data are incomplete and there is no agreed measure of severity. Variations in mortality and morbidity are nonetheless obvious, and it is often claimed by experts that no two pandemics are alike.

Of the above mentioned influenza pandemics, the Spanish flu pandemic of 1918–19 was particularly virulent, killing an estimated 40–50 fifty million people worldwide.[20] In Sweden, the death toll was around 35,000 people, 99 per cent of whom were below the age of 65. The total Swedish population was then around 5.8 million, and the rapid population increase seen in the previous years was halted during the two to three years following the pandemic. The effects on society were profound, having both political and military ramifications, and adversely affecting public trust in the authorities' ability to handle such catastrophes.

Reports on Spanish flu focused on how it impacted the military. Sweden was neutral during the First World War, but its military forces were reorganised and training increased as a consequence of it. Barracks were filled with conscripts and new cohorts were being called in each fall. Respiratory tract infections were common in crowded quarters, and when the flu struck the country in the fall of 1918, mortality rose dramatically among these new conscripts.[21]

Several local reports conveyed a state of despair and disorder, but also solidarity and local ways of coping with the hardships. Health care was affected by absenteeism, overcrowded wards, and the lack of specific treatment for serious cases. Inexperienced doctors were often sent out to the countryside to help, and some attested to their helplessness when confronted with dying patients.[22] The incidence of morbidity and mortality varied in the country; some cities and smaller communities were severely affected, with over 70 per cent of the local population falling ill and many young people dying.[23]

It would take thirty-nine years for the next pandemic to hit Sweden in 1957. During the intervening period, liberals and then social democrats were firmly in power, universal suffrage was instituted, and the welfare state was largely in place. What was to become known as the 'Swedish model' of agreement between conflicting interest groups in the labour market was signed in 1938.

The fact that influenza is a viral disease was shown conclusively in 1933. When the virus was successfully grown in embryonated eggs, the first vaccines could be manufactured. This was important for the allied war effort during the Second World War, and influenza vaccines were tested on soldiers in the 1940s.[24] Influenza vaccine production in Sweden began at the National Bacteriological Institute (SBL) in 1945–46, at a time when memory of the Spanish flu was still alive.[25] Trust in the general vaccine programme was at this time high and one of the interviewed officials (born in the early 1950s) remembered his parents' attitudes:

> I remember the older generation, they thought vaccinations were very important and it was almost kind of *solemn* to go and get vaccinated, it was not just a mundane question of routine.[26]

There were many reasons for this positive attitude towards vaccination, which had to do with the progress of modern medicine in general, and specifically with the 'revolution of the healthy body', with its roots in the 1930s, as shown in national mass movements of gymnastics, fitness, vegetarianism, and even nudism.[27] The state was considered a natural actor in promoting the well-being of its citizens, and the ties between individuals and state were mutually very strong.[28] The new institutions for social support and general welfare brought social security but also a growing individual dependence on the state and its authorities.

Asian flu was the first pandemic to occur in this era of strong ties between the state and the individual, and also in the era of virology. The pandemic was considered by the WHO as relatively mild and not a major threat to society, though the response to it was enacted as a war against the virus.[29] The attitude of the time was one of scientific optimism, and trust in vaccines and antibiotics was high. When Asian flu finally hit Sweden in October 1957, it came suddenly and with force. A large number of soldiers in some regiments fell ill, and many schools had to close. Significant absenteeism was reported in the postal service, telegraphic service, and the national railway company. The Medical Board issued general advice to the public, but responsibility was placed mainly on local authorities. Special epidemic wards opened in some larger cities.

The WHO had distributed the new virus strain to laboratories and vaccine producers around the world before the pandemic emerged, allowing time for some vaccine production. Sweden had received the A-Singapore-1/57 strain in June 1957, but it grew poorly and a new adapted strain had to be obtained from Statens Serum Institut in Denmark. Sufficient vaccine was ready for trials in October 1957, just when the pandemic struck Sweden. The efficacy and safety of the vaccine was tested on 3,000 military recruits, and between 69 and 86 per cent protection was achieved with two doses.[30]

Initially, health-care workers, in the hospitals specialised in epidemic diseases, home care personnel, and later emergency ward and ambulance drivers were given the vaccine. Some travellers were also vaccinated as well as a few in medical risk groups, mainly those with serious cardiovascular or respiratory disease.[31]

Media coverage was extensive and comparisons with the Spanish flu were common. Returning travellers infected abroad were often singled out in media reports. Scientific interest in the phenomenon of influenza pandemics seemed low, however, and very few scientific reports were written in medical journals about the pandemic. The experts that appeared publicly were often assigned by the National Bacteriological Laboratory or the National Medical Board.[32] A report in the medical literature was published afterwards, where the costs to society of Asian flu were calculated at approximately 130 million kronor (about 1,5 billion kronor today, or about €154 million),[33] and it was estimated that half of that cost would have been saved if there had been sufficient quantities of the vaccine for the whole population. The pandemic peaked in November and around 15 per cent of the population was estimated to have been affected before the season ended in April the following year. The lethality was, nevertheless, relatively low.[34]

Eleven years later, during the 1968 Hong Kong flu pandemic, the situation had changed somewhat. There was still an atmosphere of economic and scientific optimism, but trust in the omnipotence of medical science was decreasing.[35] Emphasis was placed more on influenza pandemics as natural disasters and mitigation of the consequences became a priority. However, the general tone in the media was neutral, calm, and undramatic.

The first international reports of the Hong Kong pandemic came in July 1968, when it had already been raging in Asia for some time. It began its spread among larger parts of the North American population in September 1968, and appeared at about the same time in some parts of Europe. In Sweden, there were initially sporadic cases during the fall of 1968, though the epidemic gained speed in the first months of 1969. A second, more serious wave hit the country during the next winter season, 1969/70.

The vaccine situation during the Hong Kong pandemic was similar to the one eleven years earlier. Production of the influenza vaccine at SBL was not nearly sufficient to meet the need and large quantities had to be imported from the USA.[36] The medical risk groups for serious disease were extended, including diabetics and patients with other metabolic diseases, in addition to the earlier groups of patients with cardiovascular or chronic lung diseases. As before, selected professional groups, mainly health-care workers, were vaccinated. The newly formed Board of Health and Welfare warned about the vaccine shortage but did not want to issue a priority list for vaccination. Instead, this was left to the county epidemic boards. During the second wave in late 1969, more of the vaccine was available and the national authorities issued recommendations regarding who should receive it.

After the Hong Kong flu pandemic, the national production of influenza vaccines was subsequently maintained at a relatively low level, sometimes complemented by purchases from abroad when production failed. Problems caused by shortages of staff or money, or sometimes a shortage of embryonated eggs, were not uncommon. Production was discontinued in the fall of 1982 due to run-down production facilities.[37] In 1993, the remaining vaccine production (mainly polio, diphtheria-tetanus, and measles vaccines) was separated from the diagnostic laboratories and continued as a state-owned company for about five years before it was sold off to private owners. Thus, owing to a series of political and economic decisions, there was a slow erosion of state-owned vaccine production over a period of just over a decade.[38]

Nordic vaccine production

When discussions about the need for increased pandemic preparedness intensified around the turn of the century, the question of national or regional influenza vaccine production began to appear on the agenda. It was feared that the few large companies supplying influenza vaccines would not be able to meet the needs of the market in a pandemic situation, and that smaller countries, in particular, would not be supplied. The question of joint Nordic vaccine production was brought forward, mainly by Danish authorities, with discussions starting in 2000.

In June 2005, the Nordic council of ministers decided to investigate the possibility of joint production of influenza vaccine for the Nordic region. A working group reported in November on two possible models, one with publicly controlled production and one with a public-private partnership (PPP). This was followed up by an investigation by Statens Serum Institut in Denmark of the possibilities of a public solution, and a Swedish government special commissioner explored the PPP alternative. The Swedish commissioner's conclusions were that production should be based on close collaboration with an established vaccine producer, that the emerging cell-based technology for the influenza vaccine production should be awaited, and that further negotiations with some major private producers in the meantime should be continued.[39]

This investigation resulted in the Swedish government deciding to commit themselves to a Swedish solution in cooperation with existing international pharmaceutical companies before a common Nordic agreement could be reached. The motivations for this decision have not been made public, but both strategic thinking about future influenza vaccine developments and neo-liberal ideology might have played a role. One official at the National Board of Health and Welfare reflected on whether it would have been advantageous for the Nordic countries to have their own state-controlled vaccine institutes.

> We have made everything commercial now, but I do think there would have been some advantages to have it state controlled. But still, on the other hand you never know ... the vaccine experts will not be isolated in an ivory tower, they will have contacts with the vaccine industry, so the only thing you can do in this globalized world is to describe as well as you can exactly what the connections look like.[40]

Several groups, both from the industry and medical experts, lobbied for a new production facility to be built in Sweden, whether private, state owned, or state subsidised. Since the investment costs would be high and the market uncertain, and considering the fact that EU rules on competition could be violated by state involvement, there was no government interest in such a solution.

Seasonal influenza vaccine policies

Seasonal influenza vaccines have been in use in Sweden since the 1970s, but at a low level and mainly to protect patients with chronic conditions such as cardiovascular and chronic lung diseases, as well as health-care workers. A cost–utility analysis performed in 1987 established that the costs for general vaccination did not offset the gains in direct health-care costs. A study comparing influenza vaccination in eighteen developed countries between 1980 and 1992 showed a ten-fold difference in the number of vaccine doses used among the countries studied.[41] Sweden, together with Denmark, Finland, and a few others, was at the lower end. Most countries had, by 1992, recommendations for vaccinating those aged over 65, but in the Nordic countries only Norway and Iceland had adopted this policy.

Why were the Swedish authorities reluctant to adopt the expanded use of seasonal influenza vaccination? One probable reason is the influence of studies published by Hoskins in the early 1970s, which made an impression on the Swedish Board of Health and Welfare, the authority issuing vaccination recommendations. The results of these studies, also called 'the Hoskins' paradox', seemed to show that repeated annual vaccinations would not confer protection against epidemic influenza in the long term. However, revisiting Hoskins' data reveals that this conclusion cannot be substantiated.[42] This has also been corroborated in later studies, and the conservatism in recommending annual influenza vaccination lost its strength during the 1990s. New studies on the benefits of vaccinating older persons in institutions also made a case for increasing annual vaccination. In 1997, new recommendations were finally issued on annual influenza vaccination for medical risk groups and those aged 65 and over, harmonising Swedish policy with neighbouring countries.

Around fifty mainly industrialised countries and some countries in rapid economic development vaccinated defined high-risk groups, including the elderly, in the early years of the twenty-first century. No country fully implemented its vaccine recommendations, however, and the World Health Assembly therefore set the goal of vaccination coverage for elderly people of at least 50 per cent by 2006, and 75 per cent by 2010. These goals were not reached in many European countries. In Sweden, coverage was around 65 per cent of those aged over 65 before the 2009 pandemic, but has since dwindled to 50–55 per cent for the same age group.

Some Swedish officials still doubt the cost–effectiveness of seasonal influenza vaccination and stress the importance of putting pressure on the industry to improve the vaccines:

> We have a problem that seasonal influenza vaccines are not really effective. The pandemic vaccine was quite good if you consider its effectiveness, but those that we have each autumn ... it is shown that they are not so good ... Our role here is to put pressure on the vaccine industry and tell them that now you have to come up with something that works. We are not going to give you free promotion year after year, and this is a huge source of income for the industry.[43]

Another official was similarly critical of seasonal vaccination:

> I am a little critical of those seasonal vaccinations. You shouldn't mess around too much with the immune system if you don't have to, with bad vaccines ... It is a quite bad vaccine, 60 percent protection at best. In what other cases would we tolerate that?[44]

Pandemic preparedness planning

Planning for a coming influenza pandemic had been ongoing for many years before 2009. Especially after the SARS outbreak in 2002 and the spread of A(H5N1) avian flu from 2003, the lack of a national contingency plan for a pandemic had become an issue. At the same time, the discourse on 'biosecurity' had also begun to dominate over traditional public health discourses with regard to dealing with infectious disease outbreaks. Aside from public health officials thinking in terms of epidemiology, microbiology, and risk assessments based on historical experience, a new discourse emerged related to scenario-based exercises, crisis management, and pandemic preparedness in Sweden as well as in many other western countries.[45]

In the Swedish pandemic contingency plan finalised in 2005, two strands of reasoning were elucidated: one comprising methods to protect the population using surveillance, preventive measures, and strengthened capabilities of the health-care system, the other focusing on protecting critical structures, essential services, and business continuity (or in the terms introduced by Lakoff,[46] population security versus vital systems security). The challenge was how to balance and integrate these two approaches to dealing with a pandemic. As became clear during the course of the 2009 pandemic, this was not always harmonious.

Before 2009, several large and small exercises were undertaken to examine the different aspects of dealing with a pandemic, mostly based on scenarios with a serious impact. A large EU-wide exercise 'Common Ground' focused on communication between member states and with the European Commission. National exercises dealt with crisis management and the logistics of distributing antivirals and vaccines. Obviously, mass vaccination could not be carried out; instead, computer simulations of different vaccination regimes were used. Sweden signed an advance purchase agreement with a major vaccine supplier and logistics plans were put in place for distributing the vaccine. When the WHO declared phase six of the pandemic, the trigger would be pulled to enact the agreement.

Other interventions aside from vaccination were also discussed. No strong evidence for the effectiveness of school closures was found. Other, more drastic measures, such as travel restrictions or temporary bans on social events and gatherings, were considered too costly and impractical. Much emphasis was placed on personal hygiene measures, notably hand washing. Centrally produced posters were distributed urging people to wash hands often with soap and water, to cough and sneeze into the bend of the arm, and to stay home in the case of feeling sick.

> Even at children's day care institutions, to wash their hands and sing Twinkle twinkle little star, and stop washing after singing the first verse.[47]

Nowhere in the authorities' recommendations was the use of hand sanitisers mentioned, but it appeared several times in the media as an efficient way to protect yourself and others. There was a scramble for these sanitisers and stocks were quickly emptied. The toilets of official buildings, schools, hotels, and stores were equipped with them. They were carried in pockets and handbags and publicly used in a ritualistic way. The Minister of Health proudly opened her handbag in front of TV cameras to show her sanitiser bottle, indicating that this served as a visible sign of being a responsible citizen.

For the first time in history, it was also possible to build large stockpiles of antiviral drugs for dealing with a pandemic. Although there was scepticism among some experts about the utility of such stockpiles, politicians were eager to show their determination. These drugs had earlier been sparingly used in medical treatment and prophylaxis. Now they were going to be used to protect not only those who were ill or at risk of serious disease, but also those in functions essential to society. Several examples were given, such as those working in garbage collection, elevator repair and maintenance, public transportation, and loading bank cash machines. The plan was to produce a catalogue of workplaces and employees that should be protected. However, swine flu hit Sweden before there was time to produce such a catalogue, or to reach an agreement on how to interpret the criteria for what should be considered essential functions. Aside from deciding the targets for prophylaxis, there was also the question of who should be responsible for implementing it: public health officers or crisis management administrators. The stockpiles stayed almost unused during the whole pandemic and are now require renewal or downsizing.

Preparedness put to the test

The 2009 swine flu pandemic differed from what was expected and planned for. It carried an unexpected virus (H1N1 instead of the H5N1), had an unexpected place of origin (Mexico and California instead of South East Asia), and this time it was young and healthy people who were pronounced as at risk, in addition to pregnant women, the obese, and the chronically ill.

Despite these unexpected elements, Sweden was in most respects technically well prepared to meet the pandemic. The concerned central authorities and all the county councils had some sort of pandemic planning in place. Many national level actors were involved, such as the government and government offices, the National Board of Health and Welfare, the Institute for Communicable Disease Control, the Medical Products Agency, the Swedish Civil Contingencies Agency, and the Work Environment Authority. Together they formed a National Pandemic Group that met frequently before and during the pandemic to share information. Actors at the regional and local level were the county administrative boards (which act as the regional arm of central government), county councils (which are responsible for health care), county medical officers (responsible for public health), and the municipalities (with their responsibility for social services, schools, public transport, etc.).

> We had been thinking about this for years, and this was interesting because the pandemic was one of the few things happening in the world where we actually were well prepared. For ten years we had worked out pandemic plans in Sweden and the EU. And we had a very obvious rehearsal with bird flu some years earlier. So we brought our plans and started the meetings. We did what we had said we would do.[48]

The logistics of vaccine distribution had been well designed. Shipments came to one place in southern Sweden each week, and from there were transported around the whole country within a few days. In most vaccination stations, good records were kept so that any unused vaccine lots could be redistributed. The greatest problem was that the producer was not always able to meet the promised quota, giving rise to local shortages. This created a lot of frustration among people who had queued for hours to get their shot. But all in all, this was a display of efficiency in the tradition of Swedish vaccination practices.

There were, nevertheless, difficulties when it came to the actual decisions about who should be prioritised for the vaccine. The fact that the medical risk groups in some ways differed from earlier pandemics was one. New groups shown to be at risk for serious disease were pregnant women and the pathologically obese. Children, though they seemed not to become seriously ill as often as adults, were at greater risk of being infected, and were thus important spreaders of disease. As in other influenza pandemics, there was a shift of mortality compared with seasonal influenza, from the very old to young and middle-aged adults, but they were the least willing to be vaccinated.

Here we had another panorama. Here we saw young adults in their upper teens, healthy people ... who fell very ill, we saw them in ECMO [extra-corporeal membrane oxygenation, where a machine takes over the work of the lungs and sometimes the heart], and then the risk groups sort of fail: who are the risk groups? ... All in all you had to vaccinate the young ones, because they are the ones who spread the disease. So I think you will have to reason in a correct manner. Then it happened to be such bad luck that precisely this group of young people suffered from this terrible side-effect [narcolepsy], but fundamentally it was correct scientific reasoning. It was logical.[49]

Because of the urgency, the pandemic vaccine had not been extensively tested in children. Furthermore, there was the question of whether there would be enough vaccine produced in time, and if not, should any particular risk groups be prioritised? The public health experts were not all in agreement, but the politicians decided quite early on that the only politically possible solution was to buy enough of the vaccine to immunise all Swedes with two doses. Nevertheless, some risk groups were prioritised, together with health-care workers, to receive the vaccine first. As the official Swedish evaluation has shown, there is a need to discuss concepts such as 'risk groups', 'target groups', and 'vulnerable groups' in much greater depth if the concepts are to be usable in the management of future pandemics.[50]

How was mass vaccination perceived?

When deciding quickly about measures to counter a new pandemic, authorities are often in a situation of placing a bet without knowing the odds. There is substantial risk, according to Neustadt and Fineberg, of over-simplifying the problem and of 'group think' in a network of like-minded experts. The question during the 1976 Fort Dix incident was: if this is a gamble, is it not better to gamble with money rather than people's lives? In a similar vein, the Swedish government opted for a quick mass vaccination campaign in response to the 2009 swine flu pandemic. When it was all over, it could be argued (and was by some) that it had been unnecessary and a waste of taxpayers' money.

The seriousness implied by the WHO decision to declare swine flu a pandemic without explicit judgements about its seriousness made mass vaccination a rational choice for wealthy countries with the critical infrastructure and necessary funding. Although this was the case for most countries in Europe and the north, Sweden was perhaps the most successful in implementing mass vaccination in an efficient manner and with high uptake (more than 60 per cent of the population). There were several discussions in the media, both regarding fears about the vaccine and its safety, and fears about not having enough. 'Why is the vaccine never coming, why isn't anything done, why so slow?' recalls one official about the reactions coming in to authorities.

What motivated people to get vaccinated or to vaccinate their children? Two surveys were made by the National Board of Health and Welfare during the summer before the campaign began, one in June and the other in July/August 2009.[51] In the first, 72 per cent responded that they would get vaccinated and in the second 65 per cent; the slight decrease might have been influenced by concerns about the safety of the vaccine at this time. In both polls, only a small minority said that they felt really worried about the pandemic for their own health. About half of the respondents had sought information about the risks and how they could protect themselves and a majority thought that besides vaccination, hand washing was important. This indicates a relatively reflected and calm way of looking at the pandemic, and also a concern for the health of others as much as for oneself. That altruistic motives were important for people in their decision to be vaccinated was also shown in a later study.[52]

What were the arguments used by authorities for why people should get vaccinated? In the centrally produced information material spread during the weeks preceding the start of vaccination, three arguments for vaccination were put forward with equal emphasis: for your own sake to avoid disease; to protect those near you; and to stop the spread of infection in the community. There was some debate, especially around the third argument. Can you really appeal to people's altruism in a vaccination campaign? In the end, it was decided that this was appropriate, in part based on the results of the two above-mentioned vaccination surveys.

Although the underlying beliefs guiding the decisions were not always clearly articulated, there was a conviction among many experts and decision-makers that partial herd immunity could be accomplished in the short time before the influenza wave came, and that this could change the course of the epidemic in Sweden. Of course, there were the outspoken objectives of saving lives and protecting the health-care system and other essential services from breaking down, but there was no decision to give any groups vaccination priority, with the exception of health-care workers and medical risk groups. In hindsight, this egalitarian policy could have had a positive effect on public trust in the state.

A further, often emphasised, factor was the unanimity that the different agencies, from the government down to the local municipalities, outwardly demonstrated. Even though the central authorities were playing a more dominant role than usual, local and regional governments seemed surprisingly loyal when implementing the recommendations. In general, there is an high degree of local autonomy in public health and health care in the Swedish system. Centralisation in managing the pandemic, with strong and united state guidance and local and regional implementation, was afterwards referred to as a 'Swedish model' and was regarded as one of the success factors of the vaccination campaign.

A turning point

> We had a well worked out plan with the county councils and the like and that was why we were so successful. The whole of Europe was wondering, 'How did you manage?' So what would have turned out to be a success story became an Achilles heel when it was shown that the vaccine had such serious side-effects.[53]

> I trusted them. One shot, and then my whole life changed.[54]

Both of the above quotations are important. The first concerns the trust that authorities initially had in their knowledge about how to handle the pandemic, while the second, which comes from one of the young people suffering from narcolepsy as a result of the vaccine, shows how this impacted public trust in the authorities. They illustrate important signs of a possible turning point in the Swedish public's historically deep trust in the welfare society's ability to provide health care and communicable disease prevention. Although it is too early to know if these experiences will endanger future mass vaccination efforts, it is certainly clear that this experience has caused doubt and disbelief.

When the reports about narcolepsy cases began to arrive, the first reaction from authorities and medical experts was scepticism. It was hard to believe that the vaccine could cause this unknown disorder, since influenza vaccines had been used for eighty years without similar side effects. Almost five years after the mass vaccination efforts, in 2014, it has still not been determined whether this side effect is the result of a component of the vaccine, of the influenza virus itself, is due to genetic predisposition, or a combination of all these factors. It is evident that this unexpected side effect has had a deep impact on people's thoughts about vaccination in general and mass vaccination in particular. This is felt in the expressions of parents of narcoleptic children, such as: 'We placed our children on the sacrificial altar so that you all could remain healthy', or on the other side from parents of vaccinated children who were not affected, such as: 'We had the winning lottery ticket.' In a Swedish radio interview in May 2013,[55] one young man was still hesitant about whether he had 'made it' and escaped being affected by narcolepsy, although more than three years had passed since his vaccination.

Many of the parents of narcoleptic children who were interviewed claimed that the argument for solidarity was very important in their decision to accept the vaccine. Their reasoning was that it was important to take the vaccine, that all siblings should have it, and this would be a way to protect other people or children who, for different reasons, could not take it. Among the officials interviewed, the importance of solidarity in order to reach herd immunity was also claimed, and for some this had ideological reasons.

> I think the argument holds, I think it is one of the best arguments for vaccination in society. ... And it is not only to protect other people, you don't know where you will end up next time, maybe you are in the risk group yourself. So it is not only about solidarity. I think it is a rather fine argument, so to speak.[56]

Another official answered the question of whether Sweden exaggerated the solidarity argument.

> If we signalled too strong or not? It is very hard to know ... But I think that all the work with preventing contagious diseases and the work with public health has in itself a very strong element of solidarity. You do things even if you don't know that you yourself will benefit from it.[57]

One of the interviewed officials did claim the opposite concerning solidarity, arguing that for these kinds of decisions it should never be demanded of people to have to think of others: every human being is entitled to think about him- or herself.[58]

References to solidarity are currently on the increase in public health discourse. During the 2009 pandemic, different countries emphasised the solidarity argument to different degrees. In Sweden, the argument that vaccination was both an act of solidarity as well as of individual self-interest was prominent in the authorities' communications. This seemed natural, since solidarity (in the sense of equality in a context of publicly financed health care) has traditionally been a central value in Swedish health-care policy.[59] However, despite its significance, the term solidarity has been given different, sometimes contradictory meanings, both in academic and political contexts. Prainsack and Buyx[60] are critical of the argument, claiming that state enforced public health measures such as vaccination cannot be argued for on the basis of solidarity, but require a different kind of justification, such as the duties of the state to protect vulnerable groups in a stewardship state model. Further arguments for the importance of solidarity have been proposed by Dawson and Verweij.[61]

Consequences

In preparation for a new law concerning vaccination, a Swedish governmental inquiry committee presented an analysis of the country's vaccine programmes.[62] This work began in 2008, but was completed in 2010, and was most probably influenced by the debates triggered both by the newly introduced human papilloma virus (HPV) vaccine and mass flu vaccination. The inquiry proposes several changes to achieve an 'effective vaccination activity which enjoys a high level of trust among the population and attracts high uptake by the target groups.'[63] The problem of 'heavily distorted information' is addressed, in particular 'distorted, non-objective and scaremongering information that was a great problem in the initial stage of pandemic vaccination.'[64] This inquiry and other current governmental and bureaucratic processes show the importance of deep self-reflection and afterthought to prevent polarisation or divisions arising between different sides who blame each other for spreading disinformation.

International management of the A(H1N1) 2009–10 swine flu pandemic has been subject to several evaluations concerning preparedness and response, all the way from assessing the WHO's global impact on decision-making to national, regional, and local evaluations. Forster stresses that globally and nationally, actors failed 'to correspond with more plural and variegated narratives constructed by multifarious publics, and so struggled to recruit support.'[65] He also claims that influenza is still as slippery as in 1976, that expert knowledge is 'still speculative and incomplete',[66] and that the persistence of a dominant and reductive framing of the problem constitutes the most important challenge when responding effectively to flu pandemics. The WHO, Forster argues, should be better at addressing these matters, but as it is bound to 'a reductive epistemology, and at the centre of an unreflexive, self-sustaining actor network',[67] it cannot meet this challenge.

In the Swedish authorities' own evaluation,[68] the main conclusions were that Sweden was successful in its management of the pandemic and that the mass vaccination campaign was launched and run relatively rapidly and efficiently. The authorities considered themselves basically successful in their communication with the public. The lack of a detailed plan for mass vaccination was noted as an area for improvement, as well as uncertainties about what constitutes the critical infrastructure requiring protection during a pandemic. The 2009 pandemic was officially considered a crisis in Sweden, above and beyond the everyday and familiar. In the national evaluation, the pandemic crisis was narrated as a social process, but this process was described in a very limited way and mostly from a top-down perspective, emphasising preparedness plans, governmental cooperation, and logistics.

The fact that different member states chose different paths for their vaccination strategies was embarrassing for the European Commission. The problem has long been acknowledged by EU officials, who have pushed for new legislation to strengthen the EU mandate to govern preparedness and the response to cross-border threats, be they infectious diseases or other hazards. One Swedish official remembered the procedures during the SARS epidemic.

It was shown that the EU countries handled it very differently. So if you coughed on the plane from Beijing to Frankfurt, they would take you off the plane in Frankfurt to X-ray your lungs. If you coughed on the plane from Beijing to London, you simply got off the plane and took the subway to London city. And these are matters that the EU hates, when countries handle things differently. And journalists love it of course.[69]

A strengthened EU mandate was achieved in decision 1082/2013/ EU on serious cross-border threats to health after long negotiations.[70] With this, the Commission is now able to review the preparedness plans of member states and require that they are 'inter-operable'.

Conclusions

I would think, if we would have a similar situation [again], we wouldn't be able to have mass vaccination. I think we would offer it to everyone, but focus on the special risk groups … I don't think the public would listen to a message which implies vaccinating children.
    Why would I do that? Look what happened the last time you told us to.[71]

Public health policy concerning influenza treatment remains in a delicate balance between what should be done and what can be done. We claim that the management of influenza, both as a seasonal epidemic and even more so as a pandemic, still constitutes a serious and complex problem. Historically, there have been repeated failures in protecting the public and society from influenza pandemics, both because of a lack of consciousness of the problem, a lack of tools for effective protection, and both political under- and over-reaction at times.

Facing the A(H1N1) pandemic in 2009, the Swedish response was to bring their pandemic preparedness into efficient action, with mass vaccination being the most important intervention for protecting public health. These endeavours were preceded by consensual decision-making relying on historically successful vaccination campaigns. To act in this way could be labelled a typically Swedish way of managing a medical problem when the WHO called for global solidarity. Paradoxically, both this very efficiency and consensual decision-making may have harmed instead of strengthened trust in the authorities' ability to face future pandemics.

In their media analysis, Ghersetti and Odén discuss the lack of critical evaluation by the Swedish media during and after the pandemic.[72]

Even though there were critical voices, notably in one of the major newspapers, their conclusion is that the media failed in its responsibility to undertake a critical analysis of the rationale for mass vaccination and also for the advance purchase agreement. The few critical voices were drowned out in mass consensus among authorities, experts, and journalists.

Furthermore, there is a great need for critical reflexivity among all involved political and social institutions. This work is about looking back as well as ahead. What did we know? What could we know? What will we know? One official at the Institute for Communicable Disease Control concluded in February 2013:

> I keep telling my co-workers: we did the best we could, we were not careless, we did not omit things. We have done our best and you cannot do more. And still things can happen, that's the way it is. Biology and human ... medicine is hard. We don't know everything, we have to admit that too.[73]

Acknowledgements

We are grateful for the information provided by officials at the Swedish National Board of Health and Welfare, the European Centre for Disease Prevention and Control, the Swedish Medical Products Agency, the Swedish Association of Local Authorities and Regions, and the Swedish Institute for Communicable Disease Control. We are also grateful to the Association for Narcolepsy (*Narkolepsiföreningen*) for providing information as well as the opportunity to interview parents of narcoleptic children.

This work is part of the research project 'Epidemics, Vaccination and the Power of Narratives', funded by the Marcus and Amalia Wallenberg Foundation in Sweden.

Notes

1 European Medicines Agency, '2009 (H1N1) Influenza Pandemic' (2014). http://www.ema.europa.eu/ema/index.jsp?curl=pages/special_topics/general/general_content_000461.jsp&mid=WC0b01ac05801d7bfe (accessed 29 August).

2 L. Wijnans, C. Lecomte and C. de Vries *et al.*, 'The Incidence of Narcolepsy in Europe: Before, During, and After the Influenza A(H1N1) pdm09 Pandemic and Vaccination Campaigns', *Vaccine*, 31:8 (2013), pp. 1246–54.

3 G. Nylen, A. Linde, A. A. Kettis, O. Wik, S. Stenmark and M. Erntell, 'Health Personnel the Key to High Vaccination Coverage Against Influenza', *Läkartidningen*, 109:1–2 (2012), pp. 8–9.

4 See Andrea Stöckl and Anna Smajdor, 'The MMR Debate in the United Kingdom: Vaccine Scares, Statesmanship and the Media' (Chapter 9 in this book).

5 P. Sköld, *The Two Faces of Smallpox – a Disease and its Prevention in Eighteenth- and Nineteenth Century Sweden* (Umeå: Umeå University, 1996).

6 *Ibid.*

7 *Ibid.*

8 The National Board of Health, *Allmän Hälso- och Sjukvård 1963* [*Public Health in Sweden 1963*], Annual Report of the National Board of Health (Stockholm 1965).

9 B. Zetterberg, O. Ringertz and A. Svedmyr *et al.*, 'Smallpox Outbreak and Vaccination Problems in Stockholm, Sweden 1963. II. Case Histories', *Acta Medica Scandinavica, Suppl.* 464 (1966), pp. 45–56.

10 J. Sundin, C. Hogstedt, J. Lindberg and H. Moberg, *Svenska folkets hälsa i historiskt perspektiv* [*Swedish Public Health in a Historical Perspective*] (Stockholm: Statens folkhälsoinstitut, 2005); P. Axelsson, *Höstens spöke: de svenska polioepidemiernas historia* [The Autumn Ghost: The History of Polio Epidemics in Sweden] (Stockholm: Carlsson, 2004).

11 A. Anell, A. H. Glenngård, 'Vacciner i Sverige – ett hälsoekonomiskt perspektiv [Vaccines in Sweden – a health economic perspective]: The Swedish Institute for Health Economics (2007).

12 A. R. Omran, 'The Epidemiologic Transition. A Theory of the Epidemiology of Population Change', *Milbank Memorial Fund Quarterly*, 49:4 (1971), pp. 509–38.

13 M. Singer, 'Pathogen-Pathogen Interaction: A Syndemic Model of complex Biosocial Processes in Disease', *Virulence*, 1:1 (2010), pp. 10–18.

14 R. E. Neustadt, H. V. Fineberg, 'The Swine Flu Affair: Decision-Making on a Slippery Disease (1978).

15 WHO, 'WHO/CDS/CSR/ ISR/2000.1' (2000).

16 D. Brockmann, D. Helbing, 'The Hidden Geometry of Complex, Network-Driven Contagion Phenomena', *Science*, 342:6164 (2013), pp. 1337–42; C. I. Hsu, H. H. Shih, 'Transmission and Control of an Emerging Influenza

Pandemic in a Small-World Airline Network', *Accident Analysis & Prevention*, 42:1 (2010), pp. 93–100.

17 C. A. Russell, T. C. Jones, I. G. Barr *et al.*, 'The Global Circulation of Seasonal Influenza A (H3N2) viruses', *Science*, 320:5874 (2008), pp. 340–6.

18 WHO, *The World Health Report 2007. A Safer Future. Global Health Security in the 21st Century* (Geneva, Switzerland: WHO, 2007).

19 G. Dehner, *Global Flu and You. A History of Influenza* (London: Reaktion Books, 2012).

20 WHO, 'WHO/CDS/CSR/ ISR/2000.1' (2000).

21 M. Åman. *Spanska sjukan: den svenska epidemin 1918–1920 och dess internationella bakgrund* [*The Spanish Flu: The Swedish Epidemic 1918–1920 and its International Background*] (Uppsala: Acta Universitatis Upsaliensis, 1990).

22 F. Elgh, 'Influensapandemiers påverkan på samhället' [The Impact of Influenza Pandemics on Society]', *Socialstyrelsen* (2006).

23 Åman, *Spanska sjukan*, p. 59.

24 S. A. Plotkin, W. A. Orenstein and P. A. Offit (eds), *Vaccines* (Philadelphia: Elsevier Saunders, 2013).

25 L. O. Kallings and H. Lundbäck, 'Statens Bakteriologiska Laboratorium (SBL) – en epok.' [The National Bacteriological Laboratory (SBL) – an epoch]', *Smittskydd*, 9 (1999), pp. 91–95.

26 Interview with official at the Institute for Communicable Disease Control, February 2013.

27 B. Ehn, J. Frykman and Orvar Löfgren, *Försvenskningen av Sverige. Det nationellas förvandlingar* (Stockholm: Natur och Kultur, 1993).

28 H. Berggren and L. Trägårdh, *Är svensken människa? Gemenskap och oberoende i det moderna Sverige* (Stockholm: Norstedts, 2006).

29 D. E. Blakely, *Mass Mediated Disease* (Lanham, MD: Lexington Books, 2006).

30 L. Heller, B. Körlof, J. Mörner *et al.*, 'Influensaepidemin i Sverige 1957–1958 Vaccinationsförsök' [The Influenza Pandemic in Sweden 1957–1958. Vaccination Trials]', *Nordisk Medicin*, 27:XI (1958), pp. 1706–10.

31 Elgh, 'Influensapandemiers påverkan på samhället'.

32 E. Holmer, *Samhällets reaktioner på influensapandemierna 1957–58 och 1968–70* [*Society's Reaction to the Influenza Pandemics 1957–58 and 1968–70*], Umeå Universitet (2006).

33 Heller, Körlof, Mörner *et al.*, 'Influensaepidemin i Sverige 1957–1958 Vaccinationsförsök', pp. 1706–10.

34 Elgh, 'Influensapandemiers påverkan på samhället'.

35 Blakely, *Mass Mediated Disease*, p. 145.

36 Holmer, 'Samhällets reaktioner på influensapandemierna'.
37 SBL-kommittén, 'Report Ds S 1984:7' (1984).
38 See Stuart Blume, The Erosion of Public Sector Vaccine Production: The
    Case of the Netherlands (Chapter 6 in this book).
39 L. Rekke, 'Report Concerning Vaccine Production in Sweden', Social Min-
    istry (2006).
40 Interview with official at the National Board of Health and Welfare, March
    2013.
41 D. S. Fedson, C. Hannoun, J. Leese et al., 'Influenza Vaccination in 18 Devel-
    oped Countries, 1980–1992', Vaccine, 13:7 (1995), pp. 623–7.
42 W. E. Beyer, I. A. de Bruijn, A. M. Palache et al., 'The Plea Against Annual
    Influenza Vaccination? "The Hoskins' Paradox" revisited', Vaccine, 16:20
    (1998), pp. 1929–32.
43 Interview with official at the European Centre for Disease Prevention and
    Control, March 2013.
44 Interview with official at Swedish Association of Local Authorities and
    Regions, March 2013.
45 A. Lakoff, 'The Generic Biothreat, or How we Became Unprepared', Cul-
    tural Anthropology, 23:3 (2008), pp. 399–428.
46 Ibid.
47 Interview with official at the National Board of Health and Welfare, Febru-
    ary 2013.
48 Interview with official at the National Board of Health and Welfare, March
    2013.
49 Interview with official at the Institute for Communicable Disease Control,
    February 2013.
50 National Board of Health and Welfare, 'A(H1N1) 2009. An Evaluation of
    Sweden's Preparations for and Management of the Pandemic', Stockholm
    (2009)
51 Ibid.
52 B. Rönnerstrand, 'Social Capital and Immunisation Against the 2009
    A(H1N1) Pandemic in Sweden', Scandinavian Journal of Public Health, 41:8
    (2013), pp. 853–9.
53 Interview with official at the National Board of Health and Welfare, March
    2013.
54 Daniela, 19 years, Svenska Dagbladet, 14 February 2012.
55 Sveriges Radio, 'Vetenskapsradion Forum' (2013).
56 Interview with official at the Institute for Communicable Disease Control,
    February 2013.
57 Ibid.
58 Ibid.

59 D. Michailakis and W. Schirmer, *Solidaritet som finansieringsform och som prioriteringsprincip* [*Solidarity as a Base for Funding and for Priority Setting*] (Linköping University, 2011).

60 B. Prainsack and A. Buyx, *Solidarity: Reflections on an Emerging Concept in Bioethics* (London: Nuffield Council on Bioethics, 2011).

61 A. Dawson and M. Verweij, 'Solidarity: A Moral Concept in Need of Clarification', *Public Health Ethics*, 5 (2012), pp. 1–5.

62 Statens Offentliga Utredningar (SOU [Swedish Government Official Reports]), 'Ny ordning för nationella vaccinationsprogram' [New order for national vaccine programmes] (2010:39), pp. 45–8.

63 *Ibid.*

64 *Ibid.*

65 P. Forster, *To Pandemic or Not. Reconfiguring Global Responses to Influenza* (Brighton: STEPS Centre, 2012), pp. 49–50.

66 *Ibid.*

67 *Ibid.*

68 National Board of Health and Welfare, *A(H1N1) 2009. An Evaluation of Sweden's preparations for and management of the pandemic* (Stockholm, 2009).

69 Interview with official at the European Centre for Disease Prevention and Control, March 2013.

70 EU Parliament and Council, 'Decision No 1082/2013/EU', *Official Journal of the European Union* (2013).

71 Interview with official at the National Board of Health and Welfare, March 2013.

72 M. Ghersetti and T. A. Odén, *Pandemin som kom av sig. Om svininfluensan i medier och opinion* [The pandemic that didn't come about] (Göteborg: Göteborgs universitet: Institutionen för journalistik, medier och kommunikation, 2010).

73 Interview with official at the Institute for Communicable Disease Control, February 2013.

11

Polio vaccination, political authority and the Nigerian state

Elisha P. Renne

So I told him [a soldier] that even if they are going to kill me, I will not allow the governor to enter my house ... I also said in the governor's presence that even if President Jonathan comes here, I will not allow them to immunize my child. So the governor held my hand that I should allow him to enter but I refused. I told him that this is not his house and so I will not allow him in. He pleaded with me to allow him in. He asks if I know him I said yes but I will not allow him to immunize my child.[1]

In an exchange between an elderly trader and the governor of Kaduna State in the Rigasa neighbourhood of Kaduna, in northern Nigeria, the trader-grandfather challenged the authority of his governor, and even his president, to immunise his granddaughter during a house-to-house polio vaccination exercise. This episode captures the contested nature of vaccination initiatives – between parents and the state, between individual freedom and societal benefits, between those with political authority and those resisting it. During the hour-long stand-off, which resembled something of a community drama performance with many neighbour-residents watching the proceedings, both sides – the governor and the grandfather – asserted their positions. Ultimately, the governor won, although it was not a voluntary defeat as the grandfather explained, 'When they threatened to use force against me, I threw the girl at them to immunize her. I gave them the girl. They only immunized her by force, not because I wanted.'[2]

This incident suggests the particular social relationship between those with political authority and the legitimate power of the state to use force against those who resist them. Vaccination programmes provide a useful means by which to examine this relationship since they must be run on a national basis in order to obtain herd immunity – approximately 80 per cent coverage – which prevents or reduces the spread of communicable diseases such as measles and poliomyelitis.[3] Vaccination campaigns thus rely on the political authority and police power of the state to carry out public health programmes for the benefit of its citizens. The success of these programmes, in turn, may bolster the legitimacy of state control of its citizenry – through lower infant and child morbidity and mortality rates that increase its credibility – and foster a sense of national pride in a country's progress. Through vaccination programmes, government health officials also amass a range of vital statistics that track both individuals and disease – which relates to Foucault's notion of bio-power – as a means of controlling populations and strengthening the powers of the state.[4] Indeed, the Kaduna State governor visited the Rigasa neighbourhood during the special round of the June 2013 sub-National Immunization Plus Days in Kaduna precisely because it had been identified as an area of parental non-compliance, based on data collected during earlier immunisation day exercises (Figure 11.1). Yet the specific historical context of vaccination programmes – how, by whom, and why they were implemented – and vaccine production and procurement has had consequences for such interventions and how they have been subsequently perceived.

In northern Nigeria, vaccination campaigns for smallpox and treatment camps for cerebrospinal meningitis were introduced by British health officials during the colonial period (1903–60) and vaccines used were generally imported from Great Britain. Following independence in October 1960, vaccination initiatives, such as the Smallpox Eradication Programme (SEP) and the Global Polio Eradication Initiative (GPEI), implemented by the Nigerian Ministry of Health and National Primary Health Care Development Agency (NPHCDA) with support from international NGOs, have been viewed with suspicion by some as postcolonial western interventions. In northern Nigeria, rather than legitimating state control of its citizens and promoting feelings of national pride by 'kicking polio out of Nigeria', the implementation of the GPEI has contributed to some Nigerians' resistance to state authority. While Nigerian government officials have insisted on pursuing the GPEI, some parents have resisted the programme's initial

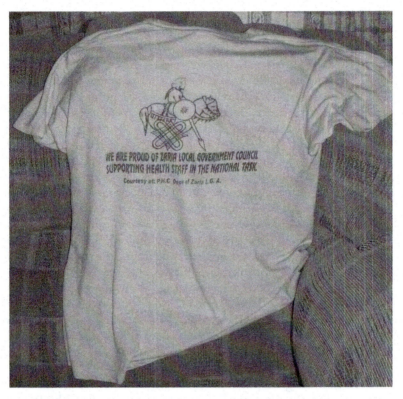

Figure 11.1 T-shirt produced for the polio vaccination team members.

single-minded concern with polio vaccination rather than on other childhood diseases, which they consider to be more life-threatening for their children.[5] Vaccination programmes thus provide insights into the relationship between citizen resistance and state power, for as Greenough has noted: 'Public health measures derive their authority from the police powers of the state, and people do not lightly offer themselves (or their immune systems) to government even when its authority is legitimate.'[6] Furthermore, the Nigerian government's focus on the polio vaccination campaign highlights its failure to provide basic primary health care and consistent provision of viable vaccines, particularly in rural areas.[7] Along with problems in the provision of other basic services such as clean water and electricity, these deficiencies have reinforced people's questions about the legitimacy of the Nigerian state and vaccination programmes promoted by its political leaders.

That GPEI implementation and purchases of imported oral polio vaccine (OPV) was funded by international organisations associated with the West (e.g., Rotary International, the European Union, the KfW Development Bank, the Gates Foundation, CDC, CIDA, UNICEF and WHO) has also led some Muslim parents, religious leaders and medical professionals in northern Nigeria to question the safety of the OPV on different grounds: fears that imported vaccines contained substances to reduce Muslim populations; beliefs that illness and cure are best addressed through prayer; and questions about the safety of vaccines, similar to concerns of some parents in the West.[8] This resistance has, nonetheless, been countered by the power of the Nigerian state in various ways – through threats of parental arrest, local government monitoring, media censorship and harassment of vaccine critics. These actions have been tempered by various sorts of health incentives and community projects as well as by plans to establish a national programme of vaccine production.[9] This particular configuration of resistance and power, which also includes many Nigerians' support for national efforts to end polio transmission in Nigeria, underscores the distinctive relationship between citizens and the state that the implementation of the GPEI in Nigeria in 1996 reveals.

This chapter begins with a discussion of the basis of state power – the political authority of officials of the Ministry of Health and related federal and INGO programmes – to carry out vaccination initiatives through immunisation campaigns, national house-to-house immunisation days, and routine immunisation provided at local clinics and hospitals.

The workings of these federal programmes are then related to the particular forms of resistance to them as expressed by parents, local political and religious leaders, university professors and, at times, by immunisation teams and clinic workers themselves. In 2013, more violent resistance to the GPEI – specifically, the murder of nine polio immunisation team members in Kano, Nigeria[10] – has hampered vaccination efforts and has led to increased insecurity and aggressive government counter-measures.[11] Continuing resistance, however, has also led to programmes and action meant to address resisters' complaints

– through improved routine immunisation at renovated clinics, special programmes for bed net distribution and measles vaccination, improved health communication about polio, programmes providing monetary awards to state governors and foodstuffs to cooperating mothers as well as community improvements. Yet despite these measures, resistance to polio vaccination efforts has continued, particularly in northern Nigeria. The chapter concludes with an examination of the state of routine immunisation in 2015, which includes clinics with erratic vaccine supplies as well as plans for new immunisation initiatives and the use of inactivated polio vaccine (IPV) for the final stages of the GPEI.[12] Despite the use of coercive, as well as appealing, measures in government's efforts to insure parents accept polio vaccination for their children, the state's ability to revitalise a national programme of primary health care, which includes the provision of early childhood vaccines, routine immunisation and basic health care for its citizens, will play an important part in the successful conclusion of the GPEI.

Vaccination programmes in colonial and independent Nigeria: state power and health agendas

In northern Nigeria, vaccination campaigns have been associated with the commencement of British colonial rule in 1903, when government officials had to address major and recurrent epidemics of smallpox and cerebrospinal meningitis on a shoestring budget.[13] While British colonial officials introduced imported lanolinated calf lymph from the British Lister Institute for smallpox vaccination in 1921, there was resistance to vaccination in the North. This resistance, which reflected a fear of Europeans and their medicine and also possibly a preference for local inoculation practice by some,[14] was compounded by the vast size of the Northern Province and inadequate health resources of the colonial medical service. This situation resulted in considerably fewer smallpox vaccinations being carried out in this area.

The colonial administration continued to try to improve immunisation levels, which included the introduction of a Vaccination Ordinance, originally enacted in 1917. In 1945, the Ordinance was amended to include a schedule for compulsory vaccination of adults and their children to be organised by local political authorities. These Native Authority officials (who would have been emirs and traditional chiefs) were also responsible for determining penalties for non-cooperation, although specific fines for non-compliance were subsequently introduced.[15] However, while colonial government officials could draft ordinances and determine fines on paper, which could be used to force traditional rulers to compel vaccination in their areas of jurisdiction, they had little means for enforcing their rules.

Along with smallpox vaccination, colonial officials also organised campaigns to treat those affected during outbreaks of cerebrospinal meningitis (CSM), which have occurred in northern Nigeria in five to ten year cycles, with recent major epidemics occurring in 1949–51, 1960–62, 1970, 1977 and 1996.[16]

Until 1969 when an effective meningitis vaccine was developed, the colonial and later Nigerian government officials encouraged measures such as sleeping with open windows or out of doors to counter the disease. Shortly after independence a large isolation camp was set up in Kano during the 1960–62 epidemic, where patients were housed in tents and fed at government expense; treatment consisted of the use of imported sulfonamide drugs.

While the measures taken during smallpox and CSM outbreaks – attempts at forced immunisation and quarantine or treatment at isolation camps – during the colonial period may have disinclined some to accept vaccination, others were sufficiently impressed with the benefits of western medicine to do so. Unlike smallpox and CSM, colonial medical officers were not concerned about poliomyelitis. Officials assumed that Nigerians had natural immunity.[17] However, Familusi and Adesina, in a study of hospital records of Nigerian children brought to University College Hospital-Ibadan from 1964 to 1973 with paralysis symptoms associated with polio, argued that polio was prevalent throughout the year in Ibadan and its surrounding areas.[18] After a short-lived polio vaccination programme in Ibadan using imported oral polio vaccine carried out by the World Health Organization (WHO) in 1974, the number of polio cases declined, leading Familusi and Adesina to advocate for routine vaccination for the disease.[19]

The smallpox and meningitis vaccines which were regularly administered by colonial government health personnel were generally imported. When an attempt was made in 1941 to manufacture smallpox vaccine in the colonial laboratory service in Yaba, Lagos, the heat-sensitive lanolinated vaccine produced there lost its potency under unrefrigerated conditions.[20] Although this vaccine continued to be produced and used by Nigerian government health staff during the Smallpox Eradication Programme, which commenced in Nigeria in 1967, the CDC recommended the use of imported freeze-dried vaccine provided by the WHO.[21] While a freeze-dried vaccine that met international standards was eventually produced at the Federal Vaccine Production Laboratories at Yaba in 1974,[22] by the time that the Expanded Programme on Immunisation was fully implemented in Nigeria, vaccines for the programme were being imported by UNICEF. Unlike countries such as Hungary and Brazil discussed by Vargha and Benchimol (Chapters 3 and 7, this volume), there has not been a large and sustained national programme of vaccine production in Nigeria, although plans to begin such a programme were announced in 2012.[23]

The expanded programme on immunisation in Nigeria

The Nigerian government took a different approach to national vaccination with the implementation of the Expanded Programme on Immunization (EPI), which began in Nigeria in 1979.

The goal of this horizontal health initiative, sponsored by WHO, was to provide vaccines for diphtheria, pertussis, tetanus, measles, polio and tuberculosis to more than 80 per cent of children worldwide through a system of primary health care centres.[24] While this goal was attained in some countries, particularly those with well-developed health infrastructures and trained personnel, in Nigeria, infrastructural, political and economic problems hampered routine immunisation.

Indeed, immunisation levels for the early 1980s were low, ranging from 5 to 10 per cent.[25] This situation was partly due to political and economic instability during the period 1979–86, when Nigerians elected a civilian president and subsequently experienced two military coups. However, during the military regime of General Ibrahim Babangida, who was anxious to gain international approval for his government, he appointed Professor Olikoye Ransome-Kuti as Minister of Health in 1986. Ransome-Kuti established a programme of primary health care centres throughout the country, with vaccines for the six early childhood diseases made widely available.[26] In March 1988, the first phase of a national immunisation exercise was held at primary health care centres, which included the distribution of free vaccines; nonetheless, nationally only fifty per cent of children under two years of age were immunised. In 1989, Ransome-Kuti pledged to achieve eighty per cent coverage by December 1990,[27] in line with the UNICEF goal of Universal Child Immunization. In Nigeria, this goal was only achieved for Bacille-Calmette-Guérin vaccine (BCG) coverage.[28]

The year 1990 was considered to be the high-point in national immunisation coverage. However, on 30 June, responsibility for primary health-care services was transferred to the local governments as part of a structural adjustment programme initiated by the International Monetary Fund, which required the federal government to curtail spending on social services;[29] in 1991, states were required to purchase their own vaccines.[30] Since imported vaccines used during the EPI drive in 1990 had been provided by UNICEF and other non-governmental organisations via the federal government without charge to local governments, the availability of these vaccines drastically declined when federal responsibility for primary health-care services was transferred to local governments. Consequently, there was a breakdown in the provision of routine immunisation through primary health-care clinics and hospitals in local governments. Overall immunisation levels, as represented by diphtheria, pertussis and tetanus (DPT3) coverage, declined and by 1993, were reported to be around 30 per cent based on government data.[31] This decline in immunisation levels, which included complete sequences of polio vaccination, may be seen in a comparison of data from the 1990, 1999 and 2003 Nigerian Demographic and Health Surveys.[32]

The reorganisation of the EPI as the National Programme on Immunization (NPI)

After a bloodless coup, led by General Sani Abacha in November 1993, government officials sought to revitalise the national immunisation programme. In July 1995, the Expanded Programme on Immunization (EPI) was renamed the National Programme on Immunization (NPI), in order to stress the nation's responsibility for immunisation and vaccine provision in Nigeria.[33]

In 1996, this programme was formally launched as part of the Family Support Programme, a project run by the First Lady, Miriam Abacha, although its staff worked closely with the Federal Ministry of Health and with international agencies and groups such as the WHO, UNICEF and Rotary International. One year after the NPI was launched, it came under the direction of Dr Dere Awosika, who continued in this position – under two successive presidents – until she was forced to resign in December 2005. Subsequently, the programme was merged with another federal parastatal, the NPHCDA, under the Ministry of Health, in 2007.

During its tenure, the NPI was responsible for the importation and distribution of vaccines to cold-store centres throughout the country. It was also responsible for promoting immunisation in Nigeria, including the provision of oral polio vaccine and the promotion of the GPEI.

The GPEI and the Nigerian state

With the decline in routine immunisation during the 1990s, NPI officials initiated a mass polio immunisation programme through the organisation of National Immunization Days when health workers went house to house, rather than relying on mothers to bring their children in for vaccination at poorly supplied clinics and hospitals. This entailed hiring and training vaccination team members as well as distributing cold chain equipment and vaccines, the latter obtained through UNICEF.[34] They also needed to establish a system for monitoring the wild poliovirus through the identification of children with acute flaccid paralysis (paralysis in one or more limbs), which included the collection, transport and analysis of stool specimens. In 1996, a laboratory at University College Hospital, Ibadan, was accredited by the WHO for the analysis of stool samples of children with acute flaccid paralysis.[35] Officials also implemented special programmes which included Sub-National Immunization Days, when efforts were directed toward states and local governments where immunisation coverage was low and 'mop-up' days, when health workers focused on specific wards and neighbourhoods to improve vaccination levels. All children under the age of 5 were given oral polio vaccine (OPV), regardless of whether they had received earlier doses in order to ensure universal coverage, since cards recording vaccination histories were not used. When the initial goal of global polio eradication by the end of year 2000 was not met, WHO officials extended the Polio Eradication Initiative goal to 2005.[36]

In northern Nigeria, these efforts were hampered by the decision of the Governor of Kano State, Alhaji Ibrahim Shekarau, to cancel National Immunization Days in Kano in October 2003. With increasing suspicions about the safety of the polio vaccine, the Federal Ministry of Health organised a health team which went to test the vaccine in South Africa.[37] At the same time, the Jama'atu Nasril Islam (JNI), the umbrella organisation for Muslims in Nigeria, sent a team of their own experts to test the vaccine in Indian laboratories. On 23 December 2003, the Minister of Health, Professor Eyitayo Lambo, announced that the 'Oral Polio Vaccine (OPV) used in Nigeria for immunisation, 'had been found to be safe and free of anti-fertility agents and HIV'.[38] One month later, the JNI team, which included two professors from Ahmadu Bello University, officially announced that they found the OPV vaccine to be contaminated.[39]

However, after additional tests were jointly carried out by MOH and JNI experts,[40] the Sultan of Sokoto, Alhaji Muhammadu Maccido, announced on 17 March 2004 that the 'Oral Polio Vaccine is safe'.[41] Nonetheless, Governor Shekarau, continued to refuse the use of the WHO-procured vaccines.[42] While the former President Ibrahim Babangida suggested that the Nigerian drug companies produce their own polio vaccine,[43] this option was not considered to be practical at the time. In July 2004, Governor Shekarau changed his position and vaccination resumed in Kano State, with health workers using polio vaccine manufactured in Indonesia.[44]

Yet even after the Kano State polio vaccination boycott was resolved, house-to-house polio immunisation continued with lacklustre results until January 2006 when the newly appointed acting director of the NPI, Dr Edugie Abebe, implemented a programme called Immunization Plus Days.[45] This programme provided parents with a range of health incentives, which included bed nets, measles vaccination and deworming tablets. The popularity of this programme contributed to a decline in the number of confirmed cases of wild poliovirus, from 1,122 cases in 2006 to 285 cases in 2007. However, political considerations again intervened and when the NPI was merged with the National Primary Health Care Development Agency (NPHCDA) in 2007, Dr Abebe resigned. The NPHCDA director, a political appointee, who took over the polio immunisation programme was inexperienced; funds ran out for bed nets and once again there was an increase in cases.

By the end of November 2008, Nigeria had 758 confirmed cases, the most cases of wild poliovirus in the world.[46]

Yet political decisions made at the end of 2008 also contributed to a significant improvement of polio vaccination efforts in Nigeria the following year. In October 2008, Dr Muhammad Ali Pate, was appointed as the new NPHCDA executive director. Not only was Dr Pate an experienced health official who had worked with the World Bank, he was also a northerner who was sympathetic to the concerns of northern Nigerian parents.[47] His organisational leadership also contributed to increased use of health incentives and new distribution methods, such as the use 'of 'transit teams' to vaccinate children on public and private transport, and the use of 'street teams' to cover children in playgrounds and other areas outside the household.'[48] While focusing on polio, health officials emphasised community communication and improvements in primary health care provision.

This change in perspective was paralleled by the Expert Review Committee's conclusion that: 'The growing national and state level commitment to polio eradication and immunisation must be taken down to local government and community level.'[49] Improved immunisation efforts in 2009 contributed to a significant decline in confirmed cases of wild poliovirus, with only twenty-one cases by the end of 2010. Although these numbers increased in 2011–13, they declined significantly in 2014 (Table 11.1).

Other factors contributing to the 2010 decline

While this significant decline in number of polio cases reflected greater levels of immunity among more Nigerian children due to changes in programme leadership and vaccination campaigns, there were other factors – social, medical, institutional, technical and legal – that contributed to an increasing number of parents who agreed to have their children vaccinated in northern Nigeria.

In June 2009, Alhaji Muhammad Sa'ad Abubakar, the Sultan of Sokoto, organised a committee of fourteen northern Nigerian traditional rulers to address the continued presence of polio in the North.[50] While his predecessor, Alhaji Muhammadu Maccido, had also supported the campaign, the new sultan's relative youth and conviction that northern Nigerians should not be seen as 'backward' energised his

Table 11.1 Cases of acute flaccid paralysis (AFP) and confirmed cases of wild poliovirus and circulating vaccine-derived poliovirus, Nigeria, 1999–2015 (as of 28 October 2015)

Year	Total confirmed polio cases	Wild-virus confirmed polio cases	Vaccine-derived confirmed polio cases
1999	981	98	–
2000	638	28	–
2001	56	56	–
2002	202	202	–
2003	355	355	–
2004	782	782	–
2005	831	830	1
2006	1144	1122	22
2007	356	285	71
2008	864	798	66
2009	542	388	154
2010	48	21	27
2011	96	62	34
2012	130	122	8
2013	57	53	4
2014	36	6	30
2015	1	0	1

Source: CDC, Global Polio Eradication website, www.polioeradication.org/ Dataandmonitoring/Poliothisweek.aspx (accessed 29 October 2015)

efforts to get traditional rulers as well as religious leaders involved. His leadership contributed to an increased acceptance of the polio eradication initiative by those who had rejected it before.

In November/December 2008, polio vaccines were given in conjunction with a national integrated measles campaign, which reflected a shift in emphasis from polio to measles. Since many northern Nigerian parents considered measles to be a greater risk to their children, this change demonstrated an acknowledgement of local concerns. Also, a more organised system for bed net distribution, developed in 2010, reflected an appreciation of parents' anxiety over malaria. Mothers who had brought their children for polio immunisation received a slip that entitled them to two bed nets, which were distributed at local sites by health officials. The popularity of bed nets contributed to increased immunisation as well. In addition to organising traditional and religious leaders and improving the distribution of health incentives, state ministers of education were encouraged to implement immunisation requirements for children attending nursery and primary schools. In Kaduna State in May 2009, for example, a letter went out to all school principals, noting that children under the age of 5 needed to to be immunised when immunisation personnel visited their schools. While some parents objected to this programme, they were allowed to write letters requesting that their children not be immunised. This effort to incorporate immunisation records as a requirement for school attendance is part of a larger process of routinising immunisation in Nigeria.[51] By the end of 2010, the decline in confirmed cases of wild poliovirus was matched by improved overall levels of immunisation. However, political events in northern Nigeria in subsequent years confounded these numbers.

Vaccination as a node of resistance to state power

Earlier examples of resistance to vaccination campaigns during the colonial period in northern Nigeria have continued in the independence era. The particular form that this resistance has taken reflects changing political and economic circumstances in which the GPEI has been implemented. As Taylor notes, 'the balance of power between state and population, contemporary to polio, has shifted dramatically', after 2009.[52]

During the early years of the twenty-first century, the GPEI has continued to face various forms of covert resistance to the campaign, which include parents misleading immunisation teams about children residing in houses, hiding children, and deceptively marking houses and children's fingers. However, in some communities, parents have become more overt in their resistance, with some demanding that polio workers provide basic amenities to their communities such as boreholes before allowing vaccination teams to proceed.[53] Indeed, parents' dissatisfaction with the failure of the federal and state governments to provide primary health care has contributed to continued resistance to the polio campaign, exemplified by an incident described in November 2011:

The only dispensary at the village [in Kano State] has been under lock and key for years, with no medical personnel attending to the health needs of the community ... All attempts to get local or state government to put the structure to use for the benefit of the community have proved abortive, residents said ... [Despite] the seeming unconcern about their health needs nonetheless, government keeps posting vaccinators with the objective of eradicating polio, whom the residents consistently [reject]. They said their rejection was in a bid to subvert the initiative so that by government failing in the cause, they will ... exact a payback for the suffered neglect.[54]

A lack of interest in polio as a public health concern, along with government officials' inability to reconstitute a working primary health-care programme, have undermined government's credibility among some northern Nigerians. Others, like the grandfather-trader in Rigasa-Kaduna, have openly refused to have their children vaccinated under any circumstances and some have threatened violence against health workers who sought to enter their houses. Some say that the vaccine is contaminated with contraceptives or HIV.[55] Similarly, two university professors from Ahmadu Bello University-Zaria, have questioned the safety of the oral polio vaccine in several nationally circulated DVDs in which they argue that western health specialists should not determine Nigerian health care priorities (Figure 11.2). They also expand on their long-standing views that OPV and other vaccines are unsafe and that some children are adversely affected by vaccination, reflecting arguments made by vaccine opponents in the West.[56] Additionally, they question the legality of threats against parents who refuse vaccination of their children.[57]

Furthermore, while some Muslim teachers (*malamai*) have accepted vaccination of students in their schools, many are still opposed to vaccination as they suspect that there is 'something in the vaccine'. As one malam explained, 'I am doing something for the children – prayers – so that they don't need the OPV.'[58]

Other religious scholars are opposed to vaccination on the grounds that Islamic medicines and medical practices obviate the need for use western medicine. These scholars have supported their position, citing the influential volume, *The Prophetic Medicine*.[59] Indeed, Mohammad Yusuf, the late leader of the radical Islamic reform group, Jama'atu Ahlus-Sunnah Lidda'Awati Wal Jihad (JASLWJ), popularly known as

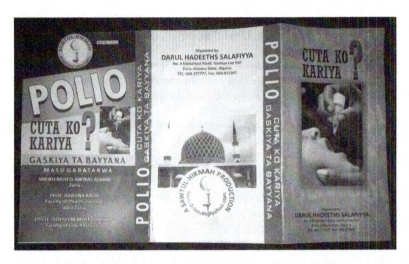

Figure 11.2 Cover of DVD, Polio: *Cuta ko Kariya?*

Boko Haram (literally, western education is forbidden), relied on *The Prophetic Medicine,* which is reflected in his assessment of western medicine and vaccines:

> For Yusuf modern vaccines are not better than Prophetic medicine ... He also stated that he had read on the Internet that modern vaccines have side effects; hence prophetic medicine is better than modern vaccines. Here Yusuf seems to be echoing the rejection of polio vaccination by some Muslims.[60]

Yusuf's views on modern vaccines as *ḥarām* (forbidden) have apparently influenced his followers in Borno and Yobe States, where low levels of immunisation in 2012 – 71 per cent and 65 per cent of children, respectively, have received no vaccinations[61] – have contributed to continued poliovirus transmission in these two states.

However, with the escalation of political violence, particularly in Borno State, associated with Boko Haram and the extrajudicial killing of Yusuf in July 2009,[62] government officials and police/military officers became the targets of Boko Haram members, not only in northeastern Nigeria but in other parts of the North as well. In February 2013, nine women health workers, who were preparing to go out for polio vaccine rounds in and near the metropolis of Kano, were shot and killed, although no group has claimed responsibility for the attack.

Government responses: sticks and carrots

Although some have associated the attack on the polio health workers in Kano with Boko Haram violence,[63] Nigerian government officials specifically blamed the killings on those involved in a programme critical of the polio campaign aired on Wazobia, a popular Kano radio station. Two radio journalists, along with the station owner, were arraigned and appeared in court in February 2013:

> The court was told that Rabo had on February 4, refused to allow polio officials to immunize his children, and that when the district head of Tarauni Local Government went to find out his reasons the following day, he conspired with the two journalists who aired a local programme called 'Sandar Girma' [literally, big stick; policemen are referred to as 'dan Sanda in Hausa]. The prosecutor added that on the programme, the duo 'discredited the polio immunization programme, defamed the character, reputation and personality of the district head in addition to instigating the attack on the polio officials'.[64]

Following the trial, the station's broadcasting licence was suspended and the station was shut down.[65]

While GPEI officials have vowed to continue their efforts and immunisation teams have been accompanied by police escorts, the insecurity associated with Boko Haram's anti-government activities and subsequent military police counter-measures have hampered house-to-house vaccination efforts. The difficulties that this situation poses for vaccination efforts in northeastern Nigeria were noted in the May 2013 Independent Monitoring Board (IMB) report on polio eradication:

> Insecurity in Nigeria is most challenging in the North East States of Borno and Yobe. These two states currently account for 69% of wild polio cases in Nigeria (and hence at the time of our meeting in the entire continent of Africa) in 2013. Population immunity has steadily declined. In Yobe, a quarter of non-polio AFP cases in quarter four of 2012 had received zero doses of polio vaccine. In Borno, over 335,000 children (32% of the target population) were missed during the April 2013 campaign.[66]

In May 2013, President Goodluck Jonathan announced that a state of emergency had been imposed on three northeastern states – Borno, Yobe and Adamawa,[67] two of which were named in the IMB report. Aside from implementing a state of emergency and closing down radio stations that broadcast shows critical of the polio vaccination campaign, critics of the GPEI have also been threatened with arrest. In some communities with low levels of immunisation where parents have continued to resist the polio initiative, more drastic measures have been implemented in some local governments. In Kano, Kwara and Niger States, parents may be arrested for failure to vaccinate their children.[68] In Gombe State, the governor announced at a primary health-care event in 2009 that 'his administration is looking into the possibility of enacting a law that would empower government to prosecute parents who do not allow their children to be immunized against the six child killer diseases'.[69] In Jamaa Local Government Area of Kaduna State, parents who do not allow their children to be vaccinated will face legal action:

> Chairman of the local government, Mr Daniel Amos, gave the warning in Gidan Waya, while flagging off six-round of the immunization. He said the immunization of children against all child-killer diseases, particularly polio is compulsory. 'There is no justification for any parent to deny children this right, especially as polio immunization is administered free. Parents should play their roles properly and avail their wards for immunization.'[70]

This pressure on local government chairmen to discipline parents and to support polio vaccination efforts has resulted in state officials such as 'the Kaduna State deputy governor, Ambassador Nuhu Audu Bajoga … lead[ing] the search into some huts in southern Kaduna to find the children and have them immunized'.[71] It has also led to statements such as that made by the Chairman of Zangon-Kataf Local Government, Christopher Haruna, who 'pledged the council's readiness to continually lend support to government on polio issues by organising the people to regularly avail their children for vaccination'.[72] The strategy to shame and to put pressure on local government officials was also advocated in the May 2013 IMB Report:

> A list of poor performing LGAs is on display in the Abuja Emergency Operations Centre. We commend the Programme for focusing their efforts on these disappointing LGAs. The LGA Chairmen responsible

should continue to receive weekly, if not daily, telephone calls from the State and Federal level.[73]

Indeed, local government chairmen in states such as Borno and Yobe are in particularly difficult positions, as they are targets both of Ministry of Health officials and anti-government Boko Haram members.

Aside from pressure on local government leaders and parents, in some areas, parental permission is circumvented altogether through the mass immunisation of children on public transport vehicles ('transport teams') or in public areas where they congregate ('street teams') – using biscuits and candy as incentives, as one vaccination team leader in Kaduna State described:[74]

> Now another strategy we have – we have a team who just immunizes children in the street. We find an elderly woman within the community, maybe she was a TBA for a long time so no one would shout at that woman if she gave OPV to the children. We used biscuits there, immediately after vaccinating she would give a biscuit to the child. That child will bring more children, without consulting the mother; they will just come.[75]

More recently, these coercive actions have been tempered by various sorts of incentives and community projects. Ministry of Health and GPEI officials have instituted other methods for addressing other, more indirect, forms of resistance. For example, in 'high-risk areas' with large numbers of 'non-compliant parents', GPEI programme officials sought to improve communications with these parents through presentations of educational films (*magaji*)[76] and through FOMWAN (Federation of Muslim Women of Nigeria) participation on immunisation teams. These efforts have also included community rallies and the solicitation of support from Muslim teachers, religious leaders and governors. Health officials organised a meeting at the offices of the Jam'atu Nasril Islam in Kaduna to encourage Muslim clerics in northern Kaduna State to advise their followers to vaccinate their children for polio.[77] In 2013, the Gates Foundation began a programme that rewards governors of states with significantly reduced polio transmission and increased immunisation levels with substantial monetary awards.[78] In June 2013, the Nigerian industrialist Aliko Dangote announced a plan to provide cooperating mothers with his products – sugar, salt and macaroni.[79]

Yet while such methods – both sticks and carrots – may work in the short term, the long-term solution to increasing levels of polio, as well as measles, BCG, DPT and yellow fever immunisation among children requires a working primary health-care system with functioning immunisation programmes. The inability of the Nigerian government to provide such a system has undermined attempts to attain sufficient levels of immunisation that would end the transmission of wild poliovirus and reduce measles cases in the country. Indeed, as one virology professor working with the GPEI observed, 'The progress they have made so far has been because of routine immunisation, not because of mass immunisation for polio.'[80]

Overall immunity and continuing problems with routine vaccination

Thus the principal problem for GPEI officials has been the dysfunctional primary health-care system, particularly in rural areas in northern Nigeria where private health clinic services are not available.[81] In some rural communities, local clinics are closed or lack personnel or provisions.[82] When parents take their children for vaccinations, they may find 'stock-outs' and are forced to return.[83] Furthermore, the irregular supply of electricity makes it difficult to maintain regular supplies of viable vaccines, while impoverished parents who want basic health care available free of charge are expected to pay for each vaccination received at clinics.[84] This situation is particularly problematic in rural areas as one journalist investigating primary health-care provision discovered:

> The correspondent, who had to disguise as a parent in search of a centre to obtain vaccination for herself and her baby, got the shock of her life when she visited a primary health centre in Ogbondoroko, a village in the outskirts of Ilorin, the Kwara State capital ...[85] When our correspondent asked if she could get her baby immunised at the centre, the nurse on duty simply told her that she would have to wait for another month, as the clinic had just finished a round of immunisation exercise.
>
> 'You should have come last Friday. We do it once every month. That is the only time you will get it here. There is no consistent power supply here. So, we cannot afford to keep the vaccines in the proper condition for long; that is why you won't get it on any other day,' the nurse said casually. Asked what measures were being taken to ensure that babies born before the earmarked day were vaccinated, one of the health workers ... said those who could not wait had to take their babies to health centres in neighbouring villages.[86]

Similar stories are reported from other parts of the country in national newspapers as well as in government documents such as a 2009 Expert Review Committee report on polio and routine immunisation:

> The ERC notes some progress in improving data quality for routine immunization but again emphasizes that there is still a massive amount of work to be done to put routine immunization [RI] on a firm footing in Nigeria. It is frustrating that basic RI activities recommended in several previous meetings have not been carried out effectively. The ERC is forced to make the same recommendations again, and urges state and local governments to make the effort to deliver this basic service.[87]

These comments were echoed three years later in the 2012 twenty-fourth ERC report which noted that, 'National efforts to strengthen routine immunization must be accelerated, with the finalization of a national immunization strategy and its endorsement by the Inter-Agency Coordinating Committee by end–2012.'[88]

Similar challenges to routine immunisation were observed in the 2011 Annual Progress Report submitted to the Global Alliance Vaccine and Immunisation (GAVI) Secretariat by the Government of Nigeria on 25 May 2012:

> The main challenges in the routine immunisation programme include some vaccines and injection supplies stock outs, repeated health workers' industrial strike actions and security challenges in several Northern States. The vaccine stock-out was due to the late release of the funds for RI (in July) and reallocation of RI vaccine funds to other priorities (measles and polio campaigns).[89]

Professor Oyewale Tomori, who has served on several polio Expert Review Committees and who is currently President of the Nigerian Academy of Science, noted that the irregular supply of vaccine, poor handling (e.g., lack of refrigeration) and inadequate supplies of syringes all contributed to declining levels of immunisation.[90]

In 2012, in order to address these concerns, President Jonathan established the 'Saving One Million Lives Initiative' programme, part of a plan to improve primary health care in Nigeria. Following his announcement, GAVI Alliance officials revealed in 2013 that they had 'approved US\$21 million (N3bn) to help improve vaccine supply chains in Nigeria as part of a partnership aimed at scaling up routine immunisation.'[91] Yet some health professionals, such as Dr Olarenwaju

Ekunjimi, the President of the Association of Resident Doctors at the Lagos University Teaching Hospital, are sceptical that such large sums of money will not be usurped by those with access to donor funds.[92] The firing in October 2013 of 'dozens of officials handling polio immunization in Kano State ... because they were using the exercise as a 'money-making venture' by the Kano State Governor, Rabiu Musa Kwankwaso,[93] suggests that Dr Ekunjimi may be correct.

This connection between immunisation, politics and corruption is also suggested by one reader, whose comments followed a brief account of the NPHCDA Executive Director's plans to improve immunisation in northern Nigeria.[94] He wrote: 'Kindly immunise us against the following killer agents: 1. Ebola Jonanthan [sic],[95] 2. Politicians, 3. JTF [Joint Task Force – the military-police force assigned to counter Boko Haram attacks], 4. Corruption, and 5. BOKO'. Professor Tomori voiced somewhat similar sentiments (more politely) when he 'stated that Nigerian leaders had only been paying lip service to issues of health – a situation that, he noted, was responsible for the "mediocre performance" in health care delivery and a near absence of accountability in national programmes of government for her citizens'.[96]

Conclusion

Vaccination campaigns ultimately rely on the power of the state but they are facilitated by trust and citizens' belief that their government is helping them.[97] When this sense of political responsibility and visible evidence of improvements in their lives – working health clinics, clean water and electricity – are lacking, some citizens may resist government vaccination programmes, particularly when they focus on a single disease such as polio, which is not viewed by parents as a major health concern.

When the Nigerian government implemented health programmes that had widespread parental approval (e.g., the Immunization Plus Program in 2006 and the Measles Immunization Campaign in 2008), immunisation levels increased in subsequent years, while confirmed cases of wild poliovirus declined. In this instance, northern Nigerian parents' support for the national task of raising levels of immunisation (and ending polio transmission) coincided with the hopes of Nigerian medical professionals for better vaccine provision and the possibility of national vaccine production as recently proposed. Yet in northern Nigeria, many residents' experience of government vaccination programmes differs from that of medical professionals and government officials. Some government vaccination programmes – particularly the Expanded Programme on Immunisation and Immunization Plus Days that offered a range of health incentives – have improved Nigerians' acceptance of polio vaccination and have contributed to an interruption in transmission of wild poliovirus in Nigeria, announced by WHO in September 2015.[98] Yet the government's inability to maintain consistent supplies of viable vaccines and of its failure to supply related basic services such as electricity and clean water, continue to undermine the political authority of the state in matters of health.

Thus an association of vaccination programmes in the West with citizens' experience of bio-power whereby they incorporate state objectives through health regimes of the body, which strengthen the power and oversight of the state contrasts with the experiences of many northern Nigerians, reflecting a distinctive historical context, particularly biomedicine's association with British colonial rule.[99] Indeed, the vaccination campaigns in northern Nigeria display a certain historical consistency in their top-down approach to public health,[100] their use of imported vaccines and the implementation of laws which hold local government officials and traditional rulers responsible for the success of vaccination initiatives. These initiatives simultaneously foster forms of resistance – such as hiding children or parents 'voting with their feet', while revealing the weakness of state in enforcing vaccination laws, providing vaccines and maintaining oversight over the running of immunisation programmes. Nonetheless, as Abu-Lughod notes, romanticising resistance to state power can be misleading,[101] as the coercive measures used in the implementation of the GPEI in recent years suggest. Such vaccination programmes can – in the short term – reduce and end wild poliovirus transmission and reinforce political authority of the state through the implementation of police powers. Yet many Nigerian health professionals believe that parents' long-term acceptance of vaccination is contingent on a viable national primary health-care system, which provides routine immunisation as well as evidence of their government's concern for their well-being, on which high levels of immunity in Nigeria ultimately rest.

Notes

1 I. Mudashir, 'Polio: Drama as Trader Turns Back Gov Yero', *Weekly Trust* (22 June 2013), www.weeklytrust.com.ng (accessed 22 June 2013).

2 *Ibid.*

3 E. Parry, R. Godfrey, D. Mabey and G. Gill (eds), *Principles of Medicine in Africa* (Cambridge: Cambridge University Press, 2004), p. 139.

4 M. Foucault, *The History of Sexuality, Vol. 1: An Introduction* (New York: Random House, 1978), p. 139.

5 L. Abu-Lughod, 'Romance of Resistance', *American Ethnologist*, 17:1 (1990), pp. 41–55.

6 P. Greenough, 'Intimidation, Coercion, and Resistance in the Final Stages of the Smallpox Eradication Campaign in Southeast Asia, 1973–1975', *Social Science & Medicine*, 41:5 (1995), p. 633.

7 B. Adebayo, 'Vaccine Delivery, Still a Mirage in Nigeria', *Punch* (23 March 2013), www.medicalworldnigeria.com (accessed 16 August 2013).

8 S. Blume, 'Anti-Vaccination Movements and Their Interpretations', *Social Science & Medicine*, 62:3 (2006), pp. 628–42.

9 C. Obinna, 'Nigeria to Begin Vaccine Production – NAFDAC', *The Vanguard* (27 March 2013), www.vanguardngr.com/2013/03/nigeria-to-begin-vaccine-production-nafdac/ (accessed 1 February 2014).

10 L. Adamu and H. Yaya, '10 Polio Workers Shot Dead in Kano: … It's an Act of Cowardice – Pate … We're Trailing the Gunmen –IG', *Daily Trust* (9 February 2013), www.dailytrust.com.ng (accessed 9 February 2013).

11 Amnesty International, *Nigeria: Trapped in the Cycle of Violence* (London: Amnesty International, 2012).

12 Adebayo, 'Vaccine Delivery, Still a Mirage in Nigeria'; R. Leo, 'GAVI Gives N3bn to Improve Vaccine Access', *Daily Trust* (13 August 2013), www.dailytrust.com.ng (accessed 13 August 2013).

13 By 1908, 'there were sixty-three medical officers in Nigeria in government service', although the primary concern of these doctors was maintaining the health of the expatriate population; R. Schram, *A History of the Nigerian Health Services* (Ibadan: University of Ibadan Press, 1971), p. 141.

14 E. Herbert, 'Smallpox Inoculation in Africa', *Journal of African History*, 16:4 (1975), p. 546.

15 F. Jakeway, 'An Ordinance to Amend the Vaccination Ordinance', *Nigerian Gazette* (No. 16 of 1945), pp. 273–5.

16 The earliest recorded outbreak of cerebrospinal meningitis in Nigeria occurred in 1906 in Sokoto; see C. Ejembi, E. Renne and H. Adamu, 'The Politics of the 1996 Cerebrospinal Meningitis Epidemic in Nigeria', *Africa*, 68:1 (1998), pp. 118–34.

17 E. Renne, *The Politics of Polio in Northern Nigeria* (Bloomington: Indiana University Press, 2010), p. 25.

18 W. R. Collis, O. Ransome-Kuti, M. E. Taylor and L. E. Baker, 'Poliomyelitis in Nigeria', *West African Medical Journal*, 10:1 (1961), pp. 217–22.

19 J. B. Familusi, J. B. and V. A. O. Adesina, 'Poliomyelitis in Nigeria: Epidemiological Pattern of the Disease among Ibadan Children', *Journal of Tropical Paediatrics and Environmental Child Health*, 23:3 (1977), pp. 120–4.

20 D. W. Horn, 'The Epidemic of Cerebrospinal Fever in the Northern Provinces of Nigeria, 1949–1950', *Journal of the Royal Sanitation Institute*, 71:5 (1951), pp. 573–88; F. Fenner, D. A. Henderson, I. Arita, Z. Jezek and I. D. Ladnyi, *Smallpox and Its Eradication* (Geneva: WHO, 1988), p. 862.

21 Fenner *et al.*, *Smallpox and Its Eradication*, p. 883.

22 However, both the CDC and WHO also sought to improve vaccine production at the Yaba laboratory and a WHO vaccine production expert, along with Nigerian laboratory staff trained in the UK, worked to produce a viable freeze-dried vaccine in 1974; *Ibid.*, p. 885.

23 An agreement by the federal government and May & Baker Nigeria PLC proposed that vaccine production begin by 2014 (S. Ogundipe, 'Nigeria: FG Domesticates Vaccine Production', *The Vanguard* (26 June 2012), http://allafrica.com/stories/201206260182.html (accessed 1 February 2014).

24 E. Ekanem, 'A 10-year Review of Morbidity From Childhood Preventable Diseases in Nigeria: How Successful is the Expanded Programme of Immunization (EPI)?', *Journal of Tropical Pediatrics*, 34:6 (1988), pp. 323–8.

25 Federal Ministry of Health, Nigeria, *Expanded Program on Immunization*: *The National Coverage Survey, Preliminary Report* (Lagos: Federal Ministry of Health, 1991), p. 3.

26 O. Olatimehin, 'Accomplishing the Goal of EPI', *National Concord* (27 April 1988), p. 3.

27 O. Orere, 'Minister Pledges to Meet Immunisation Target Next Year', *Guardian* (13 December 1989), p. 20.

28 National Planning Commission [NPC-Nigeria] & UNICEF, *Children's and Women's Rights in Nigeria: A Wake-Up Call: Situation Assessment and Analysis 2001* (Abuja: National Planning Commission and UNICEF-Nigeria, 2001), p. 84.

29 Anonymous, 'Editorial: Structural Adjustment and Health in Africa', *The Lancet*, 335:8694 (1990), pp. 885–6.

30 A. Umar, 'No Free EPI Vaccines to States from '90', *New Nigerian* (27 October 1989), p. 24.

31 Feilden Battersby Analysts (FBA), *The State of Routine Immunization Services in Nigeria and Reasons for Current Problems* (Bath: FBA Health Systems Analysts, 2005), p. 3, www.technet21.org/backgrounddocs.html (accessed 15 August 2005).

32 S. Bonu, M. Rani and O. Razum, 'Global Public Health Mandates in a Diverse World: The Polio Eradication Initiative and the Expanded Programme on Immunization in Sub-Saharan Africa and South Asia', *Health Policy*, 70:3 (2004), p. 333.

33 O. Alabi, 'Expansion on Immunisation', *Daily Sketch* (22 June 1995).

34 World Bank, 'Project Paper on a Proposed Additional Financing: Partnerships for Polio Eradication Project, Report No. 44776–NG' (Abuja: World Bank, Africa Region Office, 2008), www-wds.worldbank.org (accessed 1 November 2008).

35 This in-country testing of stool samples facilitated the rapid identification of areas with wild poliovirus cases. Samples with genomic sequencing that suggest the possibility of circulating vaccine-derived polio virus are sent to the CDC in Atlanta (Interview: Professor Festus Adu, University College Hospital, 22 February 2008, Ibadan).

36 World Health Organization, *Global Polio Eradication Initiative, Strategic Plan 2001–2005* (Geneva: WHO, 2000).

37 G. Muhammad, 'The Debate Goes On', *Weekly Trust* (13–19 December 2003), pp. 1–2.

38 I. Okpani, 'FG Declares Polio Vaccine Safe', *Daily Trust* (24 December 2003), pp. 1–2.

39 S. Babadoko and M. Kazaure, 'Polio Vaccine Contaminated-JNI Reports', *Daily Trust* (26 January 2004), pp. 1–2.

40 Okpani, 'FG Declares Polio Vaccine Safe'.

41 Anonymous, 'Oral Polio Vaccine is Safe – Sultan of Sokoto', *Daily Trust* (22 March 2004), p. 10.

42 M. Kazaure, 'Kano Rejects FG, JNI Reports', *Weekly Trust* (18 March 2004), pp. 1–2; I. Ghinai, C. Willott, I. Dadari and H. Larson, 'Listening to the Rumours: What the Northern Nigeria Polio Vaccine Boycott Can Tell Us Ten Years On', *Global Public Health*, 8:10 (2013), pp. 1138–50.

43 K. Sule, 'Polio Vaccine: IBB tasks Nigerian Drug Coys', *Daily Trust* (25 March 2004).

44 Anonymous, 'Kano Imports Polio Vaccine from Indonesia', *Daily Trust* (17 May 2004), pp. 1–2.

45 Professor Oyewale Tomori noted the importance of calling the programme Immunization Plus Days, rather than Polio Plus Days, which had been the name given to polio activities by Rotary International

(Interview, 21 February 2008, Lagos). He was making the point that general immunisation efforts had been hampered by a focus on polio.

46 Centers for Disease Control and Prevention, 'Wild Poliovirus Weekly Update' (26 November 2008), www.polioeradication.org (accessed 28 November 2008).

47 Professor Pate has been a strong supporter of routine immunisation; R. Leo, 'Preventive Medicine is the Way to Go – Pate', *Daily Trust* (20 September 2011), www.dailytrust.com.ng, (accessed 20 September 2011).

48 National Primary Health Care Development Agency (NPHCDA), Nigeria, '17th Meeting of the Expert Review Committee (ERC) on Polio Eradication & Routine Immunization in Nigeria' (Ota, Ogun State, 1–2 April 2009), www.polioeradication.org/Resourcelibrary/Advisoryand-certification/TechnicalAdvisoryGroups.aspx (accessed 25 November 2011).

49 National Primary Health Care Development Agency (NPHCDA), Nigeria, '16th Meeting of the Expert Review Committee (ERC) on Polio Eradication & Routine Immunization in Nigeria' (Abuja, 27–28 October 2008). www.polioeradication.org/Resourcelibrary/Advisory-andcertification/TechnicalAdvisoryGroups.aspx (accessed 25 November 2011).

50 I. Mudashir, 'Sultan Constitutes Committee on Polio', *Daily Trust* (16 June 2009), p. 6; The head of the Shi'a community in Nigeria, Sheikh Ibrahim El-Zakzaky, cited Islamic approval of vaccination at an immunisation day exercise in Zaria in May 2008; A. Aodu and M. Abba, 'El-Zakzaky Advocates Immunisation Against Child Killer Diseases', *Daily Trust* (20 May), www.dailytrust.com.ng (accessed 22 May 2013).

51 Technical improvements in vaccines also increased immunisation effectiveness. Beginning in March 2006, the monovalent oral polio vaccine effective against the type 1 strain of the wild poliovirus was given to children in Nigeria, resulting in significant declines of type 1 poliovirus countrywide in 2009.

52 S. Taylor, 'Political Epidemiology: Strengthening Socio-Political Analysis for Mass Immunisation – Lessons from the Smallpox and Polio Programmes', *Global Public Health*, 4:6 (2009), p. 553.

53 MM, personal communication, 2012.

54 L. Adamu, 'Polio Returns with Menace in Kano', *Daily Trust* (5 November 2011), www.dailytrust.com.ng (accessed 5 November 2011).

55 Renne, *Politics of Polio*, pp. 42–5.

56 Interview: Professor H. A. Kaita, Ahmadu Bello University, Zaria (29 August 2005).

57 Anonymous, DVD, *Polio: Cuta ko Kariya?* [Polio: Harm or Protection?] (Zaria: Darul Hadeeths Salafiyya, nd); *W.H.O. Ta Ji Tsoro* [WHO is Fearful] (Zaria: Darul Hadeeths Salafiyya, nd), purchased in Zaria in 2013.

58 See chapter 4, 'Islam and Immunization in Northern Nigeria', for a detailed discussion these views, Renne, *Politics of Polio*, pp. 51–67.

59 I. Al-Jawziyya, *The Prophetic Medicine* (Karachi: Hafiz and Sons, 2001). This book consists of a compilation of *Hadīth* (sayings of the Prophet) and portions of the *Qur'ān* pertaining to illness which stresses the power of prayer in prevention and cure. Readers are told that for every disease, God created a cure – which may consist of prayer alone or may be combined with specific medicinal substances.

60 Anonymous, 'The Popular Discourses of Salafi Radicalism and Salafi Counter-Radicalism in Nigeria: A Case Study of Boko Haram', *Journal of Religion in Africa*, 42:2 (2012), p. 125.

61 National Population Commission, Nigeria, *2013 Nigeria Demographic Health Survey – Preliminary Report* (Abuja, Nigeria: NPC, 2013), p. 25.

62 In January 2012, the Borno State government paid N100 million to the family of the Mohammad Yusuf in an out of court settlement; M. Olugbode, 'Borno Pays Deceased Boko Haram Leader's Family N100 Million', *This Day* (10 January 2012), http://allafrica.com/stories/201201100727 (accessed 14 January 2012).

63 D. McNeil, Jr, 'Gunmen Kill Nigerian Polio Vaccine Workers in Echo of Pakistan Attacks', *New York Times* (9 February 2013), p. A4; www.nytimes.com (accessed 9 Feb 2013).

64 L. Adamu and H. Yaya, 'Journalists Deny Inciting Attack on Polio Workers', *Daily Trust* (14 February 2013), www.dailytrust.com.ng (accessed 14 February 2013).

65 *Sunday Trust*, 'NBC Suspends Radio License', *Sunday Trust* (24 February 2013), www.sundaytrust.com (accessed 24 February 2013).

66 World Health Organization (WHO), *Seventh Report – May 2013, Independent Monitoring Board of the Global Polio Eradication Initiative*, Global Polio Eradication Initiative, www.polioeradication.org (accessed 6 June 2013).

67 I. Wakili, T. Hassan and H. Idris, 'President Declares State of Emergency … Fighter Jets, Troops Moved to Borno, Yobe, Adamawa', *Daily Trust* (15 May 2013), http://www.dailytrust.com.ng (accessed 15 May 2013).

68 IRIN, 'Nigeria: Jail Threat for Polio Vaccination Refuseniks' (11 August 2011), www.irinnews.org/Report/93480/NIGERIA-Jail-threat-for-polio-vaccination refuseniks (accessed 1 May 2013).

69 The uncomfortable position of traditional leaders was exemplified by the Mai of Kaltungo's admission that parents in over 200 households

in his domain had rejected polio vaccine; A. Hamagam, 'Niger Wins $750,000 from Gates Foundation', *Daily Trust* (30 April 2013), www.dailytrust.com.ng (accessed 20 April 2013). Leonard discusses a similar dilemma in Chad where local political leaders must obey federal government orders while also respecting the concerns of local community members; L. Leonard, 'Working 'Off The Record'': Polio Eradication and State Immunity in Chad', *Critical Public Health*, 21 (2011), pp. 257–71.

70 S. Isuwa, 'LG Threatens Immunisation Defaulters with Legal Action', *Daily Trust* (8 July 2013), www.dailytrust.com.ng (accessed 8 July 2013).

71 *Ibid.*

72 *Ibid.*

73 World Health Organization (WHO), *Seventh Report – May 2013, Independent Monitoring Board of the Global Polio Eradication Initiative.*

74 This method of enticement backfired in Niger State when rumours that 'children could be initiated through petty offerings of sweets and biscuits' into secret cults, a practice called *shafi milera*. This situation ended this practice in the Niger State Immunization Plus program; R. Leo and J. L. Okafor, 'Weighty Effects of Birth Control on Polio Eradication', *Daily Trust* (10 July 2012), p. 51.

75 Interview: PO-09–1, Zaria, 27 June 2009.

76 S. Nasiru, G. Aliyu, A. Gasasira, M. Aliyu, M. Zubair, S. Mandawari, H. Waziri, A. Nasidi and S. El-Kamary, 'Breaking Community Barriers to Polio Vaccination in Northern Nigeria: The Impact of a Grass Roots Mobilization Campaign (Majigi)', *Pathogens and Global Health*, 106:3 (2012), pp. 166–71.

77 C. Alabi, 'Kaduna Engages Clerics in Fight Against Polio', *Daily Trust* (1 April 2013), p. 42.

78 For example, in 2013, Niger State 'won the award for recording an appreciable improvement in the campaign for the fight of polio eradication in the state'; Hamagam, 'Niger Wins $750,000 from Gates Foundation'.

79 L. Danjuma, 'Polio: Dangote Rewards Immunised Families', *Daily Trust* (9 July 2013), www.dailytrust.com.ng (accessed 9 July 2013).

80 Interview: Professor Festus Adu, Ibadan, 22 February 2008.

81 Feilden Battersby Analysts (FBA), *The State of Routine Immunization Services in Nigeria and Reasons for Current Problems*. Bath: FBA Health Systems Analysts, 2005, www.technet21.org/backgrounddocs.html (accessed 15 August 2005); T. Omoniyi, 'Routine Immunization for Infants: Still a Battle Royale', *Daily Trust* (4 June 2012), www.dailytrust.com.ng (accessed 7 June 2012).

82 L. Adamu, 'Polio Returns with Menace in Kano'.

83 The 12th Expert Review Committee reported routine stock outs; National Primary Health Care Development Agency (NPHCDA), Nigeria, '12th Meeting of the Expert Review Committee (ERC) on Polio Eradication & Routine Immunization in Nigeria (Abuja, 3–4 May 2007), p. 8, www.polioeradication.org/Resourcelibrary/Advisoryandcertification/ TechnicalAdvisoryGroups.aspx (accessed 25 November 2011). During the federal and state elections in 2011, there were 'stock outs', with no vaccine availability in some health centres. Post-election violence in several northern Nigerian states also affected immunisation efforts.

84 According to a Nigerian National Bureau of Statistics report released in February 2012, poverty rates in northern Nigeria are estimated as having ranged from 76% to 86% in 2010; BBC, 'Nigerians Living in Poverty Rise to Nearly 61%', *BBC World News* (13 February 2012), www.bbc.co.uk/ news/world-africa-17015873 (accessed 13 February 2012).

85 'Though located in a village whose residents are mostly farmers, petty traders and cattle rearers, the health centre, painted a bright yellow and green, had just been renovated and one would expect that the services provided should be at par with its physical outlook'; Adebayo, 'Vaccine Delivery, Still a Mirage in Nigeria'. See also A. Masquelier, 'Behind the Dispensary's Prosperous Facade: Imagining the State in Rural Niger', *Public Culture*, 13:2 (2011), pp. 267–91.

86 *Ibid.*; Adebayo, 'Vaccine Delivery, Still a Mirage in Nigeria'.

87 NPHCDA, '17th Meeting of the Expert Review Committee (ERC) on Polio Eradication & Routine Immunization in Nigeria'.

88 National Primary Health Care Development Agency (NPHCDA), Nigeria, 'Final Report: 24th Meeting of the Expert Review Committee (ERC) On Polio Eradication & Routine Immunization in Nigeria, 10–11 September 2012', www.polioeradication.org/Resourcelibrary/Advisoryandcertifica-tion/TechnicalAdvisoryGroups.aspx (accessed 26 August 2013).

89 GAVI Alliance, 'Annual Progress Report 2011', submitted by the Government of Nigeria (Geneva: GAVI Alliance, 2012), www.gavialliance.org/ country/nigeria/documents/#apr (accessed 13 August 2013).

90 Tomori said, 'We should expect that there will be measles outbreak in 2013 because the government did not talk about it in 2012 … The issue of which vaccine gets which funding has been politicized'; Adebayo, 'Vaccine Delivery, Still a Mirage in Nigeria'. Unfortunately, his predicted measles outbreak was correct as in March 2013, outbreaks occurred in several northern Nigerian states, with reports of 4,000 children having contracted the disease and thirty-six deaths. This outbreak occurred despite measles vaccination campaigns in late 2008 and reported high levels of measles immunity nationally in 2011.

91 R. Leo, 'GAVI gives N3bn to Improve Vaccine Access', *Daily Trust* (13 August 2013), www.dailytrust.com.ng (accessed 13 August 2013).

92 Ekunjimi was referring specifically polio eradication initiative funding, saying that 'Corruption in the system will not allow a polio-free Nigeria by 2015'; T. Olusegun, 'The Resurgence of Polio in Nigeria', Inter Press Service (19 June 2012), www.globalissues.org/news/2012/06/19/14012 (accessed 16 August 2013).

93 H. Musa, 'Kwankwaso Fires Polio Officials Over Corruption', *Daily Trust* (8 October 2013), www.dailytrust.com.ng (accessed 8 October 2013).

94 J. Okafor, 'Polio: FG to Vaccinate 28m Children', *Daily Trust* (13 December 2012), www.dailytrust.com.ng (accessed 13 December 2013).

95 He is referring to the Nigerian president, Goodluck Jonathan (and to the Ebola virus).

96 Adebayo, 'Vaccine Delivery, Still a Mirage in Nigeria'.

97 Taylor, 'Political Epidemiology, p. 552.

98 WHO, 'WHO Removes Nigeria from Polio Endemic List', Global Polio Eradication website (25 September 2015), www.polioeradication.org (accessed 2 October 2015).

99 M. Vaughan, *Curing their Ills: Colonial Power and African Illness* (Cambridge: Polity Press, 1991).

100 Muraskin has observed a similar dynamic regarding the implementation of the GPEI in India; W. Muraskin, *Polio Eradication and its Discontents* (Hyderabad: Orient BlackSwan, 2012).

101 Lughod, 'Romance of Resistance'.

Afterword

12

The power of individuals and the dependency of nations in global eradication and immunisation campaigns

William Muraskin

At one time historians emphasised the 'Great Man in History' concept. That idea was later pushed aside by the realisation that larger, more important forces were at work. The individual's importance shrank as the role of massively expanded governments, multi-national corporations, and institutional science took centre-stage as the movers and shakers of world events. Without denying the importance of such forces and institutions, I have made it my concern to study the continued centrality and indispensability of individuals in making things happen in international public health. I have spent the better part of the last quarter-century looking at how the right men – and they tended to be men, American men in particular – in the right place, at the right time have created the conditions to radically accelerate development and delivery of vaccines for the children of the developing countries.

I have focused intensively on the International Task Force on Hepatitis B Immunisation[1] – led by James Maynard, Alfred Prince and Richard Mahoney; the Children's Vaccine Initiative[2] led by or influenced by Scott Halstead, Philip Russell and Roy Widdus; the Bill and Melinda Gates' Children's Vaccine Programme[3] led by Mark Kane and James Maynard; the Global Alliance for Vaccines and Immunization[4] created by Mark Kane, Tore Godal, Jacques-Francois Martin, Steve Landry and Amy Bateson; the Rockefeller Foundation's Public–Private Partnership project[5] single-handedly championed by Ariel Pablos-Mendez (with the support of Timothy Evans) – many of which were ultimately adopted by the Gates Foundation and (incorrectly) seen as

originating with it; and the global polio eradication campaign[6] conceived by William Foege, Alan Hinman, Ciro de Quadros and run by
Bruce Alyward. Driven by a powerful moral imperative and social consciousness, these dozen and a half men fought to make things happen
that under normal circumstances would not have happened in the fight
to save the lives of countless children using vaccines and immunisation
as their tools.

Among their supporters have been many engaged and committed
vaccine champions within the scientific community: scientist/activists
working for what they believed was clearly the 'Greater Good'. William
(Bill) Foege (former head of the American CDC and the Task force for
Child Survival, adviser to the Rockefeller and the Gates Foundations)
has talked of the importance of a 'Network of Scientists' as the people
who should be the prime movers of global initiatives – even if being
such would mean marginalising (or even undermining) the influence
of the World Health Organization (WHO).[7]

The host of global goods that have been achieved by these few men
using vaccines and immunisation as their tools is truly staggering. I
started out as a researcher enthralled by the moral fervour of the people
I was studying and their dedication to achieving their ends despite the
apparently overwhelming human, monetary and physical obstacles.
Nothing would stop them from carrying out what they saw as the
morally right thing, and I found it very difficult not to see the world as
they did: a world in which children are needlessly suffering and dying
because of uncaring, often incompetent, bureaucrats and their end-
lessly feuding organisations. These inspired men no doubt had a can-do
spirit that contrasted markedly with the prevailing ethic in international
public health.[8]

However, it has become increasingly clear to me that these great
achievements have come at a very steep price, a price which has largely
been obscured because it has been paid by people whose concerns
and needs have not been widely known, or if known, have been considered unimportant among the network of scientist-activists and influential individuals who make international public health policy their
domain. To repeat, there has been considerable but nearly invisible
'collateral damage' inflicted on the world by the good works of global
policy makers, and this damage threatens to become worse as time
passes.

The problem of power

When global leaders decide a course of action, they exercise a potent form of policy-making power. If children's lives are being saved, if the public's health improves, it is easy to focus on leaders' achievements and miss unpleasant things that are going on simultaneously. Regardless of the benefits they bring about, however, global leaders' power comes at the expense of other real or potential sources of authority. When cost–benefit analyses of vaccine campaigns and eradication programmes are prepared, the list of items to be ranked are restricted to things that can be easily quantified. Increases and decreases in power among legitimate rival stakeholders is not considered.

Since gains and losses of power are not admitted to by global policy makers, those who successfully work the levers of global health pro- grammes often conflate their personal agendas with 'global goods', allowing them to believe that what they subjectively want is objectively sought by everyone – or at least by every right-thinking person. For example, eradication campaigns have come to be seen as the ultimate and finest example of public health in action.[9]

It is widely believed that to not eradicate a disease when it is feasible to do so will be seen as a blot on our collective reputation; something for which future generations will condemn us.[10] Yet, whether admitted or not, global health power-brokers can, and regularly do, take advan- tage of this belief to subvert the priorities of developing world govern- ments, national medical professional associations, local communities and millions of families. Too often, countries' autonomy and authentic independence are the collateral damage of top-down global health. Unfortunately, this happens to a greater or less degree in most global immunisation initiatives,[11] but the most extreme and blatant loss of autonomy comes with eradication campaigns. Such campaigns literally hijack the public health agendas of the world without the sponsors even taking notice of it – blinded as they are by their deeply held personal visions of the public good. Alarmingly, we can expect a dozen or more such campaigns to be waged simultaneously in the near future through- out the developing world.

As I wrote in my book *Polio Eradication and Its Discontents*,[12] the global polio campaign is an egregious example of the often under- handed process (means) that has generally been employed to save the lives of children (ends). There was and still is a downside when a few inspired but relentless individuals successfully push through global initiatives in which vaccines are not understood as a means to help build a long-term sustainable health system but rather as indispensable weapons for winning dramatic, but short-term, wars against particular microbes.

The reality underneath the hype

The origin of the global polio eradication campaign is as astounding as it is disheartening. It is important not just as a history lesson but as a warning of the effects of power when it is exercised without accountability by self-chosen crusaders. It is a warning that is important for the future, because an all-out war on microbes is being planned right now by eradication proponents who intend to prevail regardless of developing-country governments', or their peoples', choices.

At the conclusion of the successful smallpox eradication effort in 1977, most of the world's public health communities led by the WHO took a 'no more vertical eradication programmes' position. Instead, they turned toward a new emphasis on Primary Health Care for All by the year 2000.[13] Immunisations, but not disease eradication, would be part of the new emphasis, but not pivotal to it. They would be just one component in the larger primary health care system. There were many vehement objections to this 'Health for All', especially in the United States. In particular the Rockefeller Foundation saw the WHO as dysfunctional and unable to carry out its mandate as the chief health agency in the world. The Rockefeller Foundation fired back with an 'interim' concept of 'selective primary health care' authored by Kenneth Warren and Julia Walsh which, despite its name, was aimed at undermining the new policy by emphasising immunisation systems, rather than general primary health systems, as the critical goal for policy makers.[14]

However, others were not as offended by the marginalisation of vaccines per se, as they were appalled by the negative attitude toward eradication. They feared that eradication as a tool of public health was on the verge of itself being 'eradicated'. This possibility was for them personally intolerable.

In 1980 at a National Institutes of Health conference convened by De Witt Stetten Jr, deputy director of the NIH Fogarty Centre, Stetten raised the issue of what was to be done to correct the situation.[15] The majority of participants expressed opposition to the WHO's new public health policy and talked of the need to find a disease – any disease – that could be effectively eradicated relatively quickly and cheaply to prove the continued relevance of eradication as a tool – perhaps 'the tool' – of international public health. Of the many possibilities raised, only three diseases were seen as feasible for eradication: measles, yaws and poliomyelitis. Measles was strongly favoured by Stetten and Alan Hinman, who was then the foremost measles eradication advocate.

Stetten and his colleagues were influential enough that other large-scale expert conferences on these three diseases were convened in the next few years with the hope, and expectation, that at least one of the groups would champion an eradication campaign. It quickly became clear that measles was not eradicable given existing technology, and that yaws was not a global problem, which made the next polio conference especially important.

A meeting of polio experts gathered in 1983 at the Pan American Health Organization (PAHO) in Washington, DC.[16] It was the largest meeting of its kind in twenty years and included both Jonas Salk and Albert Sabin – the rival creators of the two polio vaccines. The much anticipated conference turned out to be a major anticlimax, however, for its eradicationist organisers, De Witt Stetten and Dorothy Horstmann, and for its rapporteur, Nobel laureate Frederick Robbins. Despite Stetten's plea to the assembled group at the beginning of the conference to consider the virtue of polio eradication, by the end of the meeting Robbins declared that the experts had reached no agreement on the issue except that polio would be more difficult to eradicate than smallpox.[17]

While it is true that eradication was a non-starter, eradication was debated with great vigour at one of the sessions, where the proponents had to admit they lost ground in bitter interchanges with WHO representatives, who championed primary health care and argued compellingly against an eradication programme. The fact that most polio experts did not favour polio eradication in no way stopped its proponents from their determination to move forward. Nor did the fact that polio was a disease with a low death rate in an era of massive child mortality from other infectious diseases slow them down. Most certainly they were not deterred by the fact that polio was a low (or zero) priority for most developing countries with endemic polio and for the families and communities of which they were composed. In fact, what polio did to children was never the issue for eradicationists, rather polio was simply a 'disease of opportunity', a stalking horse, picked to showcase the power of eradication to a largely sceptical, if not downright hostile, world.

Thus a small number of men, almost all from the North and mostly Americans, in the right place, at the right time, pushed for polio eradication regardless of what anyone else thought. One of them was William (Bill) Foege, who in his capacity as head of the vital Task Force for Child Survival, had the ear of James Grant, the charismatic head of UNICEF. For Foege and Grant, the WHO's anti-eradication position was simply an obstacle to be gotten around.[18]

An even more important proponent of eradication, though not as well known at the time, was Ciro de Quadros, the head of immunisation at the Pan American Health Organization (PAHO). PAHO, although technically a regional office of WHO, was older and saw itself as both superior to, and in competition with, its so-called 'parent' in Geneva. De Quadros' position at PAHO in the 1980s uniquely gave him a laboratory to prove the continued viability of eradication as a public health tool.[19] The claim was made at the time that if a disease could be eradicated (more accurately 'eliminated') in the Americas – with their amazing range of rich and poor countries – then it could be eradicated anywhere in the world. De Quadros was psychologically committed to the idea of disease eradication in public health, as were many of those whose careers had started (and to some extent emotionally peaked) with the gruelling but often exhilarating smallpox eradication campaign, 1966–77.

Scientists and public health officials are usually not comfortable with the idea that emotions and psychological commitments have an impact in policy decisions. In the 'fact-based' community of science everything must conform to real world realities. But 'facts' often take a backseat to more human influences, because individuals matter, and individuals are not simply fact-making machines, but rather operate on a mixture of evidence and feelings. In the case of polio eradication, feelings often predominated. These were not the heart-rending emotions that many people feel when they see a crippled child; rather, it was the anguish felt by a small cadre of men who contemplated the permanent loss of a personally meaningful and cherished tool of public health: disease eradication.

In 1988 a few well-placed proponents found it relatively easily to manoeuvre the World Health Assembly (WHA) to declare for the global eradication of polio.[20] However, it is important to realise that the ministers of health at the WHA had been incapable of giving informed consent to such a far-reaching programme, because they were not provided with the type of information necessary to understand what the declaration entailed. In part this was because the proponents were themselves ignorant of conditions on the ground in the various nations of Asia and Africa. Nor, in all probability, would they have provided totally accurate information, even if they had possessed it, because they were championing an idea, a cause, not a practical project. They believed that with enough 'political will' anything could be achieved. That was the lesson, realistic or not, that they believed the success of smallpox eradication had taught.

The road to polio eradication since 1988 has been a long and rocky one. While it was sold initially as a relatively quick and cheap campaign that would have 'infinite' economic benefits once universal polio vaccination was stopped, it has turned out to be neither quick, nor cheap, nor productive of infinite economic benefits. Instead of costing approximately US$100 million (an early estimate) and ending by the year 2000, it has already reached US$15.5 billion (by 2013), and an additional estimated US$5.5 billion will be needed in the years until full eradication is declared.[21]

A continuous stream of 'unexpected' obstacles – for example, eradication proponents belatedly discovering that India is not Brazil and Nigeria is not Peru, as well as the diverse biological traits of individuals and groups and the mutagenic qualities of the live-virus Sabin vaccine – have radically slowed the eradication of wild polio.[22] Many of these 'unexpected' problems should not have come as surprises, since the polio medical literature and knowledgeable experts had warned the eradication champions of many of them from the beginning. The eradicationists' naive hope was that the campaign could be finished fast enough that the potential difficulties – especially problems from the Sabin oral vaccine itself – could be avoided. Speed was always of the essence, but speed was not always possible given the vast diversity of conditions in the developing countries. There was a lot of self-inflicted ignorance, and many important things that were unknown were things that supporters of the campaign didn't want to know. For the leaders of the polio campaign it was vital that nothing be allowed to undermine the morale of their children's crusade. Dissenters were not welcome. As Bill Foege said: invite everyone to your conferences, but don't invite back those who disagree; eradication campaigns require enthusiasm – you don't want nay-sayers around. Such a position is probably a good way to maximise organisational esprit de corps but is not compatible with 'science', which is based on constant research and adjustments to changing data. This 'hear no evil, speak no evil' requirement often trumped existing knowledge, just as it powerfully deterred support for new polio research. Inconvenient information was not desired.[23]

Is eradication the highest form of immunisation work?

It is widely assumed that the eradication of wild polio virus throughout the world will constitute an unalloyed public good. Unfortunately, this is an untrue assumption. The notion that eradication is an indispensable weapon in the arsenal of public health was already being discredited even as the polio campaign was being launched in 1988. The chronic problems of the campaign should subsequently have provided ammunition for that original critical position. In addition, the realisation that any eradicated disease for which public health immunisation ceased would automatically become a candidate biological weapon of mass destruction should have made further eradication efforts almost unthinkable. This became crystal clear after the discovery in the late 1980s that the Soviet Union had weaponised smallpox soon after it was eradicated and that smallpox was high on the list of potential terrorist weapons. On these grounds eradicationism as a tool of public health should have been as dead as a dodo. But it didn't die.

None of this happened because of the influence of those who support eradication as a tool of public health; their number has grown, and they have become more confident and aggressive. It appears that if and when polio eradication occurs, it will be used as definitive proof of the pivotal importance of eradicationism in global public health. If that occurs it will be nothing less than a disaster.

Anticipating the successful conclusion of the polio campaign, a pro-eradication conference organised by the Strüngmann Forum in Frankfurt, Germany, was held in 2010. This conference, attended by a host of prominent individuals and organisations, was in many ways radically different from the small numbers who had gathered at the Fogarty Centre in 1980 to fight for what then appeared to be a losing cause. Different, except in one regard: the emotional and philosophical commitment to eradication. At the Strüngmann conference the 'moral imperative' of eradication was not a question to be explored or debated but was rather a given, a foundational premise. No one asked: should diseases be eradicated? but rather, which ones and when?

The lessons attendees took from the ongoing polio campaign was not that unintended consequences are predictable, or that our ignorance is great, or that things often go wrong or that costs and tasks will escalate out of control, and so forth, nor that there are terrible collateral costs to developing countries when their own internally generated priorities are subordinated to outsiders. Instead, the lesson imbibed at the Strüngmann meeting was: We know what we did wrong with polio, so we will succeed in the future campaigns because we won't do things that way again.

The confidence of eradicationists seems to recognise no bounds. They seem to feel that they have learned past lessons so well, and that they are so smart and skilled, that they can start other eradication campaigns even before the polio effort has proven successful. Their argument is, we must make use of the polio infrastructure before it disappears. The polio infrastructure should be used not only to start an eradication campaign against measles, but to tackle multiple eradication campaigns, for example, mumps, rubella or what have you, piggybacking them one on top of the other. All are considered reasonable targets. In a meeting I attended at the Carter Center in Atlanta in April 2013, one CDC participant said they were looking at approximately eighteen infectious diseases with the expectation that as many as twelve of them were candidates for eradication or elimination campaigns – many of these campaigns would be conducted simultaneously.

Where one would expect humility based on the polio eradication campaign's troubled record of cost overruns and delays one finds only hubris. However, hubris at the Strüngmann conference was disguised by a show of sophisticated studies and checklists of what to do and what not to do, which is no doubt far better than what preceded the adoption of the goal of polio eradication. Nonetheless, the eradicationists are still set on seizing the public health agendas for the entire developing world for decades to come.

When an article of faith – that eradication is a moral obligation from this generation to the next – takes hold and drives a global initiative, it blinds its proponents from seeing the world from the perspective of others. Since the eradicators already know what is good, all they have to do is 'educate' the leaders and peoples of the developing world to the 'facts' on which they will surely agree. If these leaders and peoples don't agree, then they need more education – or infusions of money, which can seduce even those who don't 'educate' well. If neither of those things work, or if countries change their minds later, then governmental elites must be by definition corrupt or stupid. The eradicationists are blinded by their faith and do not see the possibility of legitimate dissent. In many places developing countries have generated their own health and development priorities which are undermined by externally driven programmes, but this possibility is not the eradicationists' chief concern, to the extent that it is a concern at all.

Unfortunately, eradication campaigns entail a problem for developing countries that other types of externally generated disease control programmes do not: they are all or nothing affairs. To achieve the desired end, every country in the world must cooperate. There is no patience for any country not doing its part. There can be no tolerance of a country's government changing its mind. National authorities have no freedom to withdraw once their consent is given, even if the cost–benefit analysis for their own populations changes radically. Eradication campaigns are inherently top-down operations in which targeted countries – usually former colonies of European empires – find themselves pressured to give up their hard-won autonomy for a 'greater good' that is determined and defined by someone other than themselves.

However, one thing is sure: no developing country has ever made the eradication of a global infectious disease its highest priority. Countries may want their endemic diseases under control, but disease eradication is not a natural concern. In addition, countries differ on which diseases they are most burdened by. In the case of polio, most countries ranked it a very low priority because other infections inflicted higher mortality on their children.

The problem of global immunisation programmes

External origination is not just an attribute of eradication programmes but of disease control as well. Even though control programmes are less binding, since withdrawal is always a possibility, the problems they cause developing countries are unfortunately very similar. For example, the choice of vaccines to be used is determined by a small group of experts primarily in the North. In fact, one man, Bill Gates, and his foundation, play an inordinate role in determining the immunisation priorities of the countries of the South. Top-down versus bottom-up priority setting is not a minor but a fundamental problem for the ex-colonial world. Most of the South is already caught in a tangle of northern economic investments, disinvestments, bi- and multi-lateral demands, controls, requirements, promises and threats that many have called neo-colonialism. The fact that global immunisation programmes are humanitarian in their aim rather than directly exploitive does not prevent their strongly destructive side effects.

The assumption made by global immunisation programmes is that the lives of children saved by a vaccine-preventable disease is a definitive good, and that those who have the power to select and supply vaccines are agents of that good. The fact that there are significant 'opportunity costs' for countries and their populations when they are pushed to accept a vaccine control programme, which may be of low priority to them, carries little weight against such a definitive act of humanitarianism. Indeed, to oppose such programmes must represent at best ignorance, and at worst an absolute evil.

One of the great virologists of the twentieth century, Alfred Prince, co-discoverer of the hepatitis B virus and creator of one of the first inexpensive hepatitis B vaccines, who was also a social activist fighting for mass hepatitis B immunisation, was an interesting dissenter from this common view found so often in the North. When I asked him why he worked on hepatitis B, he said that hepatitis B killed young and middle-aged adults who contributed to their national economies as well as to their own families, and that their deaths detracted (at some level) from whatever investments in education and resources their societies had been able to provide. This constituted, he felt, a major blow to their countries. However, if hepatitis B had killed children rather than adults, he never would have devoted his talents to developing a vaccine. There was no reason, he said, to save large numbers of children who would overwhelm their societies, strain their economies and natural resources, and result in a generation of under-employed and unemployed young people (especially males). Prince's goal was to help countries develop, not drown them in excess population or allow them to be ripped apart by angry, economically superfluous and armed young men. For him, saving children was not the ultimate goal – heresy though that might seem. The cost in economic development was too high. What passes for cost–benefit analysis in global immunisation programmes has traditionally not factored in the demographic consequences of immunisation of the sort that preoccupied Dr Prince or for that matter most ministries of finance in developing countries.[24]

Lurking under this fight between good and evil, ignorance and enlightenment, philanthropy and kleptocracy, and so on, is a lot of the old colonial mentality dressed up for modern times.[25] Developing world governments are often seen as obstacles to saving the lives of children. Like bad parents, they must be circumvented by experts for the good of the child. If global policy makers fail to convince governments to act 'correctly' then global-level nanny organisations and 'selfless' philanthropists are required to intervene. It is hard to criticise those who wage the fight for the Greater Good. But families, communities, and nations all have to find their own way. That is what being adult and independent is all about. Mistakes will be made. Deaths will occur. Children will suffer. But corrections hopefully will ultimately occur.

After the publication of my book on polio I was asked: Do you want children to be paralysed by polio or killed by measles? My reply was no, of course not. But what is the price that should be paid to save those children? How big a cost to national autonomy, community self-determination, alternative disease prevention, or alternative economic and social developmental projects is reasonable – reasonable not to me but to the people in the developing world? The cost to national self-respect is high when health policy is determined by outsiders – whether global public health officials or philanthropists who seem to daily think up brilliant new health programmes to save the children of the developing world.

Perhaps trying this thought experiment will make things clearer: If Britain or the United States were told that an Indian mega-billionaire wanted them to introduce a new vaccine that they had not prioritised, a vaccine that would push aside their own health or economic policies, how would they react? If an organisation like the WHO or THE Gates Foundation, but dominated by India, China and Kenya, set up goals for immunisation and held meetings manipulated by their nationals in which UK and US desires were subordinated to southern goals, what would the response be?

For a country like the United States with its own ghettos of poverty, sky-high minority incarceration, shocking levels of infant mortality, extreme wealth concentration and a Congress bought and sold by Wall Street banks, to tell the countries of the South how to set their priories, to condemn their unresponsive elites, corrupt rulers and unequal treatment of children, is grotesque hypocrisy. Freedom is the right to be wrong and to make mistakes. Independent countries have an inalienable right to determine their own destinies. They do not need Big Brothers intervening in the name of humanitarianism nor do they need self-appointed global elites claiming they own the routes to the greater good, as European imperialists used to intervene in the name of civilisation and Christianity. The cost to the South was too high then, and it is too high now.

An alternative to the current policies of global humanitarian assistance

What is the alternative to the present top-down system? It is simple, though unlikely to be carried out. If the northern countries and their philanthropists want to help southern countries and their children, then they must find out what the developing countries' priorities actually are. Bottom-up rather than top-down means paying attention to other people's goals rather than solipsistically pursuing one's own. Getting to know those local priorities needs slow and laborious work and requires dealing with the fact that developing countries are individually quite different.

One size doesn't fit all. For example, hepatitis B vaccine may be wanted in one country but not in another, where the vaccine might be objectively just as useful, but that country wants Japanese encephalitis immunisation instead. Global programmes constantly look for 'check lists' that try to homogenise the developing world so that the same vaccine can be introduced into all countries as part of one programme regardless of differences between them, and without any concern for what is actually desired. Global leaders must stop making vaccine and eradication policies and then trying to convince (read: force their views on) the leaders and people of the developing world. The North (and the new philanthropists as well) need to allow their money and expertise to be used by countries based on local priorities. They need to listen rather than talk. That is not the situation today, all claims notwithstanding.

Notes

1 W. Muraskin, *The War Against Hepatitis B: A History of the International Task Force on Hepatitis B Immunization* (Philadelphia: University of Pennsylvania Press, 1995).

2 W. Muraskin, *The Politics of International Health: The Children's Vaccine Initiative and the Struggle to Develop Vaccines for the Third World* (Albany: State University of New York Press, 1998).

3 W. Muraskin, *Crusade to Immunize the World's Children: the Origin of the Bill and Melinda Gates Children's Vaccine Program and the Birth of the Global Alliance for Vaccines and Immunization* (Los Angeles: University of Southern California, Marshall School, Global BioBusiness book, 2005).

4 *Ibid.*

5 W. Muraskin, *The Rockefeller Foundation's Health Sciences Division: 1977–2002, An Overview of a Quarter Century of Fighting the Infectious Diseases of the Developing World* (unpublished manuscript).

6 W. Muraskin, *Polio Eradication and Its Discontents: An Historian's Journey Through an International Public Health (Un) Civil War* (Hyderabad: Orient BlackSwan, 2012).

7 See 'Report of the Dahlem Workshop on the Eradication of Infectious Diseases, Berlin, March 16–22, 1997' in *The Eradication of Infectious Diseases,* edited by W. R. Dowdle and D. R. Hopkins (Chichester: John Wiley & Sons, 1998), pp. 187–92. According to Foege, 'The lesson may be that WHO should be seen as a scientific organisation that becomes an eradication advocate only when outside forces are sufficiently strong to make the case. That may not be a bad model to follow in the future.' For him effective polio eradication required the formation of a 'great coalition' for which 'a service organisation, Rotary International' performed the 'catalytic

role'. The WHO was not the main actor. A similar situation existed for Guinea worm eradication (a project of the Carter Center) and for onchocerciasis (Merck). For Foege it was important to foster 'tailor made structures for each eradication effort' and not try to have one organisation (WHO) be the key to such efforts. Such views were not shared by the World Health Organization. (This note uses text from Muraskin, *Polio and Its Discontents*).

8 Two examples of this writer being enthralled with his subjects can be found in *The War Against Hepatitis B* and *The Politics of International Health*.

9 See for example many of the papers in *Disease Eradication in the 21st Century: Implications for Global Health*, edited by S. L. Cochi and W. R. Dowdle (Cambridge: MIT Press, 2011).

10 This has been said to me countless times but perhaps most strongly by Scott Halstead, formerly Acting Director of Health Science, Rockefeller Foundation, and the preeminent virologist of dengue hemorrhagic fever.

11 This is made clear in Muraskin, *Crusade to Immunize the World's Children*. It was while researching this book that the hidden cost of top-down 'Great Men' global health policy became impossible to ignore.

12 Muraskin, *Polio Eradication and Its Discontents*.

13 The Alma-Ata Declaration of 1978 emerged as a major milestone of the twentieth century in the field of public health, and it identified primary health care as the key to the attainment of the goal of 'Health for All'. See WHO, 'Declaration of Alma-Ata. International Conference on Primary Health Care, Alma- Ata, USSR, 6–12 September 1978', www.who.int/ publications/almaata_declaration_en.pdf.

14 See J. A. Walsh and K. S. Warren, 'Selective Primary Health Care: An Interim Strategy for Disease Control in Developing Countries', *Social Science & Medicine* (Part C: Medical Economics), 14:2 (1980), pp. 145–63. There was nothing 'interim' about the intent of the strategy. The WHO emphasis on primary health care was seen as simply wrong-headed. It was seen as overly vague and without any targeted goals that could be measured. This strategy was a replacement for it. In addition, UNICEF, which increasingly saw itself as a rival of the WHO, was opposed to the Declaration of Alma Ata and offered itself as a white knight for its opponents. For a superb critique of UNICEF's championship of selective primary health care, see B. Wisner, 'GOBI versus PHC? Some Dangers of Selective PHC', *Social Science and Medicine*, 26:9 (1980), pp. 963–69.

15 'Report on the International Conference on the Eradication of Infectious Diseases. Can Infectious Diseases Be Eradicated?', *Reviews of Infectious Diseases*, 4:5 (September–October 1982), p. 915.

16 'Proceedings of the International Symposium on Poliomyelitis Control held at the Pan American Health Organisation, Washington, DC, 14–17 March 1983', were edited by D. M. Horstmann, T. C. Quinn and F. C. Robbins, *Review of Infectious Diseases*, 6: Supplement 2 (May–June, 1984), pp. S301–600.

17 *Ibid.*, p. S600.

18 See W. Muraskin, *Polio Eradication and its Discontents*, pp. 47–51 for a discussion of the roles of William Foege, James Grant and D. A. Henderson in championing polio eradication in the 'Declaration of Talloires', which was issued at a meeting called by Foege's Task Force for Child Survival in Talloires, France, 10–12 March 1988.

19 Muraskin, *Polio Eradication and its Discontents*, pp. 33–46.

20 David Salisbury, head of the WHO's Scientific Advisory Group of Experts, has said as much in an interview. He described a technical advisory group meeting on polio eradication that 'had been effectively outflanked after Talloires [since] polio eradication had already gone to the World Health Assembly and they had voted in favor of it before the technical advisory group had [even] considered it'. (Author interview, March 2010).

21 See The Henry J. Kaiser Family Foundation Global health Policy, 'The US Government and Global Polio Efforts', 28 May 2013, pp. 8–9, at http://kff.org/global-health-policy/fact-sheet/the-u-s-government-and-global-polio-efforts/ (accessed April 2014).

22 See 'Polio: The Problem of the Endgame Strategy' in Muraskin, *Polio Eradication and Its Discontents*, pp. 129–40.

23 Muraskin, *Polio Eradication and Its Discontents*, passim.

24 Ministries of finance have traditionally been seen as the enemy in global public health circles. The fact that they are powerful while ministries of health have been traditionally weak, has been a constant source of complaint. What has not been appreciated is that ministries of finance have to weigh many policy options: health-care interventions versus new roads, versus new schools, versus women's education, versus industry subsidies; and a host of other options. For public health practitioners, only health matters, which is a luxury many governments simply do not have.

25 I remember very well the comments made by a number of global policy makers when I first started my research: things were much easier when the world was colonised. Those men were good people who were strongly concerned about saving lives, but off the record they often sounded like unrepentant imperialists.

Index